W9-BHN-480

HEALTHWISE® HANDBOOK

A SELF-CARE GUIDE FOR YOU

FIFTEENTH EDITION

Donald W. Kemper, MPH
The Healthwise Staff

Katy E. Magee, Editor
Steven L. Schneider, MD, Medical Editor

healthwise®
for every health decision™

Healthwise, Incorporated
P.O. Box 1989
Boise, Idaho 83701

Illustrations by Nucleus Communications, Inc.

Healthwise® Handbook, Fifteenth Edition, 2001
Copyright© 1976, 1991, 1995, 1997, 1998, 1999, 2001 by Healthwise,
Incorporated, P.O. Box 1989, Boise, Idaho 83701.

All rights reserved. This book or any part thereof may not be
reproduced in any form or by any means without written permission
from the publisher.

First Edition, 1976
Fifteenth Edition, 2001

Readers may reproduce pages 1 and 2 for their personal use only.
Reproduction of those pages for resale is strictly prohibited.

15hwhb/1st/10-01
ISBN:1-877930-86-5

Healthwise and Healthwise Knowledgebase are federally registered
trademarks of Healthwise, Incorporated.

Printed in the United States of America.

Printed on recycled paper.

Table of Contents

About This Book

No book can replace the need for doctors—and no doctor can replace the need for people to care for themselves. This new edition of the *Healthwise® Handbook* contains the latest medical information to help you make the best decisions about prevention, home treatment, and when to call a doctor for over 200 common health problems. This book will also help you and your doctors work together to manage your health problems.

The guidelines in this book come from evidence-based medical information from reliable medical studies, and we have made every effort to present the information in a way that is unbiased, easy to read, and easy to use.

We recommend that you review pages 1 and 2 right away. Page 1, the Healthwise Self-Care Checklist, is a process you can follow every time a health problem arises. Page 2, the Ask-the-Doctor Checklist, will help you get the most out of every doctor visit. You may also wish to read Chapters 1 and 2 before using the rest of the book. Chapter 1, Making Wise Health Decisions, presents a process to make a health decision, ways to develop a partnership with your doctor, and information to reduce your health care costs. Chapter 2, Living Healthwise, presents information on staying healthy and detecting health problems early. The rest of the book is designed to be used on a topic-by-topic basis whenever a problem or interest develops.

 MORE INFO But this is not just a book. This icon is your link to more in-depth information on the Internet. Simply go to the Web site address listed on the back cover and "search" for the <u>text underlined in blue next to the icon</u>. This will link you to more information about the topic.

If you receive professional advice in conflict with this book, please follow your doctor's advice. Because your doctor is able to take your specific history and needs into consideration, his or her recommendations may prove to be the best. Likewise, if any self-care advice fails to provide positive results within a reasonable period, you should consult a health professional.

This book is as good as we can make it, but we cannot guarantee that it will work for you in every case. Nor will the authors or publishers accept responsibility for any problems that may develop from following its guidelines. This book is only a guide; your common sense and good judgment are also needed.

We wish you the best of health!

Donald W. Kemper, Chairman and CEO
Healthwise, Incorporated
October 2001

About Healthwise

Healthwise is a nonprofit organization whose mission is to help people make better health decisions. We create consumer health information that is based on the most current and reliable medical studies available. Expert writers and editors put this medical evidence into user-friendly terms, and a team of nationally recognized medical specialists from key centers of excellence reviews every word.

Healthwise information reaches more than 20 million families worldwide each year through our self-care handbooks, online content, and nurse call center resources. Health plans, employers, hospitals, physician groups, community organizations, government agencies, and e-health care companies trust Healthwise to support successful self-care, shared decision making, and Information Therapy™ programs. Healthwise products and consulting services have been shown to improve health and satisfaction while reducing unnecessary costs.

We publish the *Healthwise® Handbook*, *La salud en casa* (a Spanish translation of the *Healthwise Handbook*), and *Healthwise for Life* (a medical self-care guide for adults over 50).

The online content of the Healthwise® Knowledgebase is recognized by many as the most comprehensive and reliable source of consumer health information on the Web.

The "More Info" icons in this handbook link the basic self-care information in the handbook to in-depth medical information in the Healthwise Knowledgebase. People trust the Healthwise Knowledgebase for evidence-based, commercially unbiased, and referenced information on thousands of health problems, surgeries, medical tests, treatments, medications, and support groups.

Our readers often provide the best ideas for improving this book. If you have a suggestion that will make this book better, please write us at *Healthwise Handbook* Suggestions, c/o Healthwise, P.O. Box 1989, Boise, ID 83701, or e-mail us at moreinfo@healthwise.org. To learn more about our health information programs, products, and services, visit our Web site at www.healthwise.org.

Acknowledgements

This 15th edition of the *Healthwise® Handbook* comes as we enter our 27th year as a nonprofit organization. For over a quarter century our mission has been to help people stay healthy and do a better job of taking care of their health problems. This book is part of our commitment to provide the best medical information for all health decisions.

This edition of the *Healthwise Handbook* was edited by Katy E. Magee, A. Patrice Burgess, MD, and Steven L. Schneider, MD. The proofreading and editing assistance of Jo-Ann Kachigian, the layout and design work done by Terrie Britton and John Kubisiak, and the production management done by Andrea Blum are greatly appreciated. Special thanks go to the Healthwise Health Information Team for its invaluable assistance.

We are grateful to the following health professionals who reviewed this edition and shared their wisdom to make it better:

Steven N. Blair, PED

Randall D. Burr, MD

Lisa A. Cooper, MD, MPH

Alan C. Dalkin, MD

Seymour Diamond, MD

Terry J. Golden, DO

William M. Green, MD

Peter J. Kahrilas, MD

Robert B. Keller, MD

Robert A. Kloner, MD, PhD

Joy Melnikow, MD, MPH

Charles M. Myer, III, MD

Scott H. Pressman, MD

Ruth Schneider, RD, MPH

Avery L. Seifert, MD

Michael J. Sexton, MD

Peter Shalit, MD, PhD

Neil J. Stone, MD, FACC, FACP

R. Steven Tharratt, MD, FACP, FCCP

We also wish to thank the hundreds of physicians and other health professionals who have reviewed and helped to improve the previous 14 editions of the *Healthwise Handbook*.

Most of all, we would like to thank the millions of people who use the *Healthwise Handbook*. It is your actions that reward us and inspire us to look for new ways to improve this book.

The Healthwise Self-Care Checklist

Step 1. Observe the problem.

- When did it start? What are the symptoms? _____
_____
_____
_____
_____

- Where is the pain? Dull ache or stabbing pain? _____
_____

- Measure your vital signs:
  Temperature: _____   Pulse: _____/minute
  Breaths: _____/minute   Blood Pressure: _____/_____

- Think back:
  Have you had this problem before?   Yes _____   No _____
  What did you do for it? _____
  _____

  Any changes in your life (stress, medications, food, exercise, etc.)?
  _____
  _____

  Does anyone else at home or work have these symptoms?
  _____

Step 2. Learn more about it.

- *Healthwise® Handbook* (note page number): _____
- Other books or articles: _____
- Advice or opinions of others (lay or professional): _____
  _____
  _____

Step 3. Make an action plan.

- What do you think is wrong? _____
- What have you decided to do about it? _____
  _____
  _____
  _____

Step 4. Evaluate your progress.

- Are you getting better or worse? _____
  _____
  _____
  _____

Ask-the-Doctor Checklist

Before the visit:

- Complete the Healthwise Self-Care Checklist on page 1 and take it with you.
- Take a list of any medications you are currently taking. If you have seen a doctor before for a similar problem, take the record from the visit with you.

During the visit:

- State your main problem first.
- Describe your symptoms (use page 1).
- Describe past experiences with the same problem.

After the visit:

Write down:

- What's wrong: _____
- What might happen next: _____
- What you can do at home: _____
  _____

For drugs, tests, and treatments, you may want to ask:

- What's its name? _____
- Why is it needed? _____
- What are the risks? _____
- Are there alternatives? _____
- What if I do nothing? _____
- (For drugs) How do I take this? _____
- (For tests) How do I prepare? _____

At the end of the visit, ask:

- Am I to return for another visit? _____
- Am I to phone in for test results? _____
- What danger signs should I look for? _____
- When do I need to report back? _____
- What else do I need to know? _____
  _____
  _____

You, the individual, can do more for your health and well-being than any doctor, any hospital, any drug, and any exotic medical device.
Joseph Califano

I

Making Wise Health Decisions

Throughout your life you will have to make health decisions for yourself and your family. The decisions you make will influence your overall well-being as well as the quality and cost of your care. In general, people who work with their doctors to make health decisions are happier with the care they receive and the results they achieve.

Why should you help make decisions with your doctor? Aren't you paying him or her to know what to do? Well, the choices aren't always black and white. There are often several approaches to diagnosing and treating a health problem, and you are more likely to feel better about the chosen approach if it is the one best suited to your needs and values.

The best way to make health decisions is to combine the most reliable medical facts with your personal values. Among your personal values are your beliefs, fears, lifestyle, and experiences. They all play a role in helping you make decisions about your health. Put more simply:

Medical Information + Your Information = Wise Health Decisions

Skills for Making Wise Health Decisions

The following are some simple steps for you to follow when you have a health decision to make. Depending on the decision, the process may take a few minutes or hours, or as long as several weeks. Take as much time as you need to make the decision that is right for you.

1. What are your choices? Tell your doctor that you want to share in making a decision. Ask your doctor to clearly state the decision that needs to be made and what your choices are.

2. Get the facts. Learn all about each option by using resources like the library, the Internet, and your doctor. Make sure the information you collect is based on sound medical research, not the results of a single study or facts published by a company that will profit by your using its product.

MORE INFO In this book, a special icon marks some of the health problems for which more information will help you make better decisions about your care. Read the back cover of this book to learn more about where you can find reliable health information.

3. What do you think? Think about your own needs and values and what you hope for as the best possible outcome. Then sort out the information you've gathered into a list of pros and cons as you see them for each option. You may want to share your list with your doctor to make sure you have all the information you need.

4. Try on a decision. Write down what you expect will happen if you choose a particular option. Ask your doctor if what you expect is reasonable. Ask again about the side effects, pain, recovery time, or long-term outcomes of that option. Then see if you still feel it's the best choice for you.

5. Make an action plan. Once you and your doctor have made a decision, find out what you can do to make sure that you will have the best possible outcome. Write down the steps that you need to take next. Think positively about your decision, and do your part to ensure success by following your doctor's advice. Remember, when you share in making a decision, you share the responsibility for the outcome.

Work in Partnership With Your Doctor

Your relationship with your doctor greatly influences your ability to make wise health decisions and the outcome of your care. Tell your doctor that you want to be a partner in making decisions about your health. Chances are, your doctor will be happy to know that you are interested in taking an active role in your health. Common goals, shared effort, and good communication are the basis of good doctor-patient partnerships.

Skills for Becoming a Good Partner

You can hold up your end of the partnership bargain with your doctor by doing the following:

1. Take good care of yourself. Many health problems can be prevented if you protect yourself and your family by getting immunizations, being screened for health problems, and making healthy lifestyle choices. See Living Healthwise starting on page 15 for more information about how you can have more control over your health.

2. Practice medical self-care. You can manage a lot of minor problems on your own. All it takes is for you to trust your common sense and monitor how well your efforts are working. Use this book, your own experience, and advice from others to create a self-care plan.

- Use the Healthwise Self-Care Checklist on page 1 to record your self-care plan. Note whether home treatment seems to help. If you do end up calling your doctor or advice nurse, he or she will want to know what your symptoms are; what you've tried to do for the problem; and how well what you tried to do worked.

- Plan a time to call a health professional if the problem continues. If the problem seems to be getting more severe, don't wait too long before calling for help.

Calling Your Doctor

Is it okay to call your doctor? Of course it is. Often a phone call to the doctor is all you need to manage a problem at home or determine if an appointment is needed. Here's how to get the most from every call:

Prepare for your call.
Write down a one-sentence description of your problem. Then list two to three questions you have about the problem.

Have your symptom list handy.

Have your calendar handy in case you need to schedule an appointment.

Leave a clear message.
Tell your one-sentence description to the person who answers and ask to talk with your doctor.

If your doctor is not available, ask the receptionist to relay your message and have someone call you back. Ask when you might expect the return call.

Follow through.
When the doctor calls back, briefly describe your problem, ask your questions, and describe any major symptoms.

3. Prepare for office visits. Most medical appointments are scheduled to last only 10 to 15 minutes. The better organized you are, the more value you can get from the visit.

- Prepare an Ask-the-Doctor Checklist like the one on page 2 and take it with you.

- Complete a self-care checklist like the one on page 1 and take it with you.

- Write down your hunches or fears about what is wrong. These are often helpful to your doctor.

- Write down the three questions that you most want to have answered. There may not be time to ask a long list of questions.

4. Be an active participant in every medical visit.

- Be honest and straightforward. If you don't intend to take a prescribed medication, say so. If you are getting complementary treatment, such as acupuncture or chiropractic treatments, let your doctor know. To be a good partner, your doctor has to know what's going on.

- If your doctor recommends a drug, test, or treatment, get more information about the risks and benefits, costs, other alternatives, and the likely outcomes before agreeing to go through with it.

- Take notes. Write down the diagnosis, treatment and follow-up plan, and what you can do at home. Then read your notes back to the doctor to make sure you have it right. If you think it will help, take a friend along to write down what the doctor says while you listen.

5. Learn all you can about your health problem. Throughout this book, special icons mark topics for which more information will help you make better decisions about your care. The information at your disposal—whether you get it from your doctor, the library, or the Internet—is a powerful tool for helping you make wise health decisions.

If you have a complicated problem or want to know more about your health options:

- Start by asking your doctor if he or she has information about your problem that you could take home. Some doctors offer video- or audiotapes, brochures, or reprints from medical journals.

- If your health plan has an advice line, call and ask if they can help you get more information.

- If you use the Internet to find health information, start by searching sources such as the Agency for Healthcare Research and Quality (AHRQ), the Centers for Disease Control and Prevention, or a national organization that represents a particular disease (like the American Diabetes Association or the National Cancer Institute). Your health plan may also provide health information on its Web site. See Health Information at Home on page 354 for tips on finding reliable information.

- The back cover of this book offers tips to help you get more information about health problems and your testing and treatment choices.

- If you have questions or concerns about the information you find, discuss them with your doctor.

Finding a Doctor Who Will Be a Partner

A family doctor (primary care physician or internist) who knows and understands your needs can be your most valuable health partner. A host of specialists who work on separate health problems may not see your whole health picture or get a good understanding of what's important to you. In choosing a doctor there are lots of questions to ask, but these three matter the most:

- Is the doctor well trained and experienced?

- Will the doctor be available when needed?

- Will the doctor work in partnership with me?

Training and Experience

For most people, a good choice for a family doctor is a board-certified family practice doctor or an internist. For children and teens, a board-certified pediatrician or family practice doctor is a good choice. A doctor becomes board-certified by completing training in a particular specialty area and passing an examination to demonstrate that he or she has the skills and experience needed to practice that medical specialty. Most board-certified family doctors, internists, and pediatricians have broad knowledge about many common medical problems.

Availability

Because health problems rarely develop when it's convenient, it helps to have a doctor who can be contacted whenever he or she is needed. Before you select a doctor, call or visit his or her office. Tell the clinic receptionist that you are looking for a new doctor. Ask these questions:

- Is the doctor accepting new patients?

- What are the office hours?

- If I called right now for a routine visit, how soon could I be seen?

- How much time is allowed for a routine visit?

- If I cancel an appointment, will I be charged for it?

• Will the doctor discuss health problems over the phone?

• Does the doctor work with nurse practitioners or physician assistants? (These health professionals have special training in managing minor and routine health problems. They can often see you sooner, spend more time with you, and help you just as well as a doctor can.)

• Who fills in for the doctor when he or she is not available?

• What hospitals does the doctor use?

• Is the doctor eligible for maximum payments under my health plan, and will the office complete insurance forms for me?

Partner Potential

During your first visit, tell your doctor that you would like to share in making treatment decisions.

Pay attention to how you feel during the visit.

• Does the doctor listen well?

• Does the doctor speak to you in terms you can understand?

• Does the doctor spend enough time with you?

• Do you think you could build a good working relationship with the doctor?

If the answers are "no," look for another doctor. It may take more than one visit for you to decide if you will be able to work with a doctor.

Is It Time for a Change?

If you are unhappy with how your doctor treats you, it may be time for a change. Before you start looking for a new doctor, tell your current doctor how you would like to be treated. Your doctor would probably be pleased to work with you as a partner if only you would tell him or her that's what you want. Otherwise, your doctor may think that you, like many people, want him or her to do all the work.

The Advice Nurse

Many health plans and health maintenance organizations (HMOs) offer an advice nurse telephone service. Advice nurses are registered nurses who have special training to answer your questions about health problems and help you decide how to manage minor illnesses.

A call to the advice nurse can often save you a doctor visit or help you decide if you need an urgent or routine appointment.

Advice nurses can also help when your doctor diagnoses a health problem or recommends a test or treatment that you don't fully understand. Sometimes the advice nurse can answer your questions. Other times, he or she may help you come up with questions you can ask your doctor at your next visit.

Skills for Reducing Costs (But Not Quality)

Making wise health decisions can help you reduce your health care costs. The goal is to get just the care you need, nothing more, and certainly nothing less.

It is likely that you will be faced with one or more of the following health decisions at some time. Use the Skills for Making Wise Health Decisions described on pages 3 and 4 to help you decide if the services or treatments in question are right for you.

1. Should I see a doctor about a health problem? If your symptoms and the guidelines in this book suggest that you should see a doctor, don't put it off. Ignoring problems often leads to complications that are more expensive to treat.

2. Should I have a test (X-rays, blood test, CT or MRI scan, etc.) to diagnose my health problem? Don't agree to any medical test until you understand how it will help you. See page 12 for more information. The only good reason to do a test is because the benefits to you outweigh the risks and costs. No test can be done without your consent.

3. Should I take medication to treat my health problem? Always ask your doctor about any medication he or she prescribes for you. Ask what would happen if you chose not to take a medication. See page 13 for more information.

4. Should I have surgery to treat my health problem? Review the questions to ask about surgery on page 14. Get as much information about the surgery as you can and consider your needs and values. If you are not convinced that the benefits to you outweigh the risks, don't have the surgery.

5. Do I need to go to the emergency room? In life-threatening situations, modern emergency services are vital. However, emergency rooms charge two to three times more for routine services than a doctor's office would. They are not set up to care for routine illnesses, and they do not work on a first-come, first-served basis. During busy times, people with minor illnesses may wait for hours. Also, your records are not available, so emergency room doctors have no information about your medical history.

Use good judgment in deciding when to use emergency medical services. Whenever you feel you can apply home treatment safely and wait to see your regular doctor, do so. However, if you believe your situation requires urgent care, by all means go to the emergency department.

6. Do I need to be hospitalized? More than half of this country's health care dollars are spent on hospitalizations. A stay in a hospital costs far more than a vacation to most luxury resorts. (And hospitals are a lot less fun.)

Skills to Use in the Hospital

When you need to be in the hospital, there are things you can do to improve the quality of the care you receive. However, if you are very sick, ask your spouse or a friend to help watch out for your best interests.

- Ask "why?" Don't agree to anything unless you have a good reason. Agree only to those procedures that make sense for you.

- Provide an extra level of quality control. Check medications, tests, injections, and other treatments to see if they are correct. Your diligence can improve the quality of the care that you receive.

- Be friendly with the nurses and aides, and they may pay more attention to your needs.

- If you get an itemized bill, check it, and ask about any charges you don't understand.

Don't check in to the hospital just for tests. Ask your doctor if the tests can be done on an outpatient basis. If you agree to control your diet and activities, your doctor will usually support your request.

If you need inpatient care, get in and out of the hospital as quickly as possible. This will reduce costs and your risk of hospital-acquired infections.

Try to avoid additional days in the hospital by bringing in extra help at home. Ask about home nursing services to help while you recover.

Hospitals are not the only choice for people who have a terminal illness. Many people choose to spend their remaining time at home with the people they know and love. Special arrangements can be made through hospice care programs in most communities. Look up "Hospice" in the Yellow Pages directory, or ask your doctor.

7. Should I see a specialist about my health problem? Specialists are doctors who have in-depth training and experience in a particular area of medicine. For example, a cardiologist has years of special training to deal with heart problems. A visit to a specialist often costs more than a visit to your regular doctor, and the tests and treatments that you receive may be more expensive. Of course, specialists often provide the information you need to help you decide what to do about a major health problem.

When your primary care doctor refers you to a specialist, a little preparation and good communication can help you get your money's worth. Before you go see a specialist:

- Know your diagnosis or expected diagnosis.

- Learn about your basic treatment options.

• Make sure that any test results or records on your case are sent to the specialist.

• Know what your primary care doctor would like the specialist to do (take over the case, confirm the diagnosis, conduct tests, etc.).

• Ask your primary care doctor to remain involved in your care. Ask the specialist to send new test results or recommendations to both you and your regular doctor.

You Have the Right:

• To be spoken to in words that you understand.

• To be told what's wrong with you.

• To read your medical record.

• To know the benefits and risks of any treatment and its alternatives.

• To know what a treatment or test will cost you.

• To share in all treatment decisions.

• To refuse any medical procedure.

Adapted from the American Hospital Association's "Patient's Bill of Rights."

Shared Decisions About Medical Tests

Medical tests are important tools, but they have limits. Informed consumers know that medical tests have costs and risks as well as benefits.

Learn the facts:

- What is the name of the test, and why do you need it?
- If the test is positive, what will the doctor do differently?
- What could happen if you don't have the test?

Consider the risks and benefits:

- How accurate is the test? How often does it indicate a problem exists when there is none (false positive)? How often does it indicate there is no problem when there is one (false negative)?
- Is the test painful? What can go wrong?
- How will you feel afterward?
- Are there less risky alternatives?

Ask about costs:

- How much does the test cost?
- Is there a less expensive test that might give the same information?

If a test seems costly, risky, or not likely to change the recommended treatment, ask your doctor if you can avoid it. Try to agree on the best approach. No test can be done without your permission, and you have the right to refuse to have a test.

Let your doctor know:

- Your concerns about the test.
- What you expect the test will do for you. Ask if that is realistic.
- Any medications you are taking (prescription and nonprescription).
- Whether you have other medical conditions.
- Whether you prefer to accept or decline the test.

If you agree to a test, ask what you can do to reduce the risk of errors. Should you restrict food, alcohol, exercise, or medication before the test? After the test, ask to review the results. Take notes for your home records. If the results of the test are unexpected and the error rate of the test is high, consider redoing the test before basing further treatment on the results.

Shared Decisions About Medications

The first rule of medications is to know why you need each drug before you use it.

Learn the facts:

- What is the name of the medication, and why do you need it?
- How long does it take to work?
- How long will you need to take it?
- How and when do you take it (with food, on an empty stomach, etc.)?
- Are there nondrug alternatives?

Consider the risks and benefits:

- How much will this medication help?
- Are there side effects or other risks?
- Could this medication interact with other medications that you currently take?

Ask about costs:

- How much does the medication cost?
- Is a generic form of the medication available and appropriate for you?
- Is there a similar medication that will work almost as well and be less expensive?
- Can you start with a prescription for a smaller quantity to make sure the medication agrees with you?

Let your doctor know:

- Your concerns about the medication.
- What you expect it will do. Ask if that is realistic.
- About all other medications you are taking (prescription and nonprescription).
- Whether you prefer to take the medication or try other ways of treating the problem.

The chapter Your Home Health Center has more information about how to manage medications.

Shared Decisions About Surgery

Every surgery has risks. Only you can decide if the benefits are worth the risks.

Learn the facts:
- What is the name of the surgery? Get a description of the surgery.
- Why does your doctor think you need the surgery?
- Are there other options besides surgery?
- Is this surgery the most common one for this problem? Are there other types of surgery?

Consider the risks and benefits:
- How many similar surgeries has the surgeon performed? How many surgeries like this are done at this hospital?
- What is the success rate? What does success mean to your doctor? What would success mean to you?
- What can go wrong? How often does this happen?
- How will you feel afterward? How long will it be until you're fully recovered?
- How can you best prepare for the surgery and the recovery period?

Ask about costs:
- How much does the surgery cost? How can you find out?
- Can it be done on an outpatient basis, and is that less expensive?

Let your doctor know:
- How much the problem really bothers you. Are you willing to put up with symptoms to avoid surgery?
- Your concerns about the surgery.
- Whether or not you want to have the surgery at this time.
- If you want a second opinion. Second opinions are helpful if you have any doubt that the proposed surgery is the best option for your problem. If you want a second opinion, ask your primary care doctor or your surgeon to recommend another specialist. Ask that your test results be sent to the second doctor. Consider getting an opinion from a doctor who isn't a surgeon and who treats similar problems.

If I'd known I was going to live this long, I'd
have taken better care of myself.
Eubie Blake

2

Living Healthwise

Most of this book focuses on helping you deal with health problems. This chapter is meant to be used as a guide to help you prevent illness and injury by making wise health and lifestyle choices.

These basic health habits are the foundation of lifelong health and well-being:

- Stay up to date with immunizations and health screenings.

- Be physically active.

- Eat right.

- Maintain a healthy body weight.

- Be tobacco-free.

- Avoid drugs and excess alcohol.

- Manage stress.

- Take care of your teeth.

- Practice safety.

- Pursue healthy pleasures.

- Help to make a healthier world.

Maintaining these health habits will give you the best chance of staying healthy and active and feeling good about yourself throughout your life. If you have health problems, good health habits are even more important. It's never too late to make lifestyle changes that may help you recover faster or make living with a chronic disease easier.

Immunizations

Immunizations help your immune system recognize and quickly attack organisms that can cause diseases before those organisms can cause problems. Some immunizations are given in a single shot or oral dose, while others require several doses over a period of time.

Schedule your child's immunizations according to the chart on page 16. There is no need to delay immunizations because of colds or other minor illnesses. Keep good records. Children often need to show immunization records in order to attend school.

Immunization Schedule

Immunization ⇒ Age ⇓	Diphtheria Pertussis Tetanus (DTaP)	Polio (IPV)	Measles Mumps Rubella (MMR)	Chickenpox (Varicella)	Hepatitis B virus (HBV)	Haemophilus influenzae b (Hib) Booster	Pneumococcus (PCV)	Tetanus Diphtheria (TD) Booster
Birth–18 months					√(3 doses) [a]			
2 months	√	√				√	√	
4 months	√	√				√	√	
6 months	√					√	√	
6–18 months		√						
12–15 months			√			√	√	
12–18 months				√				
15–18 months	√							
4–6 years	√	√	√					
11–12 years			√ [b]	√ [c]	√ [a]			√
Adult			√ [d]					Every 10 years
50+	Influenza (flu) vaccine, annually [e]							
65+	Pneumococcal vaccine (PPV), one time only [f]							

a The age at which a baby should begin the hepatitis B vaccine series depends on his or her risk for HBV infection and the type of vaccine available. Ask your doctor when your baby should start the vaccine series. If the hepatitis B vaccine series was not given during infancy, it should be given by age 11 to 12 years.

b The second MMR should be given by age 11 to 12 years if it was not given at age 4 to 6 years.

c Those who have not been vaccinated, have not had chickenpox, or who are not immune according to a blood test should be vaccinated at this age.

d People born during or after 1956 who may not have had 2 doses of MMR vaccine should talk to their doctor about reimmunization. Women trying to get pregnant should have a blood test to check for rubella immunity.

e People younger than 50 who have chronic diseases, especially heart or lung diseases, should consider receiving an annual flu shot. Health care workers and any others who may be exposed to influenza may wish to get annual flu shots as well.

f People younger than 65 who have chronic diseases, especially diabetes, HIV, or respiratory illnesses such as emphysema, should consider receiving the pneumococcal vaccine. These people may need to receive the vaccine more than once.

Adapted from the Advisory Committee on Immunization Practices, American Academy of Pediatrics, 2001.

If you are considering not having your child immunized, talk with your health professional. There are few valid reasons for not having your child immunized.

The need for immunizations does not end with childhood. Thousands of people are hospitalized, and many die, as the result of influenza and other diseases that can be prevented by immunization. If you are in one of the high-risk groups for whom the influenza or pneumococcal vaccine is recommended (see page 19), make sure you get immunized.

 Medical experts are constantly reviewing the effectiveness of immunization programs. Therefore, immunization recommendations change periodically. Your primary care doctor or public health department can provide the most up-to-date information about immunizations.

Diphtheria, Pertussis, and Tetanus (DTaP)

Diseases like diphtheria and pertussis caused many deaths before a vaccine was developed to prevent them. This vaccine also protects against tetanus ("lockjaw"), which can result from bacterial infection of a deep cut or puncture wound.

Childhood immunizations for these diseases consist of a series of five shots starting at age 2 months. The first Td (tetanus and diphtheria)

booster is given between ages 11 and 12 years. After that, a Td booster is needed every 10 years. Follow the DTaP and Td guidelines on page 16.

Polio

Polio is a viral illness that can lead to paralysis. It is rare today because of the polio vaccine. The first dose of vaccine is given at age 2 months, and the immunization series gives life-long immunity.

Adults who have not been immunized need immunization only if they are traveling to a part of the world where new cases of polio still occur.

Measles, Mumps, and Rubella (MMR)

Measles (rubeola), mumps, and rubella (German measles) were once common childhood illnesses. Today they are quite rare, thanks to the MMR vaccine. Two shots, one given at age 12 to 15 months and one at age 4 to 6 years, provide lifelong protection (immunity).

If there is a measles outbreak in your area and your baby has not been immunized, call your doctor or health department to discuss an early MMR shot. If your child receives the vaccine before he or she is 12 months old, two additional doses are still required according to the usual schedule.

If you don't have records showing that you received two doses of MMR vaccine and you did not have these illnesses as a child, discuss your need for immunization with your doctor.

Women who are planning to get pregnant need to make sure they have been vaccinated. Rubella contracted during pregnancy, especially during the first few months, increases the risk of miscarriage, stillbirth, and severe birth defects.

Chickenpox (Varicella)

It is recommended that all children receive the chickenpox vaccine at 12 to 18 months of age. Because the chickenpox vaccine is relatively new, it is not known how long the vaccine protects a person against chickenpox. However, some people who have had the vaccine appear to be protected for as long as 20 years.

Chickenpox is more serious in teens and adults. People older than 11 or 12 years who have never had chickenpox or have not received the chickenpox vaccine should be vaccinated. Teens and adults need two doses of the vaccine. People older than 12 who aren't sure whether they have had chickenpox should discuss their need for testing and immunization with their doctor.

Hepatitis B Virus (HBV)

The hepatitis B virus (HBV) infects liver cells and can destroy them. Over time, chronic HBV infection can lead to serious, sometimes fatal liver disease. Vaccination prevents HBV infection and its possible complications. See page 94.

It is recommended that all babies be vaccinated against HBV. Three shots provide long-term immunity. Immunization is also recommended for:

• Children and teens under 18 who were not previously vaccinated, especially if they are at high risk for exposure to HBV.

• People who have more than one sex partner.

• Men who have sex with men.

• People who use intravenous drugs.

• Health care workers.

• People planning extended travel to China, Southeast Asia, Africa, and other areas where HBV infection rates are high.

Hepatitis A Virus (HAV)

Unlike other types of hepatitis, infection with the hepatitis A virus (HAV) usually does not cause long-term problems. However, it is very contagious and can cause serious illness in some cases. The vaccine consists of two shots and is extremely effective.

Vaccination against hepatitis A is recommended for:

• Anyone older than 2 who lives in or is traveling to an area where HAV infection is common. This includes parts of the United States.

• People who use intravenous drugs.

• Men who have sex with men.

- People who have liver disease.

- People who have a blood-clotting disorder, such as hemophilia.

Haemophilus influenzae Type b (Hib)

Haemophilus influenzae type b does not cause the flu. This bacterial infection can cause meningitis, pneumonia, skin and bone infections, and other serious illnesses in young children. Every child between 2 months and 5 years of age should be immunized against Hib. Children over 5 and adults need immunization only if they have sickle cell anemia or problems involving the spleen or immune system.

Influenza Virus

Annual influenza vaccinations are recommended for everyone age 50 and older, for younger people who have chronic diseases, and for women who will be in their second or third trimester of pregnancy during the flu season. Health care workers and others who are likely to be exposed to the flu virus may also wish to get the vaccine every year. The vaccine can be given to anyone older than 6 months of age. The vaccine is most effective when it is given in the autumn, well before the start of the flu season.

Pneumococcal Infection

In addition to infecting the lungs (pneumonia), pneumococcal bacteria can infect the blood (bacteremia) or the covering of the brain (meningitis). A one-time-only dose of the pneumococcal vaccine is recommended for people age 65 and older. Younger people who have chronic conditions, especially respiratory disease (except for asthma), diabetes, or HIV, should also consider getting the pneumococcal vaccine. If you received the pneumococcal vaccine before age 65 and it has been more than 5 years since you last had the shot, ask your doctor if you need a booster shot.

All babies under 2 and any children at high risk for complications from pneumococcal infection should receive the pneumococcal conjugate vaccine (PCV). This vaccine is given in a series of four shots. It is not recommended for use in adults.

Other Immunizations

Immunization against Lyme disease is recommended in some parts of North America. Talk to your health professional about this or other immunizations you or your child may need.

If you are in close contact with people who have contagious diseases or you are planning travel to areas where illnesses such as malaria, typhoid, cholera, and yellow fever are common, contact your local health department to find out if you need other immunizations.

(see page 228)

Reactions to Immunizations

Temporary, mild reactions to immunizations are common. Babies often develop a fever after the DTaP shot, and the area where the shot was given may become sore, red, or swollen. A child may develop a rash or fever 1 to 2 weeks after receiving the first dose of MMR vaccine. The rash will go away without treatment. Joint pain and swelling may also occur after the first dose of MMR vaccine, but these symptoms usually go away after about 3 days.

The chickenpox vaccine can cause soreness, redness, and swelling at the site of the injection. Fever and a mild rash also may develop. The rash will go away without treatment. However, it is possible for a person who gets a rash from the chickenpox vaccine to give chickenpox to another person.

The hepatitis B vaccine may cause pain at the injection site and nausea, a low fever, or a rash.

• Acetaminophen may soothe the discomfort and relieve fever caused by immunizations. Also see page 228. Some doctors recommend that you take acetaminophen before receiving an immunization.

• Keep written notes about any reactions you observe.

• Tell your health professional if you think the reactions are excessive.

Health Screenings

Another way to protect your health is to detect disease early, when it may be easier to treat. You can do this in two ways: by getting periodic medical exams from a health professional and by becoming a good observer of changes in your own body.

Periodic Medical Exams and Screening Tests

The schedule on page 21 will help you decide which exams and tests are right for you and your family and how often you should have them. The most appropriate schedule of preventive exams is one you and your doctor agree upon, based on your age, your risk factors for disease, how healthy you are, and how important periodic health screening is to you.

The recommendations on page 21 apply to people of average risk in each age group. You may be at higher risk for certain diseases and may therefore need more frequent exams and tests. Factors that may help your doctor determine your level of risk include your overall health, your family history (whether your close relatives have had certain diseases), and lifestyle factors, such as whether you use tobacco, how often you exercise, and your sexual history.

Health Screening Schedule

Assessment	Birth-10 years	11-24 years	25-64 years
Height and Weight	Growth chart plotted during office visit from birth on.	Periodically, or every 2 years.	Periodically.
Vision Screening	Screening between ages 3 and 4 years.		Periodically. More often if you have diabetes.
Hearing	Universal screening of infants for hearing impairment before age 3 months.		Periodically if you are regularly exposed to loud noise.
Blood Pressure, p. 243.	Screening during any office visit starting at age 3 years.	Periodically after age 21.	Periodically.
Breast Cancer Screening, pp. 245 and 247: • Mammography • Clinical breast examination			• Ages 40 to 49: discuss appropriate mammography schedule with a health professional. • From age 40: annual clinical breast exam. • From age 50: mammography every 1 to 2 years.
Cervical Cancer Screening Test (Pap test), p. 250.		Every 1 to 3 years for any female who has ever had sexual intercourse.	Every 1 to 3 years for any female who has ever had sexual intercourse.
Chlamydia		Routine for sexually active females under 20 or people at risk.	Routine for sexually active people at risk.
Cholesterol, p. 242.			Periodically. Discuss with a health professional.
Colorectal Cancer Screening, p. 98: • Fecal Occult Blood Test (FOBT) • Flexible Sigmoidoscopy			• Annual screening using FOBT after age 50. • Sigmoidoscopy after age 50.
Prostate Cancer Screening, p. 271.			Risk increases with age starting at age 50; discuss with a health professional.

Self-Exams

Periodic self-exams are also an important part of staying healthy. See the breast self-exam on page 247, the genital self-exam for women on page 249, and the testicular self-exam on page 274. Turn to page 211 to learn how to look for changes in your skin that may be early signs of skin cancer.

Other Recommended Tests and Exams

Birth to 10 years

Well-baby visits are recommended at 2 weeks and at 2, 4, 6, 9, 12, 15, 18, and 24 months of age. Your doctor may recommend a different schedule. Babies at high risk for hearing problems may be tested during this time.

Discuss the frequency of visits for a child older than 2 years with your health professional. A vision test is recommended at age 3 to 4 years. Some childhood immunizations are given at 4 to 6 years. See page 16.

Regular blood pressure checks are recommended after age 3 years and may be done during visits for other reasons.

11 to 24 years

A tetanus booster is recommended at 11 to 12 years of age. After age 21, periodic blood pressure checks are recommended and may be done during any doctor visit.

Pap tests are recommended every 1 to 3 years for any female who has ever had sexual intercourse.

25 to 64 years

The Health Screening schedule on page 21 can help you decide which tests are valuable for you and how often you should have them.

Pregnant Women

Discuss the frequency of visits and testing with your doctor. During the first prenatal visit, blood tests, urinalysis, blood pressure measurement, and screening for hepatitis B virus and HIV infection are recommended. Additional tests are needed throughout the pregnancy.

Tuberculin Test

A tuberculin test is done to determine if you have been infected with the organisms that cause tuberculosis (TB). See page 150.

Whether you need to be tested depends on how common TB is in your area and your risk of coming in contact with TB-causing organisms. If you think you may have been exposed to TB and wish to be tested, contact your doctor or the local health department.

Be Physically Active

Everyone needs regular physical activity. Along with a positive attitude and a healthy diet, your fitness level plays a major role in how well you feel, what illnesses you avoid, and how much you enjoy life. Regular physical activity:

• Lowers your risk of premature death and death caused by heart disease.

- Reduces your risk of developing diabetes, high blood pressure, colon cancer, and osteoporosis.

- Helps lower high cholesterol and blood pressure levels.

- Improves your mood, relieves stress, and promotes a sense of well-being.

- Helps build and maintain healthy bones, muscles, and joints.

- Helps you maintain a healthy body weight.

If you already make regular physical activity a part of your life, keep up the good work. If you aren't physically active, there is good news. The latest research shows that exercise doesn't have to be vigorous to improve your health. Many everyday activities raise your heart rate and, if done regularly, will keep your heart and lungs healthy, make your muscles stronger, and improve your flexibility. For more specific information about designing your personal fitness plan and staying motivated, see Fitness starting on page 285.

Eat Right

How and what you choose to eat affects many aspects of your health. Your diet plays an important role in helping you:

- Meet your nutritional needs and maintain a healthy weight.

- Have regular bowel movements.

- Prevent diseases such as heart disease, diabetes, and certain cancers.

- Treat diseases such as diabetes and high blood pressure.

Another important aspect of your diet is how carefully you prepare and handle foods. You need good food preparation and food handling habits in order to avoid food-borne illnesses. For more information about food safety, see Stomach Flu and Food Poisoning on page 98.

For more information about how you can evaluate and improve your diet, see Nutrition starting on page 293.

Maintain a Healthy Body Weight

Healthy bodies come in a variety of shapes and sizes. Weight is not the only measurement of health. In fact, your weight may say very little about your health. No matter what your shape or body size, you can improve your health by eating a balanced diet, getting regular exercise, and learning to feel good about your body.

Heredity plays a big role in your body shape and what you weigh. It would be impossible for most of us to look like fashion models or world-class athletes, but we can all learn to appreciate our bodies and treat them well to maximize our health and self-esteem.

What Is a Healthy Weight?

The Body Mass Index (see page 25) provides an estimate of your total body fat, which influences your risk for certain diseases. However, your health is determined by more than just your weight. Other measurements of health include:

• Your fitness level.

• The quality of your diet and your eating habits.

• The presence of disease indicators such as high cholesterol.

• The presence of diseases such as high blood pressure, heart disease, and diabetes.

• How fat is distributed on your body.

• Your self-esteem and body image.

If you think that your current weight puts you at risk for health problems, talk to your health professional about different ways you can manage your weight. Most people are concerned about being overweight, but for some people being underweight is a health concern. Being obese (having a body mass index of 30 or greater) can increase your risk of developing high blood pressure, high cholesterol, heart disease, type 2 diabetes, sleep apnea, some cancers, and other long-term illnesses. Losing as little as 5 percent to 10 percent of your body weight can lower your blood pressure, reduce other risk factors for heart disease, and improve your blood sugar levels.

Set Realistic Goals

Before you start a weight management program, think about your goals, your expectations, and your readiness to make lifestyle changes. A realistic weight management program should focus on the following:

• Reducing your risk of health problems.

• Increasing your fitness level by becoming more physically active.

• Making positive lifestyle changes that will become lifelong habits.

• Coming to accept the size and shape of your body.

Tools for Change

Set your body in motion.
Regular physical activity makes you feel stronger and more energetic. It also improves your overall health. Physical activity makes your body burn more calories, not just while you're exercising, but throughout the day. So if you exercise regularly and eat a healthy diet, you will find it easier to manage your weight. In addition, regular exercise builds muscle. Increasing the amount of lean muscle in your body is healthier for you and will make your body look more toned. For tips on making regular physical activity a part of your healthy lifestyle, see Fitness starting on page 285.

Plan your meals.
People who eat regular meals find it easier to maintain a healthy weight than do people who overeat, skip meals, or snack. Meals that are planned are usually more nutritious

than those that are grabbed at the last minute. Taking time to plan what you will eat will improve your diet and can help you control your weight. Skipping meals usually leads to feelings of deprivation, which can lead to overeating at the next meal or eating a less-than-nutritious snack.

Focus on reducing fat.
Eat a variety of nutritious, low-fat foods. Rather than counting calories, focus on eating more fruits and vegetables and less fat.

A low-fat diet (less than 35 percent of total calories from fat) will help you control your weight and reduce your risk of developing heart disease, high blood pressure, cancer, and other diseases. For tips on how to cut fat from your diet, see page 297.

Enjoy your food.
You can enjoy all the foods you love and still control your weight. The key is to be sensible about how much you eat and to balance calorie intake with calorie burn-off (exercise). Here are some tips:

• Enjoy your steak (or cake) twice as much: eat half in the restaurant and take the rest home to enjoy the next day.

• Have one helping of your favorite food and enjoy every bite.

• Craving an ice cream cone? Walk to the ice cream shop, have a single dip, and walk home.

All foods can fit into a healthy diet; the proper balance of those foods is what's most important.

Body Mass Index (BMI)

Your body mass index (BMI) is based on your height and weight. A healthy BMI for an adult is between 19 and 26. Disease risk increases both above and below this range. A BMI of 27 to 29 is considered overweight. A person is said to be obese when his or her BMI is 30 or higher.

Use the following table to look up the upper and lower limits of a healthy weight for your height. The height is given in inches and the weight in pounds.

Height	Healthy weight based on BMI ranging from 19 to 26
58	90-124
59	93-128
60	96-133
61	99-137
62	103-142
63	106-146
64	109-151
65	113-156
66	117-161
67	120-166
68	124-171
69	127-176
70	131-181
71	135-186
72	139-191
73	143-197
74	147-202
75	151-208
76	155-213

Be Tobacco-Free

It's never too late to quit using tobacco, even if you've been doing it for 20 or 30 years. Quitting smoking or chewing tobacco is the most important thing you can do to improve your own health and the health of those around you. Quitting is not easy. If you have already tried to quit, you know how difficult it is. But don't give up—with the right attitude and enough help, you will eventually succeed.

Tobacco use increases your risk for many health problems, including cancer, heart disease, and stroke. Your tobacco use also puts others at risk. Children who are exposed to cigarette smoke in the home have more ear infections and are prone to other health problems such as asthma. Perhaps the greatest risk to your children is that they will learn from you. Children whose parents use tobacco are more likely to use tobacco themselves.

When you stop using tobacco, it doesn't take long for your body to start to heal and for your risk of developing other health problems to decrease.

• When you quit smoking, your risk of heart attack is cut in half within 1 year after quitting. Five years after quitting, your risk is about the same as that of a person who never smoked.

Smoking Cessation Aids

Nicotine replacement products can help you break the habit of using tobacco and prevent nicotine withdrawal symptoms. The products deliver nicotine to the bloodstream without the dangerous tars, carbon monoxide, and other chemicals released by tobacco and smoke. You gradually reduce the amount of nicotine you give yourself until your body is no longer dependent on nicotine.

Nicotine replacement treatment comes in four forms: chewing gum, skin patches, nasal spray, and inhalers.

All nicotine replacement products can cause side effects. You may need to try more than one product before you find the one that works best for you.

Using a nicotine replacement product works best if you also enroll in a tobacco cessation program. Such programs help you deal with the habit of smoking or chewing tobacco, while the replacement product helps you overcome your addiction to nicotine.

A medication that does not contain nicotine is now available to help control irritability and cravings when you quit using tobacco. The medication is available only with a doctor's prescription. First try to stop using tobacco without the medication. Many people succeed without it.

• While the lung damage that smoking causes is not reversible, quitting smoking prevents more lung damage from occurring. Shortness of breath and cough will decrease.

• When you give up tobacco products, damage to your lips, tongue, mouth, and throat is reduced. Your risk for mouth and throat cancer decreases.

• If you have asthma, you will have fewer and less severe attacks after you quit smoking.

• After quitting smoking, a man may have fewer problems getting and maintaining erections.

Cigars and Smokeless Tobacco

Cigars have become popular in recent years. Many people who smoke cigars feel it is safe because they do not inhale the cigar smoke. However, holding cigars and cigar smoke in your mouth increases your risk for cancers of the mouth, tongue, throat, and larynx.

Smokeless tobacco, or snuff, can be chewed, inhaled, or held in your cheek. There is a direct link between using these products and developing mouth and throat cancer.

Facts you should know about cigars and smokeless tobacco:

• They contain nitrosamines, which cause cancer.

• They contain nicotine, which raises your heart rate and blood pressure.

• They may produce leukoplakias (wrinkled, thick, white patches) on the inside of the mouth. Leukoplakias can develop into mouth cancer.

Tips for Quitting

 No one can tell you when or how to quit smoking or chewing tobacco. Only you know why you use tobacco and what will be most difficult as you try to stop. The important thing is that you try. Believe that you will succeed, if not the first time, then the second time, or twenty-second time.

Preparation

• List your reasons for quitting: to improve your own health and your family's health, to save money, to prevent wrinkles, or whatever. Read through your list every day for a month, and your chances of success will increase.

• Figure out why you smoke. Do you use tobacco to pep yourself up? To relax? Do you like the ritual of smoking or chewing? Do you use tobacco out of habit, often without knowing why you are doing it? If specific situations trigger your desire to smoke or chew tobacco, changing your routine so that you can temporarily avoid those situations may help you stop.

- Decide how and when you will quit. About half of ex-tobacco users quit "cold turkey." The other half cut down more slowly.

- Find a healthful alternative that can replace what smoking or chewing does for you. For example, if you like to have something to do with your hands, pick up something else: a coin, worry beads, pen, or pencil. If you like to have something in your mouth, substitute sugarless gum or minted toothpicks.

- Plan a healthful reward for yourself for when you have stopped using tobacco. Take the money you save by not buying tobacco and spend it on yourself.

- Plan things to do for when you get the urge to smoke or chew. Urges don't last that long: take a walk, brush your teeth, have a mint, drink a glass of water, or chew gum.

- Choose a reliable tobacco cessation program. Good programs have at least a 20 percent success rate after 1 year. Great programs have a 50 percent success rate. A higher success rate may be too good to be true.

Action

- Set a quit date and stick to it. Choose a time that will be busy but not stressful.

- Remove ashtrays and all other reminders of using tobacco. Choose nonsmoking sections in restaurants. Avoid alcohol. Do things that reduce the likelihood of using tobacco, like taking a walk or going to a movie.

- Ask for help and support. Choose a trusted friend, preferably another former tobacco user, to give you a helping hand over the rough spots.

- Know what to expect. The worst will be over in just a few days, but physical withdrawal symptoms may last 1 to 3 weeks. After that, it is all psychological. See page 323 for relaxation tips.

- Keep low-calorie snacks handy for when the urge to munch hits. Your appetite may perk up, but most people gain fewer than 10 pounds when they quit using tobacco. The health benefits of quitting outweigh a few extra pounds. The information in the Nutrition chapter can help you plan healthy meals and snacks.

- Get out and exercise. It will distract you, help keep off unwanted pounds, and release tension. See Fitness starting on page 285.

- Don't be discouraged by slipups. It often takes several tries to quit using tobacco for good. If you do slip up and smoke or chew, forgive yourself and learn from the experience. You will not fail as long as you keep trying.

- Good luck!

Avoid Drugs and Excess Alcohol

When you say "no" to drugs and limit the amount of alcohol that you drink, you prevent accidents and several diseases and avoid a lot of other problems for yourself and your family. If drug or alcohol abuse is a problem for you or someone close to you, now is the time to seek help. For more information about drug and alcohol problems, see page 304.

Manage Stress

Stress is practically unavoidable, but it doesn't have to have a negative impact on your health and well-being. By learning how to deal with stress in ways that help you feel more in control, you may be able to improve your health, your job or school performance, your relation-ships, and your outlook on life.

 It shouldn't surprise you that some of the key factors in helping you manage stress are eating a healthy diet, getting regular exercise and enough sleep, avoiding drugs and tobacco, and drinking alcohol only in moderation. All these lifestyle factors work together.

For more information about how stress can affect your health and how you can identify and deal with the sources of stress in your life, see page 321.

Take Care of Your Teeth

Your teeth will last a lifetime if you care for them properly. Brushing and flossing regularly, eating a mouth-healthy diet, and visiting your dentist for regular checkups will help keep your teeth healthy.

Brushing

• Brush at least twice a day for 3 to 5 minutes each time.

• Use a fluoride toothpaste (young children should use only a pea-sized dab). Tartar-control toothpastes may help slow the formation of hard mineral buildup (tartar) on the teeth.

• Brush your tongue. Plaque build-up (a sticky film made of bacteria) on the tongue can cause bad breath.

Start brushing your child's teeth as soon as they come in. Brush your child's teeth for the first 4 to 5 years, until your child seems able to do it alone. A good teaching method is to have your child brush in the morning and you brush at night until your child masters the skill.

If your local water supply does not contain enough fluoride, your child may need a fluoride supplement. Discuss this with your dentist.

Flossing

Flossing properly once a day is the best way to remove plaque from below the gums and between the teeth.

Start flossing your child's teeth as soon as they touch each other. As with brushing, you will have to help with flossing until the child is old enough to manage it alone.

Diet

• Choose nutritious between-meal snacks. Avoid high-sugar foods and drinks, especially sticky, sweet foods. The longer sugar stays in touch with your teeth, the more damage it will do.

• Be sure to brush before bedtime. Food is more likely to cause cavities at night because saliva doesn't clean the mouth as well at night.

• Mozzarella and other cheeses, peanuts, yogurt, milk, and sugar-free gum (especially gum that contains xylitol) are good for your teeth. They help clear the mouth of harmful sugars and reduce plaque formation.

Dental Checkups

Choose a dentist as carefully as you choose any other doctor. See page 7 for tips on finding a dentist who meets your needs and is concerned about preventive care.

Most people who do not have serious problems with their teeth need to visit the dentist twice a year. During a dental checkup the dentist will examine your teeth and gums for signs of tooth decay and gum disease. X-rays of your teeth are usually taken once a year. If you don't have any active tooth decay or gum disease, changes in your brushing and flossing habits probably won't be necessary.

A dentist or dental hygienist will clean your teeth. He or she will scrape hard mineral buildup (tartar) off of your teeth with a small metal tool; floss your teeth thoroughly; and use a polishing compound to help clean and polish your teeth. Cleanings may be uncomfortable but usually aren't painful. Other procedures (application of sealants to prevent cavities or fluoride treatments) may be done during a routine office visit if needed.

The Academy of Pediatric Dentistry recommends that your child see a dentist either by age 1 or within 6 months after the first tooth comes in.

Practice Safety

Taking safety precautions is one of the most important things you can do to protect yourself and your family from accidents and injuries. Let common sense and these partial lists be your guides.

At Home

• Post emergency telephone numbers near telephones.

• Have an emergency plan in case of accidents, fire, or injury. Practice the plan with your family.

• Install smoke and carbon monoxide detectors in your home, and check them twice a year to make sure they work.

• Keep a working fire extinguisher in your home. Make sure everyone in the house (including the babysitter) knows how to use it.

• Keep all medications, cleaning and automotive supplies, and other hazardous products securely stored and out of the reach of children.

• Turn off appliances after use. Unplug small appliances and put them away after they have cooled.

• Store firearms unloaded and securely, out of the reach of children. Store ammunition separately.

• Prevent falls by securing rugs that slip, keeping stairs and hallways clear, and turning on lights.

• Practice safer sex. See page 282.

When On the Move

• Don't drink and drive. Don't drive if you are taking medication that may make you drowsy.

• Make sure everyone in your car is wearing a safety belt. See "Automobile Seat Restraints" on page 32.

• Obey traffic laws and speed limits.

• Keep your car, bike, skateboard, skis, and other recreational gear in good operating condition.

• Wear helmets and sport-specific padding when bicycling, in-line skating, playing baseball, etc. Wear eye protection when playing racquet sports.

• Never let children play unattended near water.

At Work

• Follow your employer's safety guidelines.

• Wear clothing and protective equipment that is appropriate for your job (hard hat, gloves, goggles, earplugs, etc.).

• Protect yourself against smoke, dangerous fumes, and exposure to chemicals.

• Know the location of fire extinguishers, first aid kits, and emergency exits nearest your workstation.

Automobile Seat Restraints

Wearing seat belts saves lives and prevents injuries. No one is strong enough to brace themselves against a sudden impact in a motor vehicle, even at very low speeds. Seat belts reduce the risk of serious injury and death.

- Wear your seat belt every time you are in a vehicle. Keep the belt snug and close to your body. Always use both the lap and shoulder belts.

- Seat belts are necessary even if your car is equipped with air bags. Air bags inflate from the steering wheel or dashboard of your car in the event of sudden impact. They are very effective in protecting front-seat riders, but they must be used with seat belts. Babies in car seats and anyone under 4' 8" should not sit in front of an air bag.

- Children younger than 12 years of age should sit in the back seat. Use child car seats for infants, children under 4 years, and those weighing less than 40 pounds. See page 231.

Pursue Healthy Pleasures

Give yourself permission to make yourself happy. The good things in life make it easier to deal with the things that aren't so good. If it's been a while since you've indulged yourself in something pleasurable, try this exercise:

- Make a list of 10 (or more) things that give you pleasure.

- Do at least one of the things on your list every day for a week.

- Enjoy and repeat!

Help to Make a Healthier World

Do what you can to make your home, your community, and your world a better place. Support a cause that is working to make positive changes. Recycle. Mentor. Tutor. Volunteer. And remember, peace on Earth begins at home: seek non-violent ways to resolve conflicts at home, at school, at work, and in your community. See pages 307 and 317.

It is by presence of mind in untried emergencies
that the native metal of man
(or woman) is tested.
James Russell Lowell

3

First Aid and Emergencies

This chapter covers both serious medical emergencies and minor first aid situations. Review this chapter before you need it. Then, when you are faced with an emergency or injury, you will know where to turn. Your confidence in dealing with both major and minor emergencies will be reassuring to an injured person.

Some of the medical emergencies covered in this chapter include:

• Bleeding, see Cuts on page 48.

• Breathing emergencies, page 38.

• Head injuries, page 53.

• Heart attack, page 55.

• Poisoning, page 65.

• Shock, page 69.

• Stroke, page 75.

• Unconsciousness, page 78.

Dealing With Emergencies

Take a deep breath. Count to 10. Tell yourself you can handle the situation.

Assess the danger. Protect yourself and the injured person from fire, explosions, or other hazards. If you suspect a spinal injury, do not move the person unless the danger is great.

If the person is unconscious or unresponsive, check the ABCs: Airway, Breathing, Circulation. If the person is not breathing, see Rescue Breathing and CPR on page 40.

Try to survey the situation as a whole. Identify and prioritize the injuries. The most obvious problem is not always the most serious. Treat the most life-threatening problems, like bleeding or shock, first. Check for broken bones and other injuries. If you need emergency assistance, call 911 or other emergency services, such as the local fire department, sheriff, or hospital.

Prepare for the Emergency Room

- If possible, call ahead to let emergency room staff know you are coming.

- Call your doctor, if possible. He or she may meet you at the emergency room or call in important information.

- If you think you may have to wait to be seen by a doctor, take this book and your medical records with you. While you are waiting you can:

  - Use page 1, the Healthwise Self-Care Checklist, to help you think through the problem and report symptoms to the doctor.

  - Use page 2, the Ask-the-Doctor Checklist, to organize questions for the doctor.

  - Review the medical test checklist on page 12.

  - Use your home medical records to prepare to discuss your medications, past test results, or treatments. Information about your allergies, medications, and health conditions may be critical.

First Aid and Emergencies

Legal Protection

If you are needed in an emergency, give what help you can. Most states have a Good Samaritan law to protect people who help in an emergency. You cannot be sued for giving first aid unless it can be shown that you are guilty of gross negligence.

Accidental Tooth Loss

If a permanent tooth is knocked out, a dentist may be able to reimplant it. Baby teeth need to come out anyway, so they are not usually reimplanted.

A chipped tooth can be repaired. A blow that was hard enough to chip a tooth may have moved several teeth out of alignment or broken the portion of bone that holds the tooth in place.

Home Treatment

If a permanent tooth is knocked out:

- Call your dentist immediately for an emergency visit. Reimplanting a tooth works best when it is done within 30 minutes. After 2 hours, it is unlikely the procedure will be successful.

- Rinse the tooth gently and place it back in the socket, between the gum and cheek (use care not to swallow the tooth), or in a small container of milk. Use tap water if milk is not available.

When to Call a Health Professional

- If a permanent tooth is knocked out or chipped.

- If a baby tooth is accidentally knocked out, schedule an appointment within 2 weeks to determine if a spacer is needed until a permanent tooth comes in.

Animal and Human Bites

After being bitten by an animal, most people want to know if they need a rabies shot. The main wild animal carriers of rabies in the U.S. are bats, raccoons, skunks, and foxes. Pet dogs, cats, and ferrets that have been vaccinated rarely have rabies. However, many stray animals have not been vaccinated. Rabies is quite rare, but it is fatal if you are not vaccinated soon after exposure. The vaccination is no more painful than a typical injection. Report all wild animal bites to your doctor and the health department or animal control department.

Bites that break the skin can cause infections. Cat and human bites are particularly prone to bacterial infection. You can get tetanus from any bite if your tetanus shots are not up to date. See page 16.

Prevention

- Vaccinate all pets against rabies. Do not keep wild animals as pets.

- Do not disturb animals—not even your pets—while they are eating.

- Teach children not to approach or play with stray animals.

- Do not touch wild animals or provoke them to attack. Do not handle sick or injured animals.

Home Treatment

- Scrub the bite immediately with soap and water. Treat it as a puncture wound. See page 67.

- If you are bitten by a pet dog, cat, or ferret, find out whether the animal has been vaccinated for rabies.

- A healthy pet that has bitten someone should be confined and observed for 10 days by a veterinarian to see if the pet develops symptoms of rabies. If you cannot locate the pet's owner, contact the health department.

- If you are bitten by a wild animal, contact your doctor and the health department. The health department can tell you whether that animal is a rabies carrier in your area, and whether treatment is needed.

When to Call a Health Professional

- If the bite is from a bat or other wild animal.

- If the bite is from a human or a cat.

straightened, heated paper clip

hot pad

Use a red-hot paper clip to relieve the pain caused by blood under a fingernail or toenail.

- If the bite is from a dog, cat, or ferret that is acting strangely or foaming at the mouth, or if the animal attacked for no apparent reason.

- If the bite is from a pet whose owner cannot be found or cannot confirm that the animal has been vaccinated for rabies.

- If there is a loss of feeling or function below the bite.

- If the bite is severe and may need stitches or if it is on your face, hand, or foot, or over a joint. If stitches are needed, they usually should be done within 8 hours.

- If signs of infection develop. See page 67.

Blood Under a Nail

Fingernails and toenails often get crunched, bashed, or smashed. These injuries usually aren't too serious, but if there is bleeding under the nail, the pressure can be very painful. The only way to relieve the throbbing and pain is by making a hole in the nail to drain the blood.

Draining is helpful only if you have severe, throbbing pain (you can feel the pulse beating under the nail) that keeps you from sleeping. This procedure is not necessary or recommended if you are not having severe pain.

Home Treatment

- Apply ice and elevate the injured area as soon as possible to minimize swelling and relieve pain. Acetaminophen or ibuprofen will also ease discomfort.

- If you have severe, throbbing pain, make a hole in the nail to relieve the pressure. (Do not do this unless you are in pain and you are confident you can do it without burning yourself. Do not do this if you have diabetes or circulation problems.) Follow these steps:

  - Straighten a paper clip and heat the tip in a flame until it is red-hot.

  - Place the tip of the paper clip on the nail and let it melt through. You do not need to push. This will not be painful, because the nail has no nerves. Go slowly and reheat the clip as necessary. A thick nail may take several tries.

First Aid and Emergencies

- As soon as the hole is complete, blood will escape and the pain will be relieved. Pain and pressure that are not relieved by this procedure may indicate a more serious injury, such as a broken finger or toe or a deep cut. In this case, you should see your doctor.

- Soak the finger twice a day for 15 minutes in warm, soapy water. Apply an antibiotic ointment and cover the nail with a Band-Aid.

- If the pressure builds up again in a few days, repeat the procedure, using the same hole.

When to Call a Health Professional

• If blood under a nail is causing severe pain and you are not willing to drain the blood from the nail yourself.

• If you drained the blood from under the nail, but your fingertip or the tip of your toe still hurts a lot.

• If you smashed your toenail and you have a condition such as diabetes or peripheral vascular disease, which decreases blood flow to the feet.

• If signs of infection develop. See page 67.

• If your nail has torn or separated from the nail bed and you need help removing it.

Blunt Abdominal Wounds

Blunt abdominal wounds caused by a blow to the stomach can cause severe bruising of the abdominal wall and bleeding from the internal organs. Such injuries are often caused by automobile, bicycle, sledding, or skiing accidents, when the victim is thrown into an object or to the ground.

An abdominal injury may cause the abdomen to become tender or rigid. The injured person may become confused and may not be able to remember what caused the injury. Signs of shock (faintness, weakness, drowsiness, or confusion; sweating and cool, clammy skin) may also develop.

Home Treatment

• Monitor the injured person's pulse and respiration rate. See pages 58 and 70. If possible, monitor the person's blood pressure as well. A rapid, weak pulse, very rapid or very slow breathing, or falling blood pressure may indicate internal bleeding. If these signs develop, **call 911** or take the person to the emergency room immediately.

• Have the injured person lie down with the feet elevated above the heart. Loosen the person's clothing and cover him or her with a blanket for warmth. Do not give the person anything to eat or drink, even though he or she may be thirsty.

- Watch for signs of shock (see page 69).

When to Call a Health Professional

- If signs of shock or internal bleeding (see page 69) develop. These may develop up to 48 hours after an abdominal injury.

- If there is bleeding from the rectum, blood in the urine, or unexpected vaginal bleeding following a blow to the abdomen.

- If the injury causes nausea, vomiting, heartburn, or loss of appetite.

- If the person's abdomen is swollen and hard, or if pressing on the abdomen causes severe pain.

- If a wound is deeper than a scratch.

Breathing Emergencies

Who needs to be trained to help a person who is having a breathing emergency? You do. If you have children, drive a car, shop at the mall, or go anyplace where a person may be in a life-threatening situation, you need to know how to respond. An added benefit is the confidence you will have when you know you can help a person when it matters most.

The guidelines presented in this book are not meant to replace formal training from a certified instructor. They are here for you to use to refresh your memory between trainings or to read aloud to a person who is performing a rescue procedure. (Note, however, that your first responsibility as a helper is to call 911 or other emergency services and to make the area safe for the victim and the rescuer.)

Choking Rescue Procedure (Heimlich Maneuver)

Choking is usually caused by food or an object stuck in the windpipe. A person who is choking cannot talk, cough, or breath, and may turn blue or dusky. The Heimlich maneuver can help dislodge the food or object.

WARNING: Do not begin the choking rescue procedure unless you are certain that the person is choking.

Adult or child older than 1 year:

- Stand behind the person and wrap your arms around his or her waist. If the person is standing, place one of your feet between his or her legs so you can support the person's body if he or she loses consciousness.

- Make a fist with one hand. Place the thumb side of your fist against the person's abdomen, just above the navel but well below the sternum.

Heimlich maneuver: Give quick upward thrusts to dislodge the object.

- Grasp your fist with the other hand. Give a quick upward thrust into the abdomen. This may cause the object to pop out. Use less force for a child.

- Repeat thrusts until the object pops out or the person loses consciousness.

- **If you choke while you are alone**, do abdominal thrusts on yourself, or lean over the back of a chair and press forcefully to pop out the object.

If the person loses consciousness, gently lower him or her to the ground. **Call 911 or other emergency services.**

- Begin standard CPR (cardiopulmonary resuscitation), including chest compressions. See page 40.

- Each time the airway is opened during CPR, look for an object in the mouth or throat. If you see an object, remove it.

- Do not perform blind finger sweeps.

- Do not perform abdominal thrusts, such as the Heimlich maneuver.

- Continue performing CPR until the person is breathing on his or her own or until an ambulance arrives.

Infant (younger than 1 year):

- Put the baby facedown on your forearm so the baby's head is lower than his or her chest.

- Support the baby's head in your palm, against your thigh. Don't cover the baby's mouth or twist his or her neck.

- To dislodge the object, use the heel of one hand to give back blows between the baby's shoulder blades. Repeat 4 times.

- If the airway remains blocked, support the infant's head and turn him or her face up on your thigh with his or her head pointing toward the floor.

To help a baby who is choking, use the heel of your hand to give back blows between the baby's shoulders.

• Place 2 or 3 fingers on the lower part of the baby's breastbone, and give up to 5 upward thrusts.

• Look for the object in the infant's mouth. If you can see it, remove it with your finger. Then give 2 rescue breaths (see page 42).

• If the back blows and chest thrusts do not dislodge the object, **call 911 or other emergency services** and begin rescue breathing (see page 42).

• Continue with back blows, chest thrusts, looking for the object, and rescue breaths until the infant coughs up the object and starts breathing on his or her own, or until help arrives.

Rescue Breathing and CPR

WARNING: CPR (cardiopulmonary resuscitation) that is done improperly or on a person whose heart is still beating can cause serious injury. Do not perform CPR unless:

1. The person has stopped breathing.

2. The person does not have signs of circulation, such as normal breathing, coughing, or movement in response to rescue breathing.

3. No one with more training in CPR is present.

For basic life support, think **ABC: A**irway, **B**reathing, and **C**irculation, in that order. You must give rescue breaths before you can begin the

Preventing Choking

• Don't drink too much alcohol before eating. It may dull your senses, and you might not chew food properly or might try to swallow too large a portion of food.

• Take small bites. Cut meat into small pieces. Chew your food thoroughly.

• Do not give popcorn, nuts, or hard candy to children younger than 3, and supervise older children when they eat these foods. Cut hot dogs and grapes lengthwise.

• Do not allow children younger than 3 to play with small objects or toys that have very small parts that could be swallowed.

• Keep balloons and plastic bags away from any child who may put them in his or her mouth.

See the Choking Rescue Procedure on page 38.

chest compressions, which will help circulate blood for a person whose heart has stopped beating.

Step 1: Check for consciousness. Tap or gently shake the person and shout, "Are you okay?" If you suspect a neck or spinal injury, do not shake the person.

If the person does not respond:

• **Adult (age 9 and older): Call 911 or other emergency services immediately** (have someone else make the call if possible). Then proceed to Step 2.

- **Infant or child through 8 years:** Check to see if the infant or child is breathing (Step 2). If the infant or child is not breathing, give rescue breaths for 1 full minute (Step 3).

Then **call 911 or other emergency services**. If the child is small enough, carry him or her to the telephone with you so you can continue to give rescue breaths. Keep the child's head and neck steady.

Step 2: Check for breathing. Look, listen, and feel for breathing for 5 seconds. Kneel next to the person with your head close to his or her head.

- Look to see if the person's chest rises and falls.

- Listen for breathing sounds, wheezing, gurgling, or snoring.

- Put your cheek near the person's mouth and nose to feel whether air is moving out.

If the person is not breathing (or if you can't tell), roll the person onto his or her back. If he or she may have a spinal injury, gently roll the person's head, neck, and shoulders together as a unit until the person is on his or her back.

CPR Ready Reference			
	Adults	**Children Age 1 through 8**	**Infants Under 1 Year**
If the person is not breathing, begin rescue breathing:	Give 2 full breaths.	Give rescue breaths for 1 full minute.	Give rescue breaths for 1 full minute.
If the person does not breathe or show signs of circulation in response to rescue breaths, locate the compression landmark:	Trace the ribs into the sternal notch; place 2 fingers on the sternum. See illustration on p. 43.	Same as for an adult.	1 finger-width below nipple line.
Do chest compressions with:	2 hands stacked; heel of 1 hand on sternum	Heel of 1 hand on sternum	2 or 3 fingers on sternum
Rate of compressions per minute:	100	100	100
Compression depth:	1½ to 2 inches	1 to 1½ inches	½ to 1 inch
Ratio of compressions to breaths:	15:2	5:1	5:1
Guidelines from the American Heart Association			

Step 3: Begin rescue breathing.

• Place your hand on the person's forehead and pinch the person's nostrils shut with your thumb and forefinger. With your other hand, continue tilting the chin forward to keep the airway open.

Airway: Position the head to open the airway.

• Take a deep breath and place your mouth over the person's mouth, making a tight seal. For an infant, place your mouth over the baby's mouth and nose. As you slowly blow air into the person, watch to see if his or her chest rises.

Breathing: Blow air in slowly; look to see if chest rises.

• If the first breath does not go in, try tilting the person's head again and give another breath.

• Slowly blow air in until the person's chest rises. Take 1½ to 2 seconds to give each breath. Between rescue breaths, remove your mouth from the person's mouth and take a deep breath. Allow his or her chest to fall and feel the air escape.

• Give the person 2 full breaths. Then check for circulation.

Step 4: Check for circulation.

Look for signs of circulation, such as breathing, coughing, or movement in response to rescue breathing.

If there are **no signs of circulation**, begin chest compressions. See Step 5.

If there are signs of circulation, continue to give rescue breaths until help arrives or until the person starts breathing on his or her own. If the person starts breathing again, he or she still needs to be seen by a health professional.

Give rescue breaths:

• Adult (age 9 and older): 2 breaths every 15 seconds

• Infant or child through 8 years: 1 breath every 3 seconds

Step 5: Begin chest compressions. Adult (age 9 and older):

• Kneel next to the person. Use your fingers to locate the end of the person's breastbone (sternum), where the ribs come together. Place 2 fingers at the tip of the sternum.

Place the heel of the other hand directly above your fingers (on the side closest to the person's face).

- Place your other hand on top of the one that you just put in position. Lock the fingers of both hands together, and raise the fingers so they don't touch the person's chest.

- Straighten your arms, lock your elbows, and center your shoulders directly over your hands.

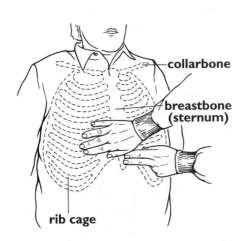

Put your hand 2 fingers'-width above the bottom of the breastbone.

- Press down in a steady rhythm, using your body weight and keeping your elbows locked. The force from each thrust should go straight down onto the sternum, compressing it 1½ to 2 inches. It may help to count "one and two and three and four...," giving 1 downward thrust each time you say a number. Lift your weight, but not your hands, from the chest each time you say "and." Give 15 compressions.

- After 15 compressions, give 2 full, slow breaths.

- Repeat the 15 compressions/2 breaths cycle 4 times (1 minute); then check again for signs of circulation. If there are still no signs of circulation, continue to give chest compressions and rescue breaths until help arrives or until signs of circulation are present and breathing is restored.

Chest Compressions: Keep your shoulders directly over your hands with your elbows straight as you give chest compressions.

Child (age 1 through 8 years):

- Position the heel of one hand 2 fingers'-width above the tip of the sternum. Press with less force than you would for an adult, compressing the sternum 1 to 1½ inches.

- Give 5 chest compressions. Then give 1 rescue breath. Repeat the 5 compressions/1 breath cycle 12 times (1 minute); then check again for signs of circulation, such as normal breathing, coughing, or

First Aid and Emergencies

movement in response to rescue breaths. If there are still no signs of circulation, continue to give chest compressions and rescue breaths until help arrives or until signs of circulation are present and breathing is restored.

Infant (younger than 1 year):

• Place 2 fingers on the baby's sternum, about 1 finger-width below an imaginary line connecting the nipples. Press with gentle force, compressing the sternum about ½ to 1 inch.

• Give 5 chest compressions. Then give 1 rescue breath. Repeat the cycle of 5 compressions and 1 breath 12 times (1 minute); then check again for signs of circulation. If there are still no signs of circulation, continue to give chest compressions and rescue breaths until help arrives or until signs of circulation are present and breathing is restored.

Bruises

Bruises (contusions) occur when small blood vessels under the skin rupture or tear. Blood seeps into the surrounding tissues, causing the black-and-blue color of a bruise.

Bruises usually develop after a bump or fall. People who take aspirin or blood thinners (anticoagulants) may bruise easily. A bruise may also develop after blood is drawn.

A black eye is a type of bruise. If you have a black eye, apply home treatment for a bruise and inspect the eye for blood. If there is any loss of or change in your vision or if you cannot move your eye in all directions, see a doctor.

Home Treatment

• Apply ice or cold packs for 10 minutes several times a day. Do this for the first 48 hours to help blood vessels constrict and to reduce swelling. The sooner you apply ice, the less bleeding there will be.

• If possible, elevate the bruised area above the level of your heart. Blood will leave the area and there will be less swelling.

• Rest the injured limb so you don't injure it further.

• If the area is still painful after 48 hours, apply heat with warm towels, a hot water bottle, or a heating pad.

When to Call a Health Professional

• If signs of infection develop. See page 67.

• If pain increases or if your ability to use or move the bruised body part decreases.

• If a blow to the eye causes:

  - Blood in the colored part of the eye or blood in the white part of the eye (see page 171).

  - Loss of or change in vision.

- Inability to move the eye normally in all directions.

- Severe pain in the eyeball rather than around the eye.

• If you suddenly begin to bruise easily, or if you have unexplained recurrent or multiple bruises.

Burns

Burns are classified as first-, second-, or third-degree depending on their depth, not on the amount of pain or the extent of the burn. A first-degree burn involves only the outer layer of skin. The skin is dry, painful, and sensitive to touch. A mild sunburn is an example of a first-degree burn.

A second-degree burn involves several layers of skin. The skin becomes swollen, puffy, weepy, or blistered.

A third-degree burn involves all layers of skin and may include any underlying tissue or organs. The skin is dry, pale white or charred black, swollen, and sometimes breaks open. Nerves are destroyed or damaged, so there may be little pain except on the edges of the burn, where there may be second-degree burns.

Prevention

• Install smoke detectors on each story of your home. Check and replace the batteries regularly.

• Keep a fire extinguisher near the kitchen. Have it inspected yearly.

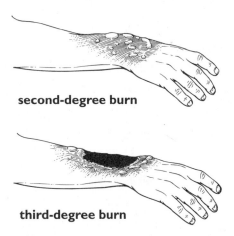

second-degree burn

third-degree burn

A second-degree burn will cause skin to swell and blister, and it may also weep fluid. A third-degree burn may cause skin to look pale white or charred black.

• Set your water heater at 120° or lower to avoid burns.

• Supervise children closely, especially in the kitchen.

• Don't smoke in bed.

• Use caution around campfires and hot appliances.

If your clothing catches fire:

• Do not run, because running will fan the flames. Stop, drop, and roll on the ground to smother the flames, or smother the flames with a blanket, rug, or coat.

• Use water to douse the fire and cool the skin.

To avoid kitchen burns:

• Use caution when handling hot foods and beverages.

• Turn pot handles toward the back of the stove.

• Smother burning food or grease with a pot or pot lid.

First Aid and Emergencies

Home Treatment

Third-degree burns require immediate medical treatment. Call a health professional and apply home treatment:

• Make sure the source of the burn has been extinguished.

• Have the person lie down to prevent shock.

• Cover the burned area with a clean sheet.

• Do not apply any salve or medication to the burn.

First- and second-degree burns can be treated at home as follows:

• Run cool tap water over the burn until the pain stops (10 to 30 minutes). Cool water is the best immediate treatment for minor burns. The cold lowers skin temperature and lessens the severity of the burn. Do not use ice or ice water, because it may further damage the injured skin.

• Remove rings, jewelry, or clothing from the burned limb. Swelling may make these items difficult to remove later.

• Clean the burn area with mild soap and water. If the burned skin or blisters have broken open, a bandage is needed. Otherwise, don't cover the burn unless clothing rubs on it. If clothing rubs the burned area, cover the burn with a nonstick gauze pad taped well away from the burn. Do not encircle a hand, arm, or leg with tape. Keep

the bandage clean and dry. Change it once a day and anytime it gets wet.

• Do not put salve, butter, grease, or oil on a burn. They increase the risk of infection and don't help the burn heal.

• After 2 to 3 days of healing, apply aloe to soothe minor burns.

If the burn causes blisters to form:

• Do not break blisters. If blisters break, clean the area by running tap water over it and applying a mild soap. Apply an antibiotic ointment, such as Polysporin or Bacitracin, and cover the burn with a nonstick sterile dressing. Don't touch the burned area with your hands or any unsterile objects. Remove the dressing every day, clean the burned area with mild soap, and cover it again.

• Take aspirin or ibuprofen to help relieve pain. Don't give aspirin to anyone younger than 20.

When to Call a Health Professional

• For all third-degree burns.

• If you are in doubt about the extent of a burn, or in doubt whether it is a second- or third-degree burn.

• If a second-degree burn involves the face, ears, eyes, hands, feet, genitals, or a joint.

• If the burn encircles an arm or leg, or if it covers more than 25 percent of the body part involved.

First Aid and Emergencies

- If the pain lasts longer than 48 hours.

- If signs of infection develop. See page 67.

- If a child younger than 5, an older adult, or a person with a weakened immune system or a chronic health problem (such as cancer, heart disease, or diabetes) is burned.

- If there is a chance the burn was caused on purpose.

Chemical Burns

Chemical burns occur when something caustic, such as a cleaning product, gasoline, or turpentine, is splashed into an eye or onto the skin.

The vapors or fumes of strong chemicals can also burn or irritate the eyes, the respiratory passages, and the lungs.

A chemically burned eye becomes red and watery and may be sensitive to light. If the damage is severe, the eye will look whitish. Chemically burned skin may become red, blistered, or blackened, depending on how strong the caustic material is.

Prevention

Wear safety glasses, goggles, or a face shield when working with chemicals. Know the location of the nearest sink or shower.

Home Treatment

Most chemical burns are treated first by rinsing.

- Immediately flush your eye or skin with a large amount of water. Use a cold shower for skin burns. For eye burns, fill a sink or dishpan with water, immerse your face in the water, and open and close your eyelids with your fingers to force the water to all parts of the eye. Or flush your eye under a running faucet or shower. A sink with a sprayer also works well.

- Continue flushing for 30 minutes or until the pain stops, whichever takes longer.

When to Call a Health Professional

Call 911 or other emergency services:

- If a strong chemical such as acid or lye is splashed into your eye.

- If you have swallowed a chemical that may cause burning or be poisonous.

Call your doctor or the local poison control center if any one of the following occurs:

- A large area of skin (more than 25 percent of any part of the body or on the face) is exposed to a strong acid, such as battery acid, or to a caustic substance, such as lye or Drano.

- A chemically burned eye still hurts after 20 minutes of home treatment.

- A chemically burned eye appears to be damaged. Symptoms include:

  - Persistent redness.

First Aid and Emergencies

- Discharge or watering.

- Any vision problems, such as double vision, blurring, or sensitivity to light.

- A gray or white discoloration over the colored part of the eye.

• Your skin shows signs of a chemical burn (see page 47).

Cuts

When you see a cut (laceration), the first steps are to stop the bleeding and determine whether stitches are needed.

If the cut is bleeding heavily or spurting blood, see "Stopping Severe Bleeding" on page 48.

Bleeding from minor cuts will usually stop on its own or after you apply a little direct pressure.

To decide whether stitches are needed, see "Are Stitches Necessary?" on page 49.

If stitches are needed, apply home treatment and seek medical care as soon as possible, certainly within 8 hours. If stitches are not needed, you can clean and bandage the cut at home.

Home Treatment

• Stop any bleeding by applying direct, continuous pressure over the wound for 15 minutes.

• Wash the cut well with soap and water. Treat an animal bite like a puncture wound. See page 67.

First Aid and Emergencies

Stopping Severe Bleeding

• Wash your hands well with soap and water. Put on medical gloves or place several layers of fabric or plastic bags between your hands and the wound.

• Elevate the site that is bleeding.

• Remove any visible objects from the surface of the wound. Do not attempt to clean out the wound.

• Press firmly on the wound with a clean cloth or the cleanest material available. If there is an object deep in the wound, apply pressure around the object, not directly over it. Do not try to remove the object.

• Apply steady pressure for a full 15 minutes. Don't peek after a few minutes to see if bleeding has stopped. If the bleeding has not slowed down or stopped after 15 minutes, **call 911 or other emergency services** and continue to apply pressure to the wound. If blood soaks through the cloth, apply another cloth without lifting the first one.

• If bleeding decreases after you apply pressure for 15 minutes, but minimal bleeding starts again once you release the pressure, apply direct pressure to the wound for another 15 minutes. Direct pressure may be applied up to 3 times (total of 45 minutes) for minimal bleeding. If bleeding (more than just oozing small amounts of blood) continues after 45 minutes of direct pressure, call a health professional.

• Watch for signs of shock. See page 69.

- Leave small cuts unbandaged, unless they will become irritated. Cuts heal best when they are left exposed to the air.

- If a cut needs bandaging, but not stitches, apply antibiotic ointment (such as Polysporin or Bacitracin). The ointment will keep the cut from sticking to the bandage. Do not use rubbing alcohol, hydrogen peroxide, iodine, or mercurochrome, which can harm tissue and slow healing.

- Use an adhesive strip (such as Band-Aid) to provide continuous pressure. Always put an adhesive strip across a cut rather than lengthwise. A butterfly bandage (see the illustration on page 49) can help hold cut skin edges together. If the cut is long, use more than one bandage.

- Apply a clean bandage at least once a day, or whenever the old bandage gets wet. Leave the bandage off whenever possible.

Butterfly bandages are best for closing a long cut.

Are Stitches Necessary?

For best results, cuts that need stitches should be sutured within 8 hours. Wash the cut well with soap and water and stop the bleeding; then pinch the sides of the cut together. If it looks better, you may want to consider stitches. If stitches are needed, avoid using an antibiotic or antiseptic ointment until after a health professional has examined the cut.

Stitches may be needed for:

- Deep cuts (more than ¼ inch deep) that have jagged edges or gape open.

- Deep cuts on a joint, such as an elbow, knuckle, or knee.

- Deep cuts on the hands or fingers.

- Cuts on the face, eyelids, or lips.

- Cuts in any area where you are worried about scarring.

- Cuts that go down to the muscle or bone.

- Cuts that continue to bleed after you have applied direct pressure for 15 minutes.

Cuts like these that are sutured usually heal with less scarring than similar cuts that are not sutured.

Stitches may not be needed for:

- Cuts with smooth edges that tend to stay together during normal movement of the affected body part.

- Shallow cuts that are less than ¼ inch deep and less than ¾ inch long.

First Aid and Emergencies

First Aid and Emergencies

When to Call a Health Professional

- If a person who has been cut goes into shock, even if bleeding has stopped. See Shock on page 69.

- If a cut continues to bleed through bandages after you apply direct pressure for 15 minutes.

- If the skin near the wound is blue, white, or cold; if you have numbness, tingling, loss of feeling; or if you are unable to move a limb normally below the wound.

- If the cut has removed all the layers of skin.

- If the cut contains, or might contain, foreign objects such as wood, glass, or gravel.

- If the cut needs stitches (see page 49). Stitches usually need to be done within 8 hours.

- If you have been cut and your tetanus shots are not up to date. See page 16. If you need a tetanus booster, you should have it within 2 days of being injured.

- If signs of infection develop. See page 67.

Electrical Burns

Electrical burns are a medical emergency. An electrical burn may look minor on the outside, but electricity can cause serious internal damage, including burns and heart rhythm disturbances.

Prevention

- Keep electrical cords out of the reach of small children and pets. Plug bare electrical sockets with plastic inserts.

- Have frayed power cords on electric appliances replaced.

- Unplug lamps before replacing light bulbs. Turn off the power at the circuit breaker when replacing bulbs in ceiling or wall lights.

- Unplug all appliances (including your computer) when making minor repairs.

- Keep appliances away from water.

- During a lightning storm, take cover inside a car, large building, or house, or seek low ground. Do not stand under a tree during a lightning storm. Get out of the water and off of boats. Stay away from metal objects.

Home Treatment

- Do not approach a victim who has been electrocuted until you are sure the area surrounding the victim is safe. Disconnect the power source if possible. If you feel tingling in your lower body, turn around and hop to a safe place.

- Do not attempt to move wires off of a victim unless you are sure the power has been disconnected.

- If it is safe to approach the victim, check ABCs (Airway, Breathing, Circulation). If necessary, begin rescue breathing and CPR. See page 40.

• To prevent shock, raise the victim's legs 8 to 12 inches and keep the victim warm.

• Cover burns with dry, sterile dressing.

When to Call a Health Professional

Call 911 or other emergency services immediately:

• If a person who has been electrocuted stops breathing, has no pulse, or has lost consciousness.

• If a person who has been electrocuted fell and may have a spinal injury.

Call your doctor for any electrical burn. Even an electrical burn that looks minor can be serious and needs to be evaluated.

Fishhook Removal

In the excitement of fishing, sometimes fingers are hooked instead of fish. It is useful to know how to remove a fishhook, especially if you are far from medical help.

Home Treatment

Remove the hook as follows:

• Use ice, cold water, or hard pressure to provide temporary numbing.

• **Step A:** Tie a piece of fishing line to the hook near the skin's surface.

• **Step B:** Grasp the eye of the hook with one hand and press down about 1/8 of an inch to disengage the barb.

• **Step C:** While still pressing the hook down (barb disengaged), jerk the line near the skin's surface so that the hook shaft leads the barb out of the skin.

Removing a fishhook

• Another option is to push the hook the rest of the way through the skin, snip off the barb, and then pull the hook out the same way it entered the skin.

• Wash the wound thoroughly with soap if possible. Treat it as a puncture wound. See page 67.

• Do not try to remove a fishhook from an eyeball. Seek medical care immediately.

When to Call a Health Professional

• If the hook is near the eye or in the eyelid or eyeball.

• If the hook is in or near a joint, in a bone or muscle, or deep in the skin.

• If you cannot remove the hook.

First Aid and Emergencies

• If your skin was punctured by a fishhook and your tetanus shots are not up to date. See page 16. If you need a tetanus booster, you should have it within 2 days of being injured.

• If signs of infection develop. See page 67.

Freeing Trapped Limbs

Fingers, arms, or legs sometimes get caught in objects such as bottles, jars, or pipes. Stay calm; panic will only make the situation worse.

Home Treatment

• Don't try to force the limb from where it is stuck, because doing so will make it swell and become more difficult to remove.

• Try to relax the limb. Relaxation alone will sometimes enable you to free the limb.

• If possible, elevate the limb.

• Apply ice around the exposed part of the limb. This may reduce any swelling and allow the limb to be released.

• If ice doesn't work, dribble soapy water or cooking oil on the limb. Turn the limb or the object so you "unscrew" it rather than pulling it out directly.

When to Call a Health Professional

Call if you are unable to free the trapped limb or if freeing the limb results in injury.

Frostbite

Frostbite is freezing of the skin or underlying tissues that occurs as a result of prolonged exposure to cold.

Frostbitten skin is pale or blue, is stiff or rubbery to the touch, and feels cold and numb. Frostbite is rated by its severity:

First degree ("frostnip"): Skin is whitish or red and tingling or burning, but there is little likelihood of blistering if it is rewarmed promptly.

Second degree: Outer skin feels hard and frozen, but tissue underneath is normal. Blistering is likely.

Third degree: Skin is white or blotchy and blue. Skin and tissue underneath are hard and frozen. Blistering always occurs.

Prevention

Stay dry and out of the wind in extreme cold, and cover areas of exposed skin. Keep your body's core temperature up:

• Wear layers of clothing. Wool and polypropylene are good insulators. Wear windproof, waterproof outer layers. Wear wool socks and waterproof boots that fit well.

- Wear a hat to prevent heat loss from your head. Wear mittens rather than gloves.

- Keep protective clothing and blankets in your car in case of a breakdown in an isolated area.

- Don't drink alcoholic or caffeinated beverages or smoke when you are out in extreme cold.

Home Treatment

- Get inside or take shelter from the wind.

- Check for signs of hypothermia (see page 58) and treat it before treating frostbite.

- Protect the frozen body part from further exposure to cold. Don't rewarm the area if refreezing is possible. Wait until you reach shelter.

- Warm small areas (ears, face, nose, fingers, toes) with warm breath or by tucking hands or feet inside warm clothing next to bare skin.

- Don't rub or massage the frozen area, because doing so will further damage tissues. Avoid walking on frostbitten feet if possible.

- Keep the frostbitten body part warm and elevated. Wrap it with blankets or soft material to prevent bruising. If possible, immerse it in warm water (104° to 108°) for 15 to 30 minutes.

- Blisters may appear as the skin warms. Do not break them. The skin may turn red, burn, tingle, or be very painful. Aspirin, ibuprofen, or acetaminophen may help relieve pain. Do not give aspirin to anyone younger than 20.

When to Call a Health Professional

- If the skin is white or blue, hard, rubbery, and cold, which indicates third-degree frostbite. Careful rewarming and antibiotic treatment are needed to prevent permanent tissue damage and infection.

- If blisters develop (second- or third-degree frostbite). Do not break blisters. The risk of infection is very high.

- If signs of infection develop. See page 67.

Head Injuries

Most bumps on the head are minor and heal as easily as bumps anywhere else. Minor cuts on the head often bleed heavily because the blood vessels of the scalp are close to the skin's surface. In children, blood loss from a scalp injury may be enough to cause symptoms of shock.

Head injuries that do not cause visible external bleeding may have caused life-threatening bleeding and swelling inside the skull. The more force involved in a head injury, the more likely a serious injury to the brain has occurred. Anyone who has experienced a head injury should be watched carefully for 24 hours for signs of a serious head injury.

Prevention

• Wear a seat belt when in a motor vehicle. Use child car seats.

• Wear a helmet while biking, motor-cycling, skating, kayaking, horseback riding, skiing, or snowboarding.

• Don't dive into shallow or unfamiliar water.

Home Treatment

• If the victim is unconscious, assume he or she has a spinal injury. Do not move the victim without first protecting the neck from movement (see page 71).

• If there is bleeding, apply firm pressure directly over the wound with a clean cloth or bandage for 15 minutes. If the blood soaks through, apply additional cloths over the first one. See "Stopping Severe Bleeding" on page 48.

• Check for injuries to other parts of the body, especially if the person has fallen. The alarm from seeing a head injury may cause you to overlook other injuries that need attention.

• Apply ice or cold packs to reduce the swelling. A "goose egg" may appear anyway, but ice will help ease the pain.

• For the first 24 hours after a head injury, watch the victim for signs of a severe head injury. Check for the following symptoms every 2 hours:

- Confusion or difficulty speaking. Ask the person his or her name, address, and age, the date, and the location.

- Inability to move the arms and legs on one side of the body, or slower movement of the limbs on one side than on the other.

- Blurred or double vision that does not clear, or significant changes in pupil size or reaction.

- Lethargy, abnormally deep sleep, or difficulty waking up.

- Vomiting that continues after the first 2 hours, or violent vomiting that persists after the first 15 minutes.

- Seizures or convulsions.

• Continue observing the person every 2 hours during the night. Wake the person up and check for any unusual symptoms. **Call 911 or go to an emergency room immediately** if you cannot wake the person or if he or she has any of the above symptoms of a severe head injury.

• A person who has a head injury should avoid contact sports until cleared by a health professional.

When to Call a Health Professional

• If the person loses consciousness at any time after being injured.

• If double vision or speech difficulty persists after the first minute.

• If weakness or numbness occurs on one side of the body.

- If blood or clear fluid drains from the ears or nose following a blow to the head (not due to a cut or direct blow to the nose).

- If the person is confused, does not remember being injured, or keeps repeating the same questions.

- If the person develops a severe headache.

- If vomiting occurs after the first 2 hours or violent vomiting persists after the first 15 minutes.

- If the person has seizures or convulsions.

- If bleeding cannot be stopped (see page 48) or the wound needs stitches (see page 49).

Heart Attack

A heart attack (myocardial infarction) is caused by a complete blockage of the blood flow to a part of the heart muscle. This usually occurs when a small blood clot forms in one of the blood vessels that supply the heart muscle.

Discomfort or pain caused by a heart attack may be felt in the chest, abdomen, upper back, neck, jaw, and/or one or both arms.

The pain of a heart attack usually lasts longer than 10 minutes and often occurs with other symptoms such as sweating, shortness of breath, or nausea. The pain of a heart attack will not usually go away with rest.

Discomfort caused by a heart attack can occur in any of the shaded areas as well as the upper back.

Many people mistake heart attack symptoms for other problems, such as indigestion, heartburn, or a pulled muscle. It is important to recognize the signals your body sends during the early stages of a heart attack and seek emergency care. Medical treatment is needed to prevent death. Sometimes, medications can be given to reduce the heart muscle damage caused by a heart attack.

When to Call a Health Professional

Call 911 or other emergency services immediately if you think you may be having a heart attack. Do not try to drive yourself to the hospital. After calling 911, chew and swallow 1 adult aspirin (unless you are allergic to or unable to take aspirin).

Symptoms of a heart attack include chest pain or discomfort that is crushing (feels like someone is sitting on your chest) or squeezing, increasing in intensity, or that occurs with any of the following symptoms:

• Sweating

• Shortness of breath

• Nausea or vomiting

• Pain in the abdomen, upper back, neck, jaw, or one or both arms

• Lightheadedness

• Rapid or irregular heartbeat

Call your doctor if you have continuous chest discomfort or pain and there is no obvious cause.

Heat Exhaustion and Heat Stroke

Heat exhaustion usually occurs when you are sweating a lot and do not drink enough to replace the lost fluids. It generally develops when you are working or exercising in hot weather. Symptoms include:

• Sweating a lot.

• Fatigue, weakness, headache, dizziness, or nausea.

• Skin that is cool, moist, pale, or flushed.

Heat exhaustion can sometimes lead to **heat stroke**, which requires emergency treatment. Heat stroke happens when your body fails to regulate its own temperature and your body temperature continues to rise, often to 105° or higher. You may stop sweating entirely if you have heat stroke. Symptoms of heat stroke include:

• Confusion, delirium, or unconsciousness.

• Skin that is red, hot, and dry, even in the armpits.

Prevention

• Drink 8 to 10 glasses of water per day. Drink even more if you are working or exercising in hot weather.

• Avoid strenuous physical activity outdoors during the hottest part of the day (10 a.m. to 4 p.m.).

• Wear light-colored, loose-fitting clothing and a hat with a brim to reflect the sun.

• Avoid sudden changes of temperature. Air out a hot car before getting into it. Never leave a child or an animal in a hot car.

• If you take diuretics (water pills), ask your doctor about taking a lower dose during hot weather.

• If you exercise strenuously in hot weather, drink more liquid than your thirst seems to require. Drink about 1 cup of water 10 to 15 minutes before you start exercising and another cup of water every 20 to 30 minutes.

Home Treatment

- Stop your activity. Get out of the sun to a cool spot, and drink lots of cool water, a little at a time. If you are nauseated or dizzy, lie down.

- If a person's temperature exceeds 102.3°, call for immediate help and try to lower the temperature as quickly as possible:

  - Remove unnecessary clothing.

  - Apply cool (not cold) water to the person's whole body; then fan the person. Apply ice packs to the groin, neck, and armpits. Do not immerse the person in ice water.

  - If you can get the person's temperature down to 102°, take care to avoid overcooling. Stop cooling the person once his or her temperature is lowered to 98.6°.

  - Do not give aspirin or acetaminophen to reduce the temperature.

  - Watch for signs of heat stroke (confusion or unconsciousness; red, hot, dry skin).

  - If the person stops breathing, start rescue breathing (see page 40).

When to Call a Health Professional

Call 911 or other emergency services if the person's body temperature reaches 102.3° and keeps rising, or if signs of heat stroke develop:

- Confusion, disorientation, unconsciousness, or seizure.

- Skin that is red, hot, and dry, even in the armpits. Sweating may be absent or excessive.

Hyperventilation

When you breathe very fast and deep (hyperventilate), the carbon dioxide (CO_2) level in your blood can drop too low. Symptoms that may occur with hyperventilation include:

- Numbness or tingling in your hands, feet, or around your mouth or tongue.

- Pounding, racing heartbeat and anxiety.

- Feeling like you can't get enough air.

- Lightheadedness (feeling like you might pass out).

- Muscle cramps or spasms.

- Chest pain.

- Loss of consciousness (if hyperventilation is severe).

Prevention

If you have hyperventilated before:

- Ask people to tell you if you start to breathe too fast.

- As soon as you notice fast breathing or other symptoms, slow your breathing to 1 breath every 5 seconds, or slow enough that symptoms gradually go away.

First Aid and Emergencies

Taking a Pulse

The pulse is the rate at which a person's heart beats. As the heart pumps blood through the body, you can feel a throbbing in the arteries wherever they come close to the skin's surface. Most of the time, the pulse is taken at the wrist, neck, or groin.

- Count the pulse after a person has been sitting or resting quietly for 10 minutes or more.

- Place two fingers gently against the wrist as shown (don't use your thumb).

- If it is hard to feel the pulse in the wrist, locate the carotid artery in the neck, just to either side of the windpipe. Press gently.

- Count the beats for 30 seconds; then double the result to calculate beats per minute.

Normal resting pulse:

- Newborn to 12 months: 100–160 beats/minute

- 1 through 6 years: 65–140 beats/minute

- 7 through 10 years: 60–110 beats/minute

- 11 years through adult: 50–100 beats/minute

Certain illnesses can cause the pulse to increase, so it is helpful to know what your resting pulse rate is when you are well. The pulse rate rises about 10 beats per minute for every degree of fever.

Home Treatment

- Sit down and concentrate on slowing your breathing. Try breathing through pursed lips or through your nose.

- Practice a relaxation technique. See page 323.

- Do not breathe in and out of a paper bag held over your nose and mouth. This technique can be dangerous.

When to Call a Health Professional

- If you are hyperventilating and cannot relieve the symptoms.

- If you have frequent or repeated episodes of hyperventilation and anxiety.

Hypothermia

Hypothermia occurs when your body temperature drops below normal. It develops when your body loses heat faster than heat can be produced by metabolism, muscle contractions, and shivering.

Early symptoms indicating mild to moderate hypothermia include:

- Shivering.

- Cold, pale skin.

- Apathy (listlessness).

- Impaired judgment.

- Clumsy movement and speech.

Later symptoms of severe hypo-thermia include:

- Cold abdomen.

- Slow pulse and breathing.

- Weakness or drowsiness.

- Confusion.

Shivering may stop if your body temperature drops below 90°.

Hypothermia is an emergency. It can quickly lead to unconsciousness and death if the heat loss continues. Hypothermia can happen at temperatures of 45° or even higher in wet and windy weather. Frail and inactive people can develop hypo-thermia indoors if they are not dressed warmly.

Early recognition is very important in the treatment of hypothermia. Often a hiker or skier will lose heat to a critical degree before others notice anything is wrong. If someone starts to shiver violently, stumble, or respond incoherently to questions, suspect hypothermia and warm the person quickly.

Prevention

Whenever you plan to be outdoors for several hours in cold weather, take the following precautions:

- Dress warmly and wear wind-proof, waterproof clothing. Wear fabrics that remain warm even when they are wet, such as wool or polypropylene.

- Wear a warm hat. An unprotected head loses a great deal of the body's total heat.

- Keep your hands and feet dry.

- Head for shelter if you get wet or cold.

- Eat well before going out and carry extra food.

- Don't drink beverages containing alcohol while in the cold. They make your body lose heat faster.

- Older or less active people can prevent indoor hypothermia by dressing warmly and keeping room temperatures above 65°.

Home Treatment

The goal of home or "in-the-field" treatment is to stop additional heat loss and slowly rewarm the person.

- For a mild case of hypothermia, get the person out of the cold and wind. Remove cold, wet clothes first, and give the person dry or wool clothing to wear.

- For a moderate case of hypother-mia, remove cold, wet clothes first. Then warm the person with your own body heat by wrapping a blanket or sleeping bag around both of you.

- Give warm liquids to drink and high-energy foods, such as candy, to eat. Do not give food or drink if the person is disoriented or uncon-scious. Do not give alcoholic or caffeinated beverages.

• Rewarming the person in warm water can cause shock or heart attack. However, in emergency situations when help is not available and other home treatments are not working, you can use a warm water bath (100° to 105°) as a last resort.

When to Call a Health Professional

Call 911 or other emergency services if the person seems confused, stumbles repeatedly, or loses consciousness and remains unconscious.

Call your doctor:

• If the victim is a child or an older adult. It's a good idea to call regardless of the severity of the symptoms.

• If the person's body temperature remains below 96° after 2 hours of warming.

Insect and Spider Bites and Stings

Insect and spider bites and bee, yellow jacket, and wasp stings usually cause a localized reaction with pain, swelling, redness, and itching. In some people, especially children, the redness and swelling may be worse, and the local reaction may last up to a few days. In most cases, bites and stings do not cause reactions all over the body.

Some people have severe skin reactions to insect or spider bites or stings, and a few have severe allergic reactions that affect the whole body (anaphylactic shock). Symptoms may include hives all over the body, shortness of breath and tightness in the throat or chest, dizziness, wheezing, or swelling of the tongue and face. If these symptoms develop, immediate medical attention is needed.

Spider bites are rarely serious, although any bite may be serious if it causes a person to have an allergic reaction.

Black widow spiders can be up to 2 inches across (although they are generally much smaller) and are shiny black with a red or yellow hourglass mark on their undersides. Bites from female black widows may cause chills, fever, nausea, and abdominal muscle pain. A person having a severe reaction may have difficulty breathing. People with high blood pressure, elderly people, and children have the greatest risk of having a severe reaction.

Brown recluse (fiddler) spiders are smaller than black widows and have long legs. They are brown with a violin-shaped mark on their heads. Their bites result in intense pain (although the bite itself may be painless), and a blister may develop that turns into a large, open sore. Their bites also may cause nausea, vomiting, headaches, and chills.

Also see Tick Bites on page 76.

Prevention

- To avoid bee stings, wear white or light-colored, solid fabrics. Bees are attracted to dark colors and flowered prints.

- Avoid wearing perfumes and colognes when you are outside.

- Apply an insect repellent containing DEET according to the directions every few hours when in insect- and spider-infested areas. Use a lower-concentration DEET product for small children and pregnant women. Wash DEET off when you come inside. Alpha Keri and Skin-So-Soft bath oils also seem to repel insects.

- Wear gloves and tuck pants into socks when working in woodpiles, sheds, and basements where spiders are found.

Home Treatment

- Remove a bee stinger by scraping or flicking it out. Don't squeeze the stinger; you may release more venom into the skin. If the stinger isn't visible, assume there isn't one.

- If you are bitten by a black widow or brown recluse spider, apply ice to the bite and call your doctor immediately. Do not apply a tourniquet.

- Apply a cold pack or ice cube to the bite or sting. Some people also find that applying a paste of baking soda or unseasoned meat tenderizer mixed with a little water helps relieve pain and decrease the reaction.

- Take an oral antihistamine (such as Benadryl or Chlor-Trimeton) to relieve pain, swelling, and itching. Calamine lotion or hydrocortisone cream may also help.

- Carry an emergency kit containing an epinephrine syringe (such as EpiPen) if you have had a severe allergic reaction to insect venom in the past. Ask your doctor or pharmacist how and when to use the kit.

- Wash the area with soap and water.

- Trim your fingernails to prevent scratching, because scratching can lead to infection.

When to Call a Health Professional

Call 911 or other emergency services if you develop signs of a severe allergic reaction soon after you are bitten or stung by an insect or spider:

- Wheezing or difficulty breathing.

- Swelling around the lips, tongue, or face, or significant swelling around the site of the bite or sting (e.g., entire arm or leg is swollen).

- Signs of shock. See page 69.

Call your doctor:

- If you develop a spreading skin rash, itching, feeling of warmth, or hives.

- If you have been bitten by the same type of spider or insect that previously caused a serious reaction.

First Aid and Emergencies

- If a blister appears at the site of a spider bite, or if the surrounding skin becomes discolored.

- If symptoms are not improving in 2 to 3 days or if signs of infection develop. See page 67.

- To talk about adrenaline kits or allergy shots (immunotherapy) for insect venom if you have had a serious allergic reaction.

Nosebleeds

Most nosebleeds are not serious and can usually be stopped with home treatment. Some common causes of nosebleeds are low humidity, colds and allergies, injuries to the nose, medications (especially aspirin), and high altitude. Blowing or picking your nose can also cause a nosebleed.

Prevention

- Low humidity is a common cause of nosebleeds. Humidify your home, especially the bedrooms, and keep the temperature cooler (60° to 64°) in sleeping areas.

- If your nose becomes very dry, breathe moist air for a while (such as in the shower) and then put a little petroleum jelly on the inside of your nose to help prevent bleeding. A saline nasal spray may also help. See page 344.

- Limit your use of aspirin, which can contribute to nosebleeds.

Home Treatment

- Sit up straight and tip your head slightly forward. Tilting your head back may cause blood to run down your throat.

- Blow all the clots out of your nose. Pinch your nostrils shut between your thumb and forefinger or apply firm pressure against the bleeding nostril for 10 full minutes. Resist the urge to peek after a few minutes to see if your nose has stopped bleeding.

Stopping a nosebleed

- After 10 minutes, check to see if your nose is still bleeding. If it is, hold it for 10 more minutes. Most nosebleeds will stop after you apply direct pressure for 10 to 30 minutes.

- Stay quiet for a few hours and do not blow your nose for at least 12 hours after the bleeding has stopped.

First Aid and Emergencies

When to Call a Health Professional

- If the bleeding hasn't stopped after you have applied direct pressure for 30 minutes.

- If blood runs down the back of your throat even when you pinch your nose.

- If your nose is deformed after an injury and may be broken.

- If nosebleeds recur often (more than four in a week).

- If you take blood thinners (anti-coagulants or high doses of aspirin) and have had more than one nosebleed in a single day.

Objects in the Ear

Children sometimes put small objects in their ears, or an insect may crawl into the ear. It may be hard to know if an insect is in the ear. Your child may say, "My ear is bumping around."

Home Treatment

- Don't try to kill an insect inside a person's ear. Pull the ear up and back and let the sun or a bright light shine into the ear. Insects are attracted to light, so the insect may crawl out.

- If the insect doesn't crawl out, fill the ear canal with warm mineral, olive, or baby oil. The insect may float out.

- To remove an object other than an insect from the ear, tilt the person's head to the side and shake it gently.

(Never shake a baby.) Gently pulling the ear up and back may straighten the ear canal and help dislodge the object.

- If you can see the object, try carefully to remove it with tweezers. Do not try this if the person will not hold very still or if the object is in the ear so far that you can't see the tips of the tweezers. Use care not to push the object in farther.

When to Call a Health Professional

- If you cannot remove the insect or object.

- If pain, fever, swelling, or drainage develop.

Objects in the Eye

A speck of dirt or small object in the eye will often wash out with your tears. If the object is not removed, it may scratch the eye (corneal abrasion). Most corneal abrasions are minor and will heal on their own in 1 to 2 days.

When an object is thrown forcefully into the eye (from a machine, for example), it is likely that the eyeball will be punctured and emergency care will be needed.

Prevention

Wear safety glasses or other protective eyewear when working with machines or tools, mowing the lawn, or cycling.

Home Treatment

- Wash your hands before touching the eye.

- Don't rub the eye; you could scratch the cornea.

- Do not try to remove an object that is over the colored part of the eye or stuck in the white of the eye. Try flushing it out with water or saline solution. If that doesn't work, call a health professional.

- If the object is at the side of the eye or on the lower lid, moisten a cotton swab or the tip of a twisted piece of tissue and touch the end to the object. The object should cling to the swab or tissue. Some minor irritation is common after you have removed the object.

- Gently wash the eye with cool water. An eyedropper helps.

- Never use tweezers, toothpicks, or other hard items to remove an object from the eye.

When to Call a Health Professional

Call 911 or other emergency services if the eyeball seems to be punctured.

Call your doctor:

- If the object is over the colored part of the eye or is embedded in the eye. Do not pull out an object that is stuck in the eye.

- If you cannot remove the object.

- If there is blood over or in front of the colored part of the eye.

- If pain is severe or persists; if it feels like there is still something in your eye; if your eye is sensitive to light; or if your vision is blurred after the object has been removed. Your cornea may be scratched. Keep your eye closed.

Objects in the Nose

Children sometimes put small objects, like beads, popcorn, or small batteries, up their noses. If the child doesn't tell you about it, your first clue may be a foul-smelling, green or yellow discharge from just one nostril. The nose may also be tender and swollen.

Home Treatment

- Have the child pinch the other nostril closed and try to blow the object out.

- If you can see the object, try to remove it with blunt-nosed tweezers. Hold the child's head still and use care not to push the object in farther. If the child resists, do not try tweezers. Minor bleeding from the nostril is not serious.

- Spray a nasal decongestant (see page 344) in the affected nostril to reduce the swelling, unless you suspect the object is a disc battery.

First Aid and Emergencies

When to Call a Health Professional

- If a disc battery is stuck in the nose. The moist tissue in the nose can cause the battery to release harmful chemicals, often in less than an hour.

- If you are unable to remove the object after several tries.

- If removing the object causes a severe nosebleed. See page 62.

Poisoning

FOR ANY POISONING: Call 911 or your local poison control center immediately.

Children will swallow just about anything, including poisons. When in doubt, assume the worst.

Always believe a child who indicates that he or she has swallowed poison, no matter how unappetizing the substance is.

If you suspect food poisoning, see page 98.

Prevention

About 80 percent of poisonings occur in children between the ages of 1 and 4. Develop poison prevention habits before your child is born or certainly before he or she is crawling. Infants grow so fast that sometimes they are crawling and walking before you have time to protect them.

- Never leave a poisonous product unattended, even for a moment.

Lead Poisoning

Infants and young children who inhale or eat dust, food, or other things that contain lead are at risk for developing learning disabilities and growth problems. Lead poisoning can cause serious problems in adults as well.

Lead is present in old paint, water pipes, and other substances. Lead-based paint may be a hazard in older homes, especially if the paint is flaking or peeling and a child eats the paint flakes.

To reduce the risk of lead poisoning:

- Keep painted surfaces in good repair. Clean paint flakes and chips from older painted surfaces (such as floors and windowsills) carefully.

- Keep young children away from home remodeling and refinishing projects.

- If your home has lead or lead-soldered water pipes, use cold water and let the water run for a few minutes before using it for drinking, cooking, or making baby formula.

- Have your child's blood tested for lead at about 1 year of age.

- Call your local health department for more information about preventing lead poisoning.

First Aid and Emergencies

• Lock all drugs and vitamins away from children. Aspirin is a common source of childhood poisoning, especially flavored baby aspirin. Lock up drugs between doses.

• Do not keep poisons, such as drain opener, dishwasher detergent, oven cleaner, or plant food, under your kitchen sink. Keep them completely out of the reach of children. Dishwasher detergent is especially dangerous.

• Keep products in their original containers. Never store poisonous products in food containers.

• Use childproof latches on your cupboards.

• Use "Mr. Yuk" stickers and teach your children to recognize them.

• Purchase syrup of ipecac (see page 348), and keep the poison control center number near your phone.

Home Treatment

• Call a poison control center, hospital, or health professional immediately. Have the poison container with you so you can describe the poison. You will be told whether it is safe to make the person vomit.

• Do not have the person vomit if he or she:

  - Is having convulsions.

  - Is unconscious.

  - Has a burning sensation in the mouth or throat.

Carbon Monoxide Poisoning

Carbon monoxide is a colorless, odorless, tasteless gas produced from burning fuels such as natural gas, gasoline, fuel oil, or wood. If fuel-burning appliances are not used properly, dangerous levels of carbon monoxide can build up in enclosed areas.

When a person inhales carbon monoxide, the carbon monoxide begins to replace the oxygen in the blood. This condition is called carbon monoxide poisoning. Symptoms include headache, dizziness, and nausea. If the exposure to carbon monoxide continues, the person may lose consciousness and even die. Infants, small children, older adults, and people with chronic health problems are more easily affected by high amounts of carbon monoxide in the blood, and their symptoms may be more severe.

A good way to protect yourself and your family from carbon monoxide poisoning is to install a carbon monoxide detector in your home. Also, have your heating appliances, chimneys, and vents inspected each year. Do not leave your car's engine running when the car is in an enclosed area such as a garage, even if the garage door is open.

If you know or suspect that someone has carbon monoxide poisoning, seek medical care immediately.

- Has swallowed a corrosive agent or petroleum product (dishwasher detergent, lye, bleach, disinfectant, drain opener, floor wax, kerosene, grease remover).

• If suggested by the poison control center, induce vomiting by:

  - Giving syrup of ipecac, if available. See page 348.

  - Placing a spoon or finger at the back of the person's throat.

• When vomiting begins, place the person's head lower than his or her chest to keep vomited material from entering the lungs.

Puncture Wounds

Puncture wounds are caused by sharp, pointed objects that penetrate the skin. Nails, tacks, ice picks, knives, needles, and teeth can all cause puncture wounds. Puncture wounds become infected easily because they are difficult to clean and provide a warm, moist place for bacteria to grow.

Home Treatment

• If the object that caused the wound is small, such as a tack or sewing needle, remove it, checking to make sure it is intact. If the object is large or caused a deep wound, leave it in place and call a health professional immediately.

Signs of Infection

Infection can develop after a wound to the skin or mucous membranes, especially if the wound is not cleaned well. Cuts, scrapes, puncture wounds, burns, blisters, stings, bites, and rashes can all become infected. Bruises, sprains, broken bones, and other conditions can lead to infection under the skin.

Signs of infection include:

• Increased pain, swelling, redness, warmth, or tenderness.

• Red streaks extending from the affected area.

• Discharge of pus.

• Swollen lymph nodes in the neck, armpits, or groin.

• Fever of 100° or higher with no other cause.

Call a health professional if signs of infection develop after a wound or injury. You may need to be treated with antibiotics.

• Allow the wound to bleed freely for up to 5 minutes to clean itself out, unless there has been a large loss of blood or the blood is squirting out. If bleeding is heavy, see "Stopping Severe Bleeding" on page 48.

First Aid and Emergencies

• Clean the wound thoroughly with soap and water. Do not use alcohol, hydrogen peroxide, iodine, or mercurochrome.

• Watch for signs of infection (see page 67). If the wound closes, an infection under the skin may not be detected for several days.

When to Call a Health Professional

• If severe bleeding cannot be controlled. See page 48.

• If the wound is in your head, neck, chest, or abdomen, unless it is minor.

• If the skin near the wound is blue, white, or cold; if there is numbness, tingling, or loss of feeling; or if you are unable to move a limb below the wound.

• If an animal bite is severe and may need stitches, or if it is on your face, hand, or foot. Stitches usually need to be done in 8 hours.

• If you are unable to remove an object from the wound or if you think part of the object may still be in the wound.

• If the wound was caused by a cat or human bite.

• If the wound was caused by an injection of a substance under high pressure (such as from a paint sprayer).

• If you have a puncture wound and your tetanus shots are not up to date (see page 16).

• If a deep wound to the foot occurred through a shoe.

• If signs of infection develop. See page 67.

Removing Splinters

Try using scotch tape first. Simply put the tape over the splinter, then pull it up.

If that doesn't work, you can grasp the end of the splinter with tweezers and try to gently pull it out. If the splinter is embedded in the skin, clean a needle with alcohol and make a small hole in the skin over the end of the splinter. Then lift the splinter with the tip of the needle until it can be grasped with the tweezers and pulled out.

After the splinter has been removed, wash the area with soap and water. Apply a bandage if needed to keep the wound clean; otherwise, leave the wound open to the air. Watch for signs of infection.

Call a health professional if the splinter is very large or deeply embedded and cannot be easily removed, or if the splinter is in the eye.

Scrapes

Scrapes or abrasions happen so often that they seem unimportant. Good home treatment will reduce scarring and prevent infection.

Home Treatment

- Scrapes are usually very dirty. Remove large pieces of debris with tweezers. Then scrub well with soap and water and a washcloth. The injured person will probably complain loudly, but cleaning is necessary to prevent infection and scarring. Scrubbing may cause some minor bleeding. Using a water sprayer from the kitchen sink is a good way to wash a scrape.

- Apply steady pressure with a clean bandage or cloth to stop bleeding.

- Applying ice may help reduce swelling and bruising.

- If the scrape is large or in an area that may be rubbed by clothing, apply an antibiotic ointment (such as Polysporin or Neosporin) to the scrape and cover it with a nonstick bandage (such as Telfa).

When to Call a Health Professional

- If bleeding continues after 30 minutes of pressure.

- If your tetanus shots are not up to date. See page 16.

- If you cannot clean the scrape well because it is too large, deep, or painful or has dirt and debris embedded under the skin.

- If signs of infection develop. See page 67.

Shock

Shock may develop as a result of sudden illness or injury. When the circulatory system is unable to get enough blood to the vital organs, the body goes into shock. Sometimes even a mild injury will lead to shock.

The signs of shock include:

- Cool, pale, clammy skin.

- Weak, rapid pulse.

- Shallow, rapid breathing.

- Low blood pressure.

- Thirst, nausea, or vomiting.

- Confusion or anxiety.

- Faintness, weakness, dizziness, or loss of consciousness.

Shock is a life-threatening condition. Prompt home treatment can save the person's life.

Home Treatment

- Have the person lie down and elevate his or her legs 12 inches or more. If the injury is to the head, neck, or chest, keep the legs flat. If the person vomits, roll the person to one side to let fluids drain from the mouth. Use care if there could be a spinal injury (see page 71).

Counting Respiration Rates

The respiration rate is the rate at which a person breathes. It increases with fever and some illnesses. The best time to count the respiration rate is when a person is resting, perhaps after taking the person's pulse while your fingers are still on the person's wrist. The person's breathing is likely to change if he or she knows you are counting it.

- Count the number of times the chest rises in 1 full minute.

- Notice whether there is any sucking in beneath the ribs or any apparent wheezing or difficulty breathing.

Normal resting respiration rate:

- Newborn to 1 year:
  40–60 breaths/minute

- 1 through 6 years:
  18–26 breaths/minute

- 7 years through adult:
  12–24 breaths/minute

- Control any bleeding (see page 48) and splint any fractures (see page 73).

- Keep the person warm, but not hot. Place a blanket underneath the person, and cover the person with a sheet or blanket, depending on the weather. If the person is in a hot place, try to keep the person cool.

- Take and record the person's pulse every 5 minutes. See page 58.

- Comfort and reassure the person to relieve anxiety.

When to Call a Health Professional

Call 911 or other emergency services if a person develops signs of shock.

Snake Bites

While thousands of people are bitten by snakes every year in the United States, only about 10 people die as a result. Rattlesnakes inflict most poisonous snake bites. Other poisonous snakes in North America are copperheads, cottonmouths (also called water moccasins), and coral snakes. If you are bitten by a snake you know or suspect is poisonous, call for emergency medical care.

If you are bitten by a snake and it is safe for someone who is with you to kill the snake, have the person do so, and take the dead snake with you when you get medical care. By knowing what kind of snake has bitten you, a health professional can quickly select the correct treatment. Be very careful when handling the dead snake. The snake's biting reflex remains for up to 60 minutes after it has died.

Get medical care as quickly as possible. Medication for snake bites is most effective when given within 4 hours and is less effective after more than 12 hours have passed.

Prevention

- Find out what the local snakes look like, whether they are poisonous, and where you are likely to encounter them.

- Wear high leather boots and long pants when you are in areas that snakes inhabit.

- Do not put your hands or feet anywhere until you can see that it is safe to do so. Do not step over logs or rocks if you cannot see the other side.

- Avoid walking in snake-infested areas at night.

- Do not handle snakes, even if they are dead, unless you know how to identify snakes and know their habits.

Home Treatment

Call 911 or other emergency services if you think you have been bitten by a poisonous snake. While you are waiting for help to arrive (or if help is not available):

- Keep calm. Frantic activity will cause the poison to spread faster.

- If possible, lie down and keep the area of the bite lower than your heart.

- Splint the arm or leg that was bitten at or below heart level. See page 73.

- Drink nonalcoholic beverages in frequent, small amounts to reduce the risk of shock.

- Snake bite kits (such as the Extractor) may be of temporary benefit while you wait for medical help to arrive. Use them only if you have been instructed how and when to do so by an expert.

When to Call a Health Professional

Call 911 or other emergency services if you think that you or someone you are with has just been bitten by a poisonous snake.

Spinal Injuries

Injury to the spine must be considered anytime there has been an accident involving the neck or back. Permanent paralysis may be avoided if the injured person is immobilized and transported correctly.

Signs of a spinal injury include:

- Severe pain in the neck or back.

- Bruises on the head, neck, shoulders, or back.

- Weakness, tingling, or numbness in the arms or legs.

- Loss of bowel or bladder control.

- Loss of consciousness.

Home Treatment

- If you suspect a spinal injury, do not move the person unless there is an immediate threat to life, such as fire. Don't drag victims from automobile accidents.

• If the person is in immediate danger, and must be moved, do whatever you can to move the person's head, neck, and shoulders together as a unit while you move him or her to safety.

• If the person was injured in a diving accident, don't pull the injured person from the water, because you may cause permanent damage. Float the person face up in the water until help arrives. The water will act as a splint and keep the person's spine immobile.

When to Call a Health Professional

Call 911 or other emergency services to transport the injured person if you suspect a spinal injury.

Strains, Sprains, Fractures, and Dislocations

A **strain** is an injury caused by over-stretching or tearing a muscle or tendon. A **sprain** is an injury to the ligaments or soft tissues around a joint. A **fracture** is a broken bone. A **dislocation** occurs when one end of a bone is pulled or pushed out of its normal position.

All four injuries cause pain and swelling. Unless a broken bone is obvious, it may be difficult to tell if an injury is a strain, sprain, fracture, or dislocation. Injuries often involve all four. Rapid swelling often indicates a more serious injury. If a bone

is poking through the skin, or if a limb turns white, cold, or clammy below the injured area, immediate medical care is needed.

Most minor strains and sprains can be treated at home, but severe sprains, fractures, and dislocations need professional care. Apply home treatment while you wait to see your doctor.

A **stress fracture** is a weak spot or small crack in a bone caused by repeated overuse. Stress fractures in the small bones of the foot are common during intensive training for basketball, running, and other sports. The most common symptom is persistent pain at the site of the fracture. The pain may improve during exercise but will be worse before and after activity. There may not be any visible swelling.

Prevention

It may not always be possible to prevent accidents that cause strains, sprains, fractures, or dislocations. However, if you train properly for activities, try not to push too hard during activities, wear protective gear, and use equipment that is in good condition, you will improve your chances of avoiding serious injury.

Other tips for preventing accidents include the following:

• Make sure you can always see where you are going.

• Don't carry objects that are too heavy.

Splinting

Splinting immobilizes a limb that you suspect is fractured to prevent further injury until you can see a health professional. Splinting may also be helpful after a snakebite while you wait for help to arrive. There are two ways to immobilize a limb: tie the injured limb to a stiff object, or fasten it to some other part of the body.

For the first method, tie rolled-up newspapers or magazines, a stick, a cane, or anything that is stiff to the injured limb with a rope, a belt, or anything else that will work. Do not tie too tightly.

Position the splint so the injured limb cannot bend. A general rule is to splint from a joint above the suspected fracture to a joint below it. For example, splint a broken forearm from above the elbow to below the wrist.

For the second method, tape a broken toe to the next toe, or immobilize an injured arm by tying it across the chest.

Note: These splinting methods are for short-term, emergency use only. Your doctor will provide you with a splint or cast that is appropriate for the specific joint and the type of injury.

- Use a step stool to reach objects that are above your head. Don't stand on chairs, countertops, or unstable objects.

- Keep toddlers away from objects that may cause injuries if the child falls on them (coffee tables, stairs, and fireplaces).

- See the prevention tips for Sports Injuries on page 136.

Home Treatment

Generally speaking, whether the injury affects soft tissue or bone, the basic treatment is the same: **RICE**, which stands for rest, ice, compression, and elevation, to treat the acute pain or injury. Begin the RICE process immediately for most injuries.

R. Rest. Do not put weight on the injured joint for at least 24 to 48 hours.

- Use crutches to support a badly sprained knee or ankle.

- Support a sprained wrist, elbow, or shoulder with a sling, which will help the injury heal faster.

- Rest a sprained finger by taping it to the healthy finger next to it (this works for toes too). Always put padding between the two fingers or toes you are taping together.

Injured muscle, ligament, or tendon tissue needs time and rest to heal. Stress fractures need rest for 2 to 4 months.

I. Ice. Cold will reduce pain and swelling and promote healing. Heat feels nice, but it does more harm than good if it is applied too soon (less than 48 hours) after an injury.

First Aid and Emergencies

Removing a Ring

If you did not remove a ring before an injured finger started to swell, try the following method to remove the ring:

- Stick the end of a slick piece of string, such as dental floss, under the ring toward your hand.

- Starting at the side of the ring closest to the middle knuckle, wrap the string snugly around your finger, wrapping beyond the middle knuckle. Each wrap should be right next to the one before it.

- Grasp the end of the string that is stretched under the ring and start unwrapping it. Push the ring ahead of the unwrapped string as you go, until the ring passes the middle knuckle.

Wrap toward the end of the finger.

Pull the ring over the wrapped joint.

Apply ice or cold packs immediately to prevent or minimize swelling. For difficult-to-reach injuries, a cold pack works best. See "Ice and Cold Packs" on page 133.

C. Compression. Wrap the injured area with an elastic (Ace) bandage or compression sleeve to immobilize and protect the area. Don't wrap it too tightly, because doing so can cause more swelling. Loosen the bandage if the area below the wrap feels numb, tingles, or feels cool. A tightly wrapped sprain may fool you into thinking you can keep using the joint. With or without a wrap, the joint needs total rest for 1 to 2 days.

E. Elevation. Elevate the injured area on pillows while you apply ice and anytime you are sitting or lying down. Try to keep the injury at or above the level of your heart to help minimize swelling and bruising.

Heat (hot water bottle, warm towel, heating pad) may be used after 48 to 72 hours of cold treatments if the swelling is gone. Some experts recommend going back and forth between heat and cold treatments.

You may be able to prevent further damage with some of the following:

- Splint an arm, leg, finger, or toe that you suspect is broken. Use a splint or a sling for a short period of time (a few hours) while waiting to see your doctor. See page 73.

- Apply a sling to support an injured arm. Do not put an arm sling on a baby.

- Remove all rings immediately if the sprain is to a finger or part of the hand. Swelling is likely to occur, making removal of the ring more difficult later. See "Removing a Ring" on page 74.

- Aspirin, ibuprofen, naproxen sodium, or ketoprofen may help ease inflammation and pain. Do not give aspirin to anyone younger than 20.

- Gentle exercise can be started as soon as the initial pain and swelling have gone away. If you have a broken bone or a severe sprain, your doctor may put the limb in a cast.

When to Call a Health Professional

- If the injured limb or joint is deformed or out of its normal position.

- If the skin over the site of an injury is broken.

- If there are signs of nerve or blood vessel damage:

  - Numbness, tingling, or a "pins-and-needles" sensation.

  - Skin that is pale, white, or blue, or feels colder than the skin on the limb that is not hurt.

  - Inability to move the limb normally because of weakness, not just pain.

- If you cannot bear weight on or straighten an injured limb, or if an injured joint wobbles or feels unstable.

- If pain is severe or lasts longer than 24 hours.

- If swelling:

  - Develops within 30 minutes of the injury.

  - Does not improve after 48 hours of home treatment.

- If signs of infection develop following an injury. See page 67.

Stroke

A stroke occurs when a blood vessel (artery) supplying blood to the brain bursts or becomes blocked by a blood clot. Within minutes, the nerve cells in that area of the brain are damaged and die. As a result, the part of the body controlled by those cells cannot function properly.

Call 911 or other emergency services immediately if you think you may be having a stroke. Do not try to drive yourself to the hospital. If medical treatment is sought as soon as stroke symptoms are noticed, fewer brain cells may be permanently damaged by the stroke.

The effects of a stroke may range from mild to severe and may be temporary or permanent. A stroke can affect vision, speech, behavior, thought processes, and the ability to move parts of the body. Sometimes it can cause a coma or death. The effects of a stroke depend on:

- Which brain cells are damaged.

- How much of the brain is affected.

First Aid and Emergencies

First Aid and Emergencies

• How quickly blood supply is restored to the affected area.

 A person may have one or more <u>transient ischemic attacks</u> (TIAs) before having a stroke. TIAs are often called mini strokes because their symptoms are similar to those of a stroke. The difference between a TIA and a stroke is that TIA symptoms usually disappear within 10 to 20 minutes; however, TIA symptoms may last up to 24 hours. A TIA can occur months before a stroke occurs. It is a warning signal that a stroke may soon follow. The first TIA should always be treated as an emergency, even if the symptoms go away after just a few minutes.

When to Call a Health Professional

Call 911 or other emergency services immediately if you have any of the following symptoms of stroke:

• Any new weakness, numbness, or paralysis in your face, arm, or leg, especially on only one side of your body.

• Blurred or decreased vision in one or both eyes that does not clear with blinking.

• New difficulty speaking or understanding simple statements.

• Sudden, unexplainable, and intense headache that is different from any headache you have had before.

• Severe dizziness, loss of balance, or loss of coordination, especially if another warning sign is present at the same time.

If a symptom was definitely there and then went away after a few minutes, call your doctor immediately. Symptoms that go away in a few minutes may be caused by a TIA. A TIA is a strong sign that a major stroke may soon occur and should be treated as an emergency.

Tick Bites

Ticks are small, spiderlike insects that bite into the skin and feed on blood. Ticks live in the fur and feathers of many birds and other animals. Tick bites occur more often from early spring to late summer.

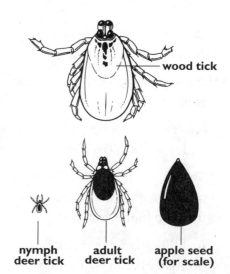

Lyme disease is usually spread by nymph deer ticks, which are difficult to see. Adult deer ticks are about the size of an apple seed. All ticks grow larger as they fill up with blood.

 For more information, see the back cover.

Most ticks do not carry diseases, and most tick bites do not cause serious health problems. However, it is important to remove a tick as soon as you find one.

Many of the diseases ticks may pass to humans (including Rocky Mountain spotted fever, relapsing fever, Colorado tick fever, and Lyme disease) have the same flulike symptoms: fever, headache, muscle aches, and a general feeling of illness. Sometimes a rash or craterlike sore (ulcer) may accompany the flulike symptoms. An expanding red rash is an early symptom of Lyme disease. It may appear 1 day to 1 month after you have been bitten by a deer tick. If you develop flulike symptoms or a rash after being bitten by a tick, be sure to tell your health professional.

Prevention

Before going outdoors in a tick-infested area:

- Put on light-colored clothing and tuck pant legs into socks.

- Apply an insect repellent containing DEET to exposed areas of skin or to clothing. Apply carefully around eyes and mouth.

  - Children and pregnant women should use a lower-concentration DEET product.

  - Don't put repellent on small children's hands, because they often put their hands in their mouths.

  - After returning indoors, wash the repellent off with soap and water.

Home Treatment

- Check regularly for ticks when you are out in the woods, and thoroughly examine your skin and scalp when you return home. Check your pets too. The sooner ticks are removed, the less likely they are to spread infection.

- Remove a tick by gently pulling on it with tweezers, as close to the skin as possible. Fine-tipped tweezers may work best. Pull straight out and try not to crush the body. Save the tick in a jar for tests in case you develop flulike symptoms after you have been bitten.

- Wash the area and apply an antiseptic.

When to Call a Health Professional

- If you are unable to remove the entire tick.

- If you develop a red rash that expands over several days, especially if you know you were recently exposed to ticks. The rash may or may not be in the area where you were bitten and may be accompanied by flulike symptoms, such as fatigue, headache, stiff neck, fever, chills, or body aches.

 Your doctor will probably be able to tell if you have Lyme disease based on your symptoms and whether you may have been exposed to deer ticks. In most cases, blood tests to diagnose Lyme disease are not useful.

Unconsciousness

An unconscious person is completely unaware of what is going on and is unable to make purposeful movements. Fainting is a brief form of unconsciousness; a coma is a deep, prolonged state of unconsciousness.

Causes of unconsciousness include stroke, epilepsy, heat stroke, diabetic coma, insulin shock, head injury, suffocation, alcohol or drug overdose, shock, bleeding, irregular heartbeat, and heart attack.

Fainting is a short-term loss of consciousness, usually lasting only a few seconds. It is most often caused by a momentary drop in blood flow to the brain. When you fall or lie down, blood flow is improved and you regain consciousness. Fainting is a mild form of shock and is usually not serious. If it happens often, there may be a more serious problem. Dizziness and fainting can also be brought on by sudden emotional stress or injury. See page 176.

Home Treatment

- Make sure the unconscious person can breathe. Check for breathing, and if necessary, open the airway and begin rescue breathing. See page 40.

- Check the person's pulse. See page 58. If there is no pulse, call for help and start cardiopulmonary resuscitation (CPR). See page 40.

- Keep the person lying down on his or her side.

- Look for a medical alert bracelet, necklace, or card that identifies a medical problem such as epilepsy, diabetes, or drug allergy.

- Treat any injuries.

- Do not give the person anything to eat or drink.

When to Call a Health Professional

Call 911 or other emergency services if a person remains unconscious for longer than a few seconds.

Call your doctor:

- If a person completely loses consciousness, even if the person is now awake.

- If unconsciousness follows a head injury and the victim is now awake. A person with a head injury needs to be carefully observed. See page 53.

- Whenever a person with diabetes loses consciousness, even if he or she is now awake. He or she may have insulin shock (low blood sugar) or be in a diabetic coma (too much sugar in the blood).

A great step towards independence is a
good-humored stomach.
Seneca

4

Digestive and Urinary Problems

The cause of problems with the digestive and urinary systems can be hard to pinpoint. Sometimes serious and minor problems start with the same symptoms. Fortunately, most digestive and urinary problems are minor and home treatment is all that is needed.

Use the chart on page 80 to find the symptoms that most closely match the ones you are having. Some illnesses that can cause digestive and urinary problems are covered more thoroughly in other chapters. Use the chart or the index to find those topics.

Abdominal Pain

You can get clues about the cause of abdominal pain and how serious the problem may be by noting the following:

• The severity of the pain. A visit to a health professional is usually needed when severe abdominal pain comes on suddenly and continues, or when new or different pain becomes more severe over several hours or days.

• The location of the pain. See illustration on page 79.

If you have abdominal pain, it helps to tell your doctor exactly where the pain is.

Digestive and Urinary Problems

Symptoms	Possible Causes
Nausea or vomiting	Nausea and Vomiting, p. 95; Hepatitis, p. 94; Medication reaction—call your doctor or pharmacist; Adverse Drug Reactions, p. 351.
Bowel Movements	
Frequent, watery stools	Diarrhea, p. 86; Stomach Flu and Food Poisoning, p. 98; Antibiotics, p. 349.
Stools are dry and difficult to pass	Constipation, p. 82.
Bloody or black, tarry stools	Ulcers, p. 100; Diarrhea, p. 86.
Pain during bowel movements; bright red blood on surface of stool or on toilet paper	Hemorrhoids, p. 96; Anal fissure, p. 97; Constipation, p. 82.
Abdominal Pain	
Pain and tenderness localized to one place with possible nausea, vomiting, and fever	Appendicitis, p. 81; Urinary Tract Infections, p. 103; Ovarian cyst, p. 81; Gallstones, p. 92; Kidney Stones, p. 90; also see p. 79.
Bloating and gas with diarrhea, constipation, or both	Irritable Bowel Syndrome, p. 91.
Burning or discomfort behind or below breastbone	Heartburn, p. 87; Ulcers, p. 100; Chest Pain, p. 152.
Pain in lower abdomen and lower back just before menstrual period	Menstrual Cramps, p. 259; Ovarian cyst, p. 81.
Pain on one side of lower abdomen with possible pregnancy	Ectopic Pregnancy, p. 255.
Urination	
Pain or burning while urinating	Urinary Tract Infections, p. 103; Kidney Stones, p. 90; Prostate problems, pp. 269 to 272; Sexually Transmitted Diseases, p. 278.
Difficulty urinating or weak urine stream (males)	Prostate problems, pp. 269 to 272.
Leaking urine or loss of bladder control	Urinary Incontinence, p. 101.
Blood in urine	Urinary Tract Infections, p. 103; Kidney Stones, p. 90; also see p. 105.
Abdominal Lumps or Swelling	
Painless lump or swelling in groin that comes and goes	Hernia, p. 89.
Very rigid or distended abdomen	Blunt Abdominal Wounds, p. 37; Appendicitis, p. 81; Watch for shock, p. 69.

Generalized pain is pain that occurs in more than half of the abdomen. Generalized pain can occur with many different illnesses, most of which will go away without medical treatment. Heartburn (indigestion) and stomach flu are common problems that can cause generalized abdominal pain. **Cramping**, which can be very painful, is rarely serious if passing gas or a stool relieves it. Many women have cramping pain with their periods. Unless it is significantly different than usual, or it localizes to one area of the abdomen, generalized pain is usually not a cause for concern.

Localized pain is pain that is most intense in one part of the abdomen. Localized pain that comes on suddenly and persists, that gradually becomes more severe, or that gets worse when you move or cough may indicate a problem in an abdominal organ, such as appendicitis, pancreatitis, diverticulitis, an ovarian cyst, or gallbladder disease.

Any new abdominal pain that lasts more than a few days needs to be evaluated by a health professional.

Home Treatment

Most of the time, abdominal pain improves with home treatment and does not require a visit to a health professional.

Specific home treatment for abdominal pain often depends on the symptoms that accompany the pain, such as diarrhea or nausea and vomiting. Be sure to review the home treatment guidelines for any other symptoms you have that are covered in this or other chapters.

Appendicitis

The appendix is a small sac attached to the large intestine. (See illustration on page 87.) Sometimes the appendix becomes inflamed or infected (appendicitis). If not treated, appendicitis can cause the appendix to burst and spread infection throughout the abdomen (peritonitis). This can cause a rigid or distended abdomen.

Typical symptoms of appendicitis include:

• Pain in the abdomen that begins around the navel or a little higher. The pain becomes more intense and then moves (localizes) to the lower right part of the abdomen below the navel. The pain is steady and gets worse when you walk or cough.

• Loss of appetite, nausea, vomiting, and constipation.

• Fever and chills.

Call your health professional:

• If you think you have appendicitis.

• If continuous pain in the lower right abdomen lasts longer than 4 hours.

Also see When to Call a Health Professional on page 82.

If you have mild abdominal pain without other symptoms, try the following:

• Rest until you are feeling better.

• Drink plenty of fluids to avoid dehydration. You may find that taking small, frequent sips of a beverage is easier on your stomach than trying to drink a whole glass at once.

• Try eating several small meals instead of two or three large ones. Eat mild foods, such as rice, dry toast or crackers, bananas, and applesauce. Avoid spicy foods, other fruits, alcohol, and drinks that contain caffeine until 48 hours after all symptoms have gone away.

When to Call a Health Professional

Call 911 or other emergency services if you have any of the following:

• Signs of shock (see page 69).

• Pain in the upper abdomen with chest pain that is crushing or squeezing, feels like a heavy weight on your chest, or occurs with any other symptoms of a heart attack (see page 55).

• Signs of severe dehydration (see page 84).

• Severe abdominal pain following an injury to the abdomen.

• Severe abdominal pain and fainting.

Call your doctor if you have:

• Ongoing severe abdominal pain.

• Localized pain that lasts longer than 4 hours.

• Generalized abdominal pain or cramping pain that has lasted longer than 24 hours and is not improving.

• Inability to keep down fluids.

• Pain that gets worse when you move or cough and does not feel like a pulled muscle.

• Any abdominal pain that has lasted longer than 3 days.

Constipation

Constipation occurs when stools are difficult to pass. Some people are overly concerned with stool frequency because they have been taught that a healthy person has a bowel movement every day. This is not true. Most people pass stools anywhere from 3 times a day to 3 times a week. If your stools are soft and pass easily, you are not constipated.

Constipation may occur with cramping and pain in the rectum caused by straining to pass hard, dry stools. There may be some bloating and nausea. There may also be small amounts of bright red blood on the stools caused by slight tearing as the stools are pushed through the anus. The bleeding should stop when the constipation is relieved.

If a stool becomes lodged in the rectum (impacted), mucus and fluid may leak out around the stool, which sometimes leads to leakage of fecal material (fecal incontinence). You may experience this as constipation alternating with diarrhea.

Lack of fiber and too little water in the diet are common causes of constipation. Other causes include inactivity, delaying bowel movements, medications, pain caused by a tear (fissure) in the lining of the rectum, and laxative overuse. Irritable bowel syndrome (see page 91) may also cause constipation.

Toilet training may contribute to constipation in young children. Children who are involved in play or other activities and ignore the urge to pass stools may become constipated. Children and adults who are reluctant to use toilets away from home may become constipated.

Prevention

- Eat plenty of high-fiber foods such as fruits, vegetables, and whole grains. You can also add fiber to your diet in the following ways (also see page 296):

  - Eat a bowl of bran cereal with 10 grams of bran per serving.

  - Add 2 tablespoons of wheat bran to cereal or soup.

  - Try a product, such as Citrucel, FiberCon, or Metamucil, that contains a bulk-forming agent. Start with 1 tablespoon or less and drink extra water to avoid bloating.

- Avoid foods that are high in fat and sugar.

- Drink at least 6 to 8 glasses (1½ to 2 quarts) of water and other fluids every day. Drink extra fluids in the morning.

- Be more physically active. A walking program is a good start. See Fitness starting on page 285.

- Set aside relaxed times for having bowel movements. Urges usually occur sometime after meals. Establishing a daily routine (after breakfast, for example) may help.

- Go when you feel the urge and encourage your children to do the same. Your bowels send signals when a stool needs to pass. If you ignore the signal, the urge will go away and the stool will eventually become dry and difficult to pass.

Home Treatment

- Follow the diet outlined in Prevention to help relieve and prevent constipation.

- If necessary, use a stool softener or a very mild laxative such as milk of magnesia. Do not use mineral oil or any other laxative for more than 2 weeks without consulting your doctor.

- If an infant or child up to age 10 is having rectal pain because he or she is unable to have a bowel movement, put the child in a warm bath with 2 ounces of baking soda in the tub. This may help relax the muscles that normally keep stool inside the rectum, allowing the child to pass the stool.

- If your child is 6 months old or older and the warm bath does not work, use 1 or 2 glycerin suppositories to make the stool easier to pass. Use glycerin suppositories only once or twice. If constipation is not relieved or develops again, discuss the problem with your doctor.

- Do not give laxatives or enemas to a child without talking to your child's doctor first.

When to Call a Health Professional

- If constipation persists after home treatment has been followed for several days for an adult or according to a doctor's recommendation for an infant.

- If rectal bleeding is heavy (more than a few bright red streaks) or if the blood is reddish brown or black.

- If rectal bleeding lasts longer than 2 to 3 days after constipation has improved, or if bleeding occurs more than once.

- If you have sharp or severe abdominal pain.

- If you have rectal pain that either continues after you pass a stool or keeps you from passing stools at all.

- If you experience stool leakage (fecal incontinence).

- If your stools have become consistently more narrow (they may be no wider than a pencil).

- If you are unable to have bowel movements without using laxatives.

Dehydration

Dehydration occurs when your body loses too much water. When you stop drinking water or lose large amounts of fluids because of diarrhea, vomiting, or sweating, your body's cells reabsorb fluid from the blood and other tissues. Severe dehydration can lead to shock, which can be life-threatening.

Dehydration is very dangerous for infants, small children, and older adults. Watch closely for its early signs anytime there is an illness that causes high fever, vomiting, or diarrhea. The early symptoms are:

- Dry mouth and sticky saliva.

- Urinating smaller amounts than usual.

- Dark yellow urine.

Prevention

- Prompt home treatment for illnesses that cause diarrhea, vomiting, or fever will help prevent dehydration. See the chart on page 80.

- To prevent dehydration during hot weather or exercise, drink 8 to 10 glasses of fluid (water and/or sport drinks) each day. Drink extra water before, during, and after exercise.

Rehydration Drinks

Diarrhea and vomiting can cause your body to lose large amounts of water and essential minerals called electrolytes. If you are unable to eat for a few days, you are also losing nutrients. This happens faster and is more serious in infants, young children, and older adults.

A rehydration drink (Pedialyte, Lytren, Rehydralyte) will replace fluids and electrolytes in amounts that are best used by your body. Sports drinks and other sugared drinks will replace fluid, but most contain too much sugar (which can make the diarrhea worse) and not enough of the other essential ingredients. Plain water won't provide any necessary nutrients or electrolytes.

Rehydration drinks won't make diarrhea or vomiting go away faster, but they will prevent serious dehydration from developing.

You can make an inexpensive rehydration drink. However, do not give this homemade drink to children under age 12.

Measure all ingredients precisely. Small variations can make the drink less effective or even harmful. Mix:

- 1 quart water
- ½ teaspoon baking soda
- ½ teaspoon table salt
- 3 to 4 tablespoons sugar
- ¼ teaspoon salt substitute ("lite" salt), if available

Home Treatment

Treatment of mild dehydration is simple: stop the fluid loss and restore lost fluids as soon as possible.

- To stop vomiting or diarrhea, do not eat any solid foods for several hours or until you are feeling better. During the first 24 hours, take frequent, small sips of water or a rehydration drink.

- Once the vomiting or diarrhea is controlled, drink water, diluted broth, or sport drinks a sip at a time until your stomach can handle larger amounts. Drinking too much fluid too soon can cause vomiting to recur.

- If vomiting or diarrhea lasts longer than 24 hours, sip a rehydration drink to replace lost minerals.

- Watch for signs of more severe dehydration (see When to Call a Health Professional below).

For home treatment of vomiting or diarrhea in infants and children, see page 226.

When to Call a Health Professional

Call a health professional immediately if the following signs of severe dehydration develop:

- Sunken eyes, no tears, dry mouth and tongue.

- Sunken soft spot on an infant's head.

- Little or no urine for 8 hours.

- Extreme dizziness or lightheaded-ness when moving from lying down to sitting upright.

- Rapid breathing and heartbeat.

- Sleepiness, difficulty awakening, listlessness, and extreme irritability.

Also call a health professional:

- If vomiting lasts longer than 24 hours in an adult.

- If a person is unable to hold down even small sips of fluid, and there-fore cannot drink enough to replace lost fluids.

- If severe diarrhea (large, loose stools every 1 to 2 hours) lasts longer than 2 days in an adult.

Diarrhea

Diarrhea occurs when the intestines push stools through before the water in the stools can be reabsorbed by the body. This causes bowel movements to occur more frequently and stools to become watery and loose. A person who has diarrhea may also have abdominal cramps and nausea.

The exact cause of diarrhea is often difficult to pinpoint. Viral stomach flu (gastroenteritis) or food poison-ing often causes diarrhea. Many medications, especially antibiotics, can cause diarrhea; so can laxatives, if they are overused. Sorbitol (a sugar substitute) and olestra (a fat substitute used in some processed foods) may cause diarrhea. For some

people, emotional stress, anxiety, or food intolerance may bring on this problem. Irritable bowel syndrome (see page 91) may also cause diarrhea.

Drinking untreated water that con-tains parasites, viruses, or bacteria is another cause of diarrhea. Symp-toms may develop a few days to a few weeks after you drink the contaminated water.

Home Treatment

To treat diarrhea in infants and children under age 11, see Home Treatment on page 226.

- Don't eat any food for several hours or until you are feeling better. Take frequent, small sips of water or a rehydration drink.

- Avoid antidiarrheal drugs for the first 6 hours. After that, use them only if there are no other signs of illness, such as fever, cramping or discomfort, or bloody stools. Stop taking antidiarrheal medica-tions as soon as stools thicken. See antidiarrheal preparations on page 343.

- After the first 24 hours (or sooner, depending on how you feel), begin eating mild foods, such as rice, dry toast or crackers, bananas, and applesauce. Avoid spicy foods, other fruits, alcohol, and drinks that contain caffeine until 48 hours after all symptoms have disap-peared. Avoid dairy products for 3 days after symptoms disappear.

- Take care to avoid dehydration. See page 84.

When to Call a Health Professional

- If you develop signs of dehydration (see page 84).

- If you have severe diarrhea (large, loose bowel movements every 1 to 2 hours).

- If diarrhea lasts longer than 2 weeks.

- If stools are bloody or black.

- If abdominal pain increases or localizes, especially to the lower right or lower left part of the abdomen.

- If diarrhea occurs with a fever.

- If your symptoms become more severe or frequent.

- If diarrhea occurs after drinking untreated water.

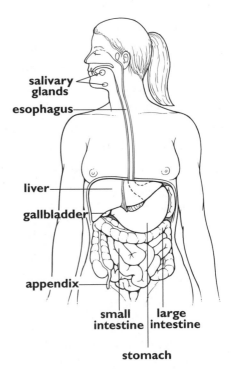

Organs of the digestive tract

Heartburn

Heartburn occurs when there is an abnormal backflow of stomach juices into the esophagus, the tube that leads from the mouth to the stomach. The backflow (reflux) causes a feeling of burning, warmth, or heat beneath the breastbone. The discomfort may spread in waves upward into your neck, and you may get a sour taste in your mouth. Heartburn can last up to 2 hours or longer. Symptoms often start after you eat. They grow worse when you lie down or bend over and improve when you sit or stand up.

MORE INFO Don't be concerned if you have heartburn now and then; nearly everyone does. Following the home treatment tips can prevent most cases of heartburn. However, if backflow of stomach acid into your esophagus happens regularly, you may have gastroesophageal reflux disease (<u>GERD</u>). GERD can cause continuous irritation of the lining of the esophagus, which can lead to other health problems. It is important to visit a health professional if you have frequent heartburn and home treatment does not relieve the discomfort.

Home Treatment

Try other home treatment measures before taking antacids or stomach acid reducers to relieve heartburn. If you take medications to relieve your heartburn without doing other home treatment, your heartburn is likely to keep coming back. If symptoms are not relieved by home treatment, or if symptoms last longer than 2 weeks, call your doctor.

- Eat smaller meals, and avoid late-night snacks. Don't lie down for 2 to 3 hours after eating.

- Avoid foods that bring on heartburn. These may include chocolate, fatty or fried foods, peppermint- or spearmint-flavored foods, coffee, alcohol, and carbonated drinks.

- Limit acidic foods that can irritate your esophagus. These include citrus fruits and juices such as orange juice and tomato juice. Limit spicy foods.

- Avoid clothes with tight belts or waistbands.

- Stop smoking. Smoking promotes heartburn.

- Lose weight if you are overweight. Being overweight can worsen heartburn, and the loss of even a few pounds can help prevent heartburn.

- If you get heartburn at night, raise the head of your bed 6 to 8 inches by putting blocks underneath your bed frame or placing a foam wedge under the head of your mattress. (Adding extra pillows does not work well.)

- Avoid aspirin, ibuprofen, naproxen sodium, and other anti-inflammatory drugs. These can cause heartburn. Try acetaminophen instead.

- Take a nonprescription product for heartburn. Antacids, such as Maalox, Mylanta, Tums, and Gelusil, neutralize stomach acid. Stomach acid reducers, such as Pepcid AC, Tagamet HB, and Zantac, reduce the production of stomach acid. Ask your pharmacist to help you choose one of these medications, and follow the package instructions and your doctor's advice for its use.

When to Call a Health Professional

Call 911 or other emergency services if you have any of the following:

- Pain in the upper abdomen with chest pain that is crushing or squeezing, feels like a heavy weight on your chest, or occurs with any other symptoms of a heart attack (see page 55).

- Signs of shock (see page 69).

Call your doctor:

- If there is blood in your vomit or stools.

• If you suspect that a medication is causing heartburn. Antihistamines, central nervous system depressants, birth control pills, and anti-inflammatory drugs, including aspirin, ibuprofen, and naproxen sodium, can sometimes cause heartburn.

• If you are routinely having pain or difficulty when swallowing solid foods.

• If you are losing weight and you don't know why.

• If heartburn persists for more than 3 weeks despite home treatment. Call sooner if symptoms are severe or are not relieved at all by antacids or acid reducers. See Ulcers on page 100.

Hernia

A hiatal hernia is a common problem that occurs when a portion of the stomach bulges into the chest cavity. Hiatal hernias often do not cause symptoms. However, sometimes a hiatal hernia will cause a backflow of stomach acid into the esophagus (the tube leading from the mouth to the stomach), which can cause heartburn and a sour taste in the mouth. See Heartburn on page 87.

An inguinal hernia occurs when abdominal tissue bulges through a weak spot in the abdominal wall in the groin area. Inguinal hernias are more common in men than in women. In a man, an inguinal hernia may bulge into the scrotum.

A person with an inguinal hernia may sense that something has "given way." Other symptoms may include:

• A tender bulge in the groin or scrotum. The bulge may appear gradually, or it may form suddenly after heavy lifting, coughing, or straining. The bulge may disappear when the person lies down.

• Groin discomfort or pain that may extend into the scrotum. Discomfort may increase with bending or lifting.

• Nausea and abdominal swelling.

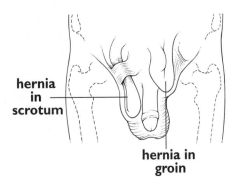

hernia in scrotum

hernia in groin

A hernia can cause a bulge or lump in the groin or scrotum.

Inguinal hernias can be caused by increased abdominal pressure resulting from lifting heavy weights, coughing, or straining to pass stools or urine. Sometimes a weak spot in the abdominal wall is present at birth. An inguinal hernia is called reducible if the bulging tissue can be pushed back into place in the abdomen. If the tissue cannot be pushed back into place, the hernia is called irreducible.

Kidney Stones

 MORE INFO Kidney stones can form from the minerals in urine. The most common cause of kidney stones is not drinking enough water.

As long as they stay in the kidneys, kidney stones usually cause no problems. A stone may move out of the kidney into the tube that leads to the bladder (ureter). If the stone blocks the flow of urine, there may be severe pain.

Symptoms that may develop when a kidney stone moves through a ureter include:

• Pain in the side, groin, or genital area that begins suddenly and gets worse over 15 to 60 minutes until it is steady and nearly unbearable. The pain may stop for a while when the stone is not moving, and pain often vanishes suddenly when the stone moves into the bladder.

• Nausea and vomiting.

• Blood in the urine.

• Feeling like you need to urinate often or pain when urinating.

• Loss of appetite, diarrhea, or constipation.

• Inability to find a comfortable body position.

Call your doctor immediately if you suspect that you are passing a kidney stone. Most small kidney stones pass without the need for any medical treatment other than pain medication. In rare cases, surgery may be needed.

If an inguinal hernia is irreducible, the tissue may become trapped outside the abdominal wall. If the blood supply to the tissue is cut off (strangulated hernia), the tissue will swell and die. The dead tissue will quickly become infected, requiring immediate medical attention. Rapidly increasing pain in the groin or scrotum is a sign that a hernia has become strangulated.

A hernia can develop anywhere there is a weakness in the abdominal wall. Common places for hernias to develop are the bellybutton (umbilical hernia) and at the site of an incision from abdominal surgery (incisional hernia).

Prevention

• Use proper lifting techniques (see page 110), and avoid lifting weights that are too heavy for you.

• Lose weight if you are overweight.

• Avoid constipation and do not strain during bowel movements and urination.

• Stop smoking, especially if you have a chronic cough.

When to Call a Health Professional

Call a health professional immediately if a testicle swells and is painful, particularly in a child or adolescent.

Also call a health professional:

- If mild groin pain or an unexplained bump or swelling in the groin continues for more than 1 week.

- If the skin over a hernia or bulge in the groin or abdomen becomes red.

- If heartburn persists for more than 3 weeks despite home treatment. Call sooner if symptoms are severe or are not relieved at all by antacids or acid reducers. See Heartburn on page 87.

If you have been diagnosed with a hernia, call a health professional:

- If you have sudden, severe pain in the groin area, along with nausea, vomiting, and fever.

- If the hernia cannot be pushed back into place with gentle pressure when you are lying down.

 If you suspect that you have a hernia, see your doctor to confirm the diagnosis and discuss your treatment options.

Irritable Bowel Syndrome

Irritable bowel syndrome (IBS) is one of the most common disorders of the digestive tract. Symptoms of IBS often increase with stress or after eating and include:

- Abdominal bloating, pain, and gas.

- Mucus in the stool.

- Feeling as if a bowel movement hasn't been completed.

- Irregular bowel habits, with constipation, diarrhea, or both.

The cause of IBS is unknown. Symptoms are thought to be related to abnormal muscle contractions in the intestines. However, when tests are done, they find no changes (such as inflammation or tumors) in the physical structure of the intestines.

IBS can persist for many years. An episode may be more severe than the one before it, but the disorder itself does not worsen over time or lead to more serious diseases such as cancer. Symptoms tend to get better over time.

If you have not yet been diagnosed with IBS, try to rule out other causes of stomach problems, such as eating a new food, nervousness, or stomach flu. Try home treatment for 1 to 2 weeks. If there is no improvement, or if your symptoms worsen, call your doctor for an appointment.

 Your doctor may prescribe medication for you to take in addition to doing home treatment. There are no tests that can diagnose irritable bowel syndrome, but your doctor may recommend testing to rule out other possible causes of your symptoms. The amount of testing your doctor will do depends on your age, the pattern and severity of your symptoms, and your response to initial treatment.

Gallstones

Gallstones are tiny stones (usually made of cholesterol) that form in the gallbladder. Most people who have gallstones do not have any symptoms.

Sometimes gallstones cause the gallbladder to become inflamed. The main symptom is a dull aching or cramping pain that starts in the upper right abdomen and may radiate to the center of the upper abdomen or to the right upper back or shoulder blade. The pain may be severe and usually lasts several hours. Fever and vomiting also may be present.

Symptoms often occur at night, usually at about the same time every night. Pain may or may not be related to a meal.

Risk factors for gallstones include a high-fat, high-sugar diet; obesity; lack of exercise; rapid weight loss; estrogen replacement therapy; diabetes; high cholesterol; and high blood pressure. Gallstones are more common in women than in men.

 MORE INFO Gallstones that don't cause symptoms don't require treatment. If you have gallstones that cause pain or infection, you may want to consider having gallbladder surgery.

If you have mild symptoms, it is safe to wait until symptoms recur several times before seeking treatment. See When to Call a Health Professional on page 82 to decide what to do if your symptoms become more severe.

Prevention

There is no way to prevent IBS. However, symptoms often worsen or improve because of changes in your diet, your stress level, medications, the amount of exercise you are getting, and other reasons that may or may not be known. Identifying the things that trigger your symptoms may help you avoid or minimize attacks.

Home Treatment

If constipation is your main symptom:

• Eat more fruits, vegetables, legumes, and whole grains. Add these fiber-rich foods to your diet slowly so they do not worsen gas or cramps. See page 296.

• Add unprocessed wheat bran to your diet. Start by using 1 tablespoon per day, and gradually increase to 4 tablespoons per day. Sprinkle bran on cereal, soup, and casseroles. Drink extra water to avoid becoming bloated.

• Try a product, such as Citrucel, FiberCon, or Metamucil, that contains a bulk-forming agent. Start with 1 tablespoon or less per day, and drink extra water to prevent bloating.

• Use laxatives only if your doctor recommends them.

• Be more physically active. Exercise helps the digestive system work better.

If diarrhea is your main symptom:

- Using the fiber-rich food and wheat bran suggestions for relieving constipation can sometimes help relieve diarrhea by absorbing liquid in the large intestine.

- Avoid foods that make diarrhea worse. Try eliminating one food at a time; then add it back gradually. If a food doesn't seem to be related to symptoms, there is no need to avoid it. Many people find that the following foods or drinks make their symptoms worse:

  - Alcohol, caffeine, nicotine

  - Beans, broccoli, cabbage, apples

  - Spicy foods

  - Foods high in acid, such as citrus fruit

  - Fatty foods, including bacon, sausage, butter, oils, and anything deep-fried

- Avoid dairy products that contain lactose (milk sugar) if they seem to worsen symptoms. However, be sure to get enough calcium in your diet from other sources. See "Lactose Intolerance" on page 300.

- Avoid sorbitol (an artificial sweetener found in some sugarless candies and gum) and olestra (a fat substitute used in some processed foods, such as potato chips).

- Add more starchy food (bread, rice, potatoes, pasta) to your diet.

- If diarrhea persists, a non-prescription medication such as loperamide (the active ingredient in products such as Imodium) may help. Check with your doctor if you are using loperamide twice a month or more.

To reduce stress:

- Keep a record of the life events that occur with your symptoms. This may help you see any connection between your symptoms and stressful occasions.

- Get regular, vigorous exercise such as swimming, jogging, or brisk walking to help reduce tension.

- See page 323 for more tips on managing stress.

When to Call a Health Professional

- If you have been diagnosed with irritable bowel syndrome and your symptoms get worse, begin to disrupt your usual activities, or do not respond as usual to home treatment.

- If you are becoming increasingly fatigued.

- If your symptoms frequently wake you.

- If your pain gets worse with movement or coughing.

- If you have abdominal pain and a fever.

- If you have abdominal pain that does not get better when you pass gas or stools.

- If you are losing weight and you don't know why.

- If your appetite has decreased.

- If there is blood in your stools. See page 98.

Hepatitis

Hepatitis means "liver inflammation." Viruses cause hepatitis A, B, and C, the most common types of hepatitis.

Most people in the U.S. get hepatitis A after having intimate contact with someone who is infected with the hepatitis A virus (HAV). Large groups of people can become infected with HAV if someone who has hepatitis A prepares food for them. HAV infection goes away without medical treatment, causing no long-term problems.

The hepatitis B virus (HBV) lives in blood and other body fluids. It is commonly spread during sexual contact and when people share needles to inject drugs. A pregnant woman who is infected with HBV can pass the virus to her baby. Young people who become infected with HBV are more likely to develop chronic HBV infection and long-term liver problems than are people who become infected later in life.

The hepatitis C virus (HCV) is spread when HCV-infected blood enters a person's body. Blood transfusions were once a common means of spreading HCV. The virus is also spread among people who share needles to inject drugs. Many people develop chronic HCV infection, which can lead to severe liver damage after many years.

Hepatitis symptoms are similar to flu symptoms. They include nausea, headache, sore muscles, and fatigue. Some people have pain in the upper right side of the abdomen. Jaundice may develop, causing the skin and whites of the eyes to turn yellow and making the urine dark. Call a health professional if you develop hepatitis symptoms or if you may have been exposed to hepatitis. Because all three types of viral hepatitis have similar symptoms, blood tests are needed to determine which hepatitis virus is causing the infection.

Vaccines can prevent hepatitis A and B, but there is no vaccine for hepatitis C. If you are exposed to HAV or HBV before you have been vaccinated, getting a shot of immune globulin is likely to keep you from becoming infected.

 MORE INFO Drug treatment is available for people with chronic hepatitis infection (HBV or HCV) who are likely to develop liver problems.

Nausea and Vomiting

Nausea is a very unpleasant feeling in the pit of the stomach. A person who is nauseated may feel weak and sweaty and produce lots of saliva. Intense nausea often leads to vomiting, which forces stomach contents up the esophagus and out of the mouth. Home treatment will help ease the discomfort.

Nausea and vomiting may be caused by:

- Viral stomach flu or food poisoning (see page 98).

- Stress or nervousness.

- Medications, especially antibiotics and anti-inflammatory drugs, such as aspirin, ibuprofen, and naproxen sodium.

- Pregnancy (see "Morning Sickness" on page 252).

- Diabetes.

- Migraine headache (see page 190).

- Head injury (see page 53).

Nausea and vomiting can also be signs of other serious illnesses involving abdominal organs such as the liver (hepatitis, see page 94), pancreas, gallbladder (see page 92), stomach (ulcers, see page 100), or appendix (appendicitis, see page 81).

Home Treatment

Home treatment may be all that is needed to treat occasional vomiting. For home treatment of vomiting in children under age 4, see page 225. For older children and adults:

- Watch for and treat early signs of dehydration. See page 84. Older adults and young children can quickly become dehydrated from vomiting.

- After vomiting has stopped for 1 hour, drink 1 ounce of a clear liquid every 20 minutes for 1 hour. Clear liquids include apple or grape juice mixed to half strength with water, rehydration drinks, weak tea with sugar, clear broth, and gelatin dessert. Avoid citrus juices.

- If vomiting lasts longer than 24 hours, sip a rehydration drink to restore lost fluids and nutrients. See page 85.

- When you are feeling better, begin eating clear soups, mild foods, and liquids until all symptoms have been gone for 12 to 48 hours. Gelatin dessert, dry toast, crackers, and cooked cereal are good choices.

- Rest in bed until you are feeling better.

When to Call a Health Professional

• If signs of severe dehydration develop (see page 84).

• If vomiting occurs with:

- Severe headache, sleepiness, lethargy, or stiff neck. See "Encephalitis and Meningitis" on page 162.

- Chest pain. See Heart Attack on page 55.

- Fever and increasing pain in the lower right abdomen.

- Fever and shaking chills.

- Abdominal swelling.

- Pain in the upper right or upper left abdomen. See illustration on page 79.

• If vomit contains blood or material that looks like coffee grounds. See Shock on page 69.

• If vomiting and fever last longer than 48 hours.

• If you suspect that a medication is causing the problem. Antibiotics and anti-inflammatory medications (aspirin, ibuprofen, naproxen sodium, etc.) may cause nausea or vomiting. Learn which of your medications can cause these symptoms.

• If vomiting occurs after a head injury. See page 53.

• If any vomiting lasts longer than 1 week.

Rectal Problems

The rectum is the lower part of the large intestine. At the end of the rectum is the anus, where stools pass out of the body.

Rectal problems are common. Most everyone experiences itching, pain, or bleeding in the rectal or anal area at some time. These problems are often minor and will go away on their own or with home treatment.

Anal itching can have many causes. Skin around the anus may become irritated because of stool leakage. Anal itching can also be a sign of pinworms (see page 233), especially in households with children. Caffeine and spicy foods can irritate the lining of the rectum, causing anal itching and discomfort. If the anus is not kept clean, itching may result. However, trying to keep the area too clean by rubbing it with dry toilet paper or using harsh soap may injure the skin.

Hemorrhoids are enlarged and inflamed veins that may develop inside or outside of the anus. Straining to pass hard stools, being overweight or pregnant, and prolonged sitting or standing can all cause hemorrhoids.

Hemorrhoids generally last several days and often come back (recur). The symptoms of hemorrhoids include bright red streaks of blood on stools or blood dripping from the anus; leakage of mucus from the anus; irritation or itching around the anus; and feeling as if a bowel movement hasn't been completed. Sometimes an internal hemorrhoid will actually stick out of the anus, and it may have to be pushed back into place with a finger.

Pain is not usually a symptom, unless a blood clot forms in a hemorrhoid or the blood supply to a hemorrhoid is cut off (strangulated). A clotted hemorrhoid may be extremely painful but is not dangerous. However, a strangulated hemorrhoid may need emergency treatment.

 You may want to consider surgery if you have hemorrhoids that bleed persistently, are very uncomfortable, or make it difficult to keep your anal area clean. Talk to your doctor about your options for surgery.

An **anal fissure** may cause pain during bowel movements and streaks of blood on stools. Anal fissures are long, narrow sores that usually develop when the tissue in the anal area is torn during a bowel movement.

Prevention

- Keep your stools soft. Include plenty of water, fresh fruits and vegetables, and whole grains in your diet. Include up to 2 tablespoons of bran or a commercial stool softener, such as Citrucel, in your diet each day. Regular exercise promotes smooth bowel movements. Also see Constipation on page 82.

- Try not to strain during bowel movements, and never hold your breath. Take your time, but don't sit on the toilet too long.

- Avoid sitting or standing too much. Take short walks to increase blood flow in your pelvic region.

- Keep the anal area clean, but be gentle when cleansing it. Use water and a fragrance-free soap, such as Ivory, or use baby wipes or Tucks pads.

Home Treatment

- Take warm baths. They are soothing and cleansing, especially after you have a bowel movement. Sitz baths (warm baths with just enough water to cover the anal area) are also helpful for hemorrhoids but may worsen anal itching.

- Wear cotton underwear and loose clothing to decrease moisture in the anal area.

- Apply a cold compress on the anus for 10 minutes, 4 times a day.

- Ease itching and irritation with zinc oxide, petroleum jelly, or hydrocortisone (1%) cream. Use medicated suppositories (such as Preparation H) to relieve pain and lubricate the anal canal during bowel movements. Ask your doctor before using any product that contains a local anesthetic (these products have the suffix "-caine" in the name or ingredients). Such products cause allergic reactions in some people.

Flexible Sigmoidoscopy

Flexible sigmoidoscopy is a screening test for precancerous growths and cancers of the colon and rectum. The sigmoidoscope is a flexible viewing instrument that is inserted into the rectum to examine the lower bowel. The exam takes about 10 to 30 minutes, is only mildly uncomfortable, and is very safe.

 MORE INFO Having flexible sigmoidoscopy exams reduces your risk of dying from colorectal cancer. Most experts recommend that you have a flexible sigmoidoscopy exam around age 50. However, experts disagree about how often you should have repeat exams. Recommendations usually range from every 3 years to every 10 years. In addition to screening for cancer, doctors sometimes wish to examine the colon to check for the cause of rectal bleeding or persistent diarrhea or constipation.

When to Call a Health Professional

- If rectal bleeding occurs for no apparent reason and is not associated with trying to pass stools.

- If rectal bleeding continues for more than 1 week or occurs more than once.

- If stools become more narrow than usual (may be no wider than a pencil).

- If pain caused by hemorrhoids is severe, or if moderate anal pain continues after a full week of home treatment.

- If any unusual material or tissue seeps or sticks out of the anus.

- If a lump near the anus gets bigger or becomes more painful and you develop a fever.

- If fever accompanies bloody stools.

Stomach Flu and Food Poisoning

Stomach flu and food poisoning are different ailments with different causes. However, many people confuse the two because the symptoms are so similar.

Stomach flu is usually caused by a viral infection in the digestive system. To prevent stomach flu, you must avoid contact with the virus, which is not always easy to do.

Food poisoning is usually caused by a toxin produced by bacteria in food that is not handled or stored properly. Bacteria can grow rapidly when certain foods, especially meats, dairy products, and sauces, are not handled properly during preparation or are kept at temperatures between 40° and 140°.

Suspect food poisoning when symptoms are shared by others who ate the same food, or when symptoms develop after eating unrefrigerated foods. Symptoms of food poisoning may begin as soon as 1 or 2 hours or

MORE INFO **For more information, see the back cover.**

as long as 48 hours after eating. Nausea, vomiting, and diarrhea may last from 12 to 48 hours.

Botulism is a rare but often fatal type of food poisoning. It is generally caused by improper home canning methods for low-acid foods like beans and corn. Bacteria that survive the canning process may grow and produce toxins in the jar. Symptoms include blurred or double vision and difficulty swallowing or breathing.

Prevention

To prevent food poisoning:

- Keep hot foods hot and cold foods cold.

- Follow the 2-40-140 rule. Don't eat meat, dressings, salads, or other foods that have been kept for more than 2 hours between 40° and 140°.

- Use a thermometer to check your refrigerator. It should be between 34° and 40°.

- Defrost meats in the refrigerator or microwave, not on the kitchen counter.

- Keep your kitchen clean. Wash your hands, cutting boards, and countertops frequently. After handling raw meats, especially chicken, wash your hands and utensils before preparing other foods.

- Cook hamburger until it is well done. Cook chicken until the juices run clear.

- Do not eat raw eggs or uncooked sauces made with raw eggs.

- Discard any cans or jars with bulging lids or leaks.

- Follow home canning and freezing instructions carefully. Contact your county agricultural extension office for advice.

Home Treatment

- Viral stomach flu and food poisoning will usually go away within 24 to 48 hours. Good home care can speed recovery. For adults and older children, see Nausea and Vomiting on page 95 and Diarrhea on page 86. For infants and young children, see page 225.

- Watch for and treat early signs of dehydration (see page 84). Older adults and young children can quickly become dehydrated from diarrhea and vomiting.

When to Call a Health Professional

- If vomiting lasts longer than 1 day in an adult.

- If severe diarrhea (large, loose stools every 1 to 2 hours) lasts longer than 2 days in an adult.

- If signs of severe dehydration develop. See page 84.

- If you suspect food poisoning from a canned food or have symptoms of botulism (blurred or double vision, difficulty swallowing or breathing). If you still have a sample of the food you suspect caused your symptoms, take it to the doctor for testing.

Ulcers

An ulcer (peptic ulcer) is a sore or crater in the lining of the digestive tract. Most ulcers develop in the stomach (gastric ulcers) or in the upper part of the small intestine (duodenal ulcers).

Until recently, the cause of ulcers was not well understood. It is now believed that most people who develop ulcers are infected with *Helicobacter pylori (H. pylori)* bacteria. Most people who are infected with *H. pylori* do not develop ulcers unless other factors are also present. Such factors may include:

• Use of certain medications.

• Excessive alcohol use.

• Smoking.

• Stress.

• Other illnesses.

Most ulcers that are not caused by *H. pylori* infection are caused by frequent use of aspirin or other non-steroidal anti-inflammatory drugs (such as ibuprofen, indomethacin, naproxen sodium, and clinoril), which can damage the digestive tract's lining.

The symptoms of an ulcer are often similar to symptoms of other common stomach problems like heartburn (indigestion) or inflammation of the stomach lining (gastritis). Symptoms may include a burning or gnawing pain between the navel and the breastbone. The pain often occurs between meals and may wake you during the night. Eating something or taking an antacid usually relieves the pain. Ulcers may also cause bloating, nausea, or vomiting after meals.

Ulcers can cause bleeding in the stomach and small intestine, which may cause stools to appear dark red, black, or tarry. Without treatment, ulcers may occasionally cause a blockage between the stomach and the small intestine. An ulcer occasionally may break through (perforate) the stomach wall, caus-ing severe abdominal pain and a rigid abdomen. Ulcers that bleed or perforate the stomach wall require immediate medical treatment.

 If you think you have an <u>ulcer</u> and your symp-toms do not improve after 10 to 14 days of home treat-ment, make an appointment with your doctor. He or she can evaluate your symptoms and prescribe a treatment plan that may include antacids or other medications.

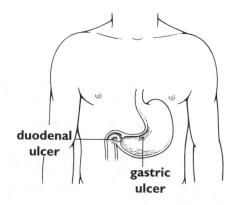

Most ulcers occur in the stomach (gastric ulcer) or in the opening to the small intestine (duodenal ulcer).

For more information, see the back cover.

Home Treatment

- Avoid foods, especially spicy or greasy foods, that seem to bring on symptoms. It isn't necessary to eliminate any particular food from your diet if it doesn't cause you problems.

- Avoid coffee, tea, cola, and other products that contain caffeine. Many people find that caffeine makes their pain worse.

- Try eating smaller, more frequent meals. If it doesn't help, return to a regular diet.

- Stop smoking. Smoking slows healing of ulcers and increases the likelihood that they will come back.

- Limit your alcohol intake. Excessive amounts of alcohol may make an ulcer heal more slowly and may make symptoms worse.

- Do not take aspirin, ibuprofen, or naproxen sodium. Try acetaminophen instead.

- Antacids (such as Tums, Maalox, and Mylanta) reduce the amount of acid in your stomach. Acid reducers (such as Pepcid AC, Tagamet HB, Zantac 75, and Axid AR) decrease the amount of acid your stomach produces. Reducing the amount of acid in your stomach helps your ulcer heal. If you are taking antacids, you may need frequent, large doses to do the job. Talk with your doctor about the best dose. Also see page 341.

- Learn to relax and manage stress. Too much stress may slow ulcer healing. Practice the relaxation techniques on page 323.

When to Call a Health Professional

- If you have pain in the upper abdomen with chest pain that is crushing or squeezing, feels like a heavy weight on your chest, or occurs with any other symptoms of a heart attack (see page 55).

- If you have been diagnosed with an ulcer and you have severe, continuous abdominal pain, severe vomiting, blood in vomit or stools, dizziness or lightheadedness, or signs of shock (see page 69).

- If your symptoms continue or get worse after 10 to 14 days of treatment with antacids or acid reducers.

- If you are losing weight and you don't know why.

- If nausea or vomiting often occurs right after meals.

- If abdominal pain awakens you from sleep.

- If you have pain or difficulty when swallowing.

Urinary Incontinence

If you suffer from loss of bladder control (urinary incontinence), you are not alone. Many people are coping with this problem.

Many cases of incontinence can be controlled or cured if the underlying problem is corrected. Water pills (diuretics) and many other common medications can cause temporary incontinence. Constipation, urinary tract infections, stones in the urinary tract, multiple pregnancies, and being overweight are other causes of incontinence.

The two most common types of persistent or chronic loss of bladder control are described here.

Stress incontinence occurs when small amounts of urine leak out during exercise or when you cough, laugh, or sneeze. It is more common in women than in men, but it may affect some men after prostate surgery. Kegel exercises often help relieve stress incontinence. See page 103. Ask your doctor about devices that can be used to prevent urine from leaking.

Urge incontinence happens when the need to urinate comes on so quickly that there is not enough time to get to the toilet. Causes include bladder infection, prostate enlargement, tumors that press on the bladder, Parkinson's disease, and nerve-related disorders such as multiple sclerosis or stroke.

Home Treatment

- Don't let incontinence keep you from doing the things you like to do. Absorbent pads or briefs, such as Attends and Depend, are available in pharmacies and supermarkets. No one will know you are wearing an absorbent pad.

- Avoid beverages that contain caffeine, which overstimulates the bladder. Do not cut down on fluids overall; you need fluids to keep the rest of your body healthy.

- Stop smoking. This may reduce your coughing, which may in turn reduce your problem with incontinence.

- Lose weight if you are overweight.

- Practice "double-voiding." Empty your bladder as much as possible, relax for a minute, and then try to empty it again.

- If you have stress incontinence, practice Kegel exercises daily. See "Kegel Exercises" on page 103.

- Urinate on a schedule, perhaps every 3 to 4 hours during the day, whether the urge is there or not. This may help you restore control.

- Wear clothing that can be removed quickly, such as pants with elastic waistbands.

- Clear a path from your bed to the bathroom, or consider placing a portable commode by your bed.

- Keep skin in the genital area dry to prevent rashes. Vaseline or Desitin ointment will help protect the skin from irritation caused by urine.

- Incontinence is sometimes caused by a urinary tract infection. If you feel pain or burning when you urinate, see Urinary Tract Infections on page 103.

• Pay special attention to any medications you are taking, including nonprescription drugs, since some affect bladder control.

 Don't let <u>incontinence</u> embarrass you. Take charge and work with your doctor to treat any underlying condition that may be causing the problem.

For more information about urinary incontinence, contact the National Association for Incontinence, P.O. Box 8310, Spartanburg, SC 29305, 1-800-252-3337.

When to Call a Health Professional

• If you suddenly become incontinent.

• If you are urinating frequently, but only passing small amounts of urine.

• If your bladder feels full even after you urinate.

• If you have difficulty urinating when your bladder feels full.

• If you feel burning or pain while urinating. See Urinary Tract Infections on page 103.

• If your urine looks bloody. See "Blood in the Urine" on page 105.

• If your urine has an unusual odor.

• If urinary incontinence interferes with your life in any way.

Kegel Exercises

Kegel exercises can help cure or improve stress incontinence by strengthening the pelvic muscles that control the flow of urine. No one will know you are doing them except you.

• Locate the muscles by repeatedly stopping your urine in midstream and starting again.

• Practice squeezing these muscles while you are not urinating. If your stomach or buttocks move, you are not using the right muscles.

• Hold the squeeze for 3 seconds, then relax for 3 seconds.

• Repeat the exercise 10 to 15 times per session. Do at least three Kegel exercise sessions per day.

Urinary Tract Infections

The urinary tract includes the kidneys, ureters, bladder, and urethra. The kidneys filter the blood, and the waste products from the blood become urine. The ureters carry urine from the kidneys to the bladder. The bladder holds the urine until the urine is expelled from the body through the urethra.

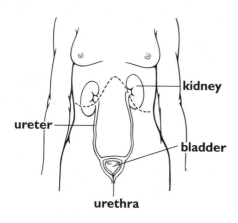

Infections can occur in any of the structures of the urinary tract.

Urinary tract infections (UTIs), including bladder infections (cystitis) and kidney infections (pyelonephritis), are generally caused by bacteria that are normally present in the digestive system. Females get UTIs more often than males do.

Early symptoms of a UTI may include burning or pain during urination and itching or pain in the urethra. The urine may be cloudy or reddish in color and may have an unusual odor. There may also be discomfort in the lower abdomen or back and a frequent urge to urinate without being able to pass much urine. Chills and fever may be present if the infection is severe, especially if it has spread to the kidneys.

Men with symptoms similar to those caused by a UTI may have an infection of the prostate gland or the epididymis (the tube that transports sperm from the testicle). See Prostate Infection on page 269 and Testicular Problems on page 272.

Men who have enlarged prostates, women who have had multiple pregnancies, people with kidney stones or diabetes, and those who are paralyzed from the waist down may be at higher risk for chronic urinary tract infections.

Other causes of irritation to the genital area that may be associated with UTIs include having sexual intercourse, using a diaphragm or spermicide for birth control, wearing tight pants, riding a bike, using perfumed soaps and powders, or even eating spicy foods.

If urinary pain or vaginal burning and redness occur in a young girl, consider the possibility of an allergy to bubble bath or soap. Urinary pain or vaginal burning may also be a symptom of a sexually transmitted disease (STD) or a sign of sexual abuse. If you are concerned about possible sexual abuse of a child, call a health professional.

Prevention

• Drink plenty of fluids; water is best. Aim for at least 2 quarts per day.

• Urinate frequently.

• Females should wipe from front to back after going to the toilet. This will reduce the spread of bacteria from the anus to the urethra. Teach young girls this habit during toilet training.

- Avoid douching and bubble baths, and don't use vaginal deodorants or perfumed feminine hygiene products.

- Stay out of hot tubs if you are prone to UTIs.

- Wash the genital area once a day with plain water or mild soap and water. Rinse well and dry the area thoroughly.

- Drink extra water before sexual intercourse and urinate promptly afterwards. This is especially important if you tend to get UTIs.

- Wear cotton underwear, cotton-lined panty hose, and loose clothing.

- Avoid alcohol, caffeine, and carbonated beverages, which can irritate the bladder.

- Include cranberry and blueberry juice in your diet. These may protect against UTIs, especially in females.

Home Treatment

Start home treatment at the first sign of genital irritation or painful urination. A day or so of self-care may clear up a minor infection. However, if your symptoms last longer than 1 or 2 days or worsen despite home treatment, call your doctor. Because the organs of the urinary tract are connected, untreated UTIs can spread, which may lead to kidney infections and other serious problems.

- Drink extra fluids (think in terms of gallons) as soon as you notice symptoms and for the next 24 hours. This will help dilute the urine, flush bacteria out of the bladder, and decrease irritation.

- Urinate frequently and follow the other tips outlined in Prevention.

- Check your temperature twice daily. Fever may indicate a more serious infection.

- A hot bath may help relieve pain. Avoid using bubble bath and harsh soaps. Apply a heating pad over your genital area to help relieve the pain. Never go to sleep with a heating pad in place.

- Avoid sexual intercourse until symptoms improve. Do not use a diaphragm. It may put pressure on your urethra and slow down or prevent complete emptying of the bladder.

Blood in the Urine

A blow to the kidneys, kidney stones, excessive running, or a urinary tract infection can cause blood in the urine. Blood in the urine can be a sign of a serious illness and should always be discussed with a health professional.

Eating foods such as beets, blackberries, and foods containing red artificial food colorings can temporarily color the urine pink or red. Certain medications can also discolor the urine.

When to Call a Health Professional

• If painful urination occurs with any of the following symptoms:

  - Fever of 101° or higher and chills.

  - Inability to urinate when you feel the urge.

  - Pain in the back, side, groin, or genital area.

  - Blood or pus in the urine.

  - Unusual vaginal or penile discharge.

  - Nausea and vomiting.

• If symptoms get worse despite home treatment.

• If symptoms do not improve after 1 to 2 days of home treatment.

• If you are pregnant or have diabetes and you have symptoms of a urinary tract infection.

• If you suspect that your child has a urinary tract infection or has been sexually abused.

Stand up straight!
Mom

5

Back and Neck Pain

Although back and neck pain are usually preventable, most of us will suffer from one or both at some time in our lives. Fortunately, most acute back injuries will heal on their own within 6 to 12 weeks.

By following the prevention and home treatment guidelines in this chapter, you can recover from most back and neck pain and prevent it from recurring.

Back Pain

Your back includes the area from below your head to your tailbone. It is composed of the bones of the spine (vertebrae); the joints that guide the direction of movement of the spine; the discs that separate the bones of the spine and absorb shock as you move; and the muscles

and ligaments that hold them all together. One or more of these structures can be stressed or injured, causing back pain.

Most back pain is the result of overuse injuries caused by prolonged or repeated movements or postures that strain the back. A sudden improper movement that twists the back can result in strain or sprain of the spinal ligaments, the muscles in the back, or the sacroiliac joints (the joints between the spine and the pelvic bones).

You can damage your discs the same way so that they stretch, tear, or rupture. If the tear is large enough, the jellylike material inside the disc may leak out and press against a nerve. The nerve may also become irritated due to swelling or inflammation in other parts of the spine.

First Aid for Back Pain

When you first feel a catch or strain in your back, try these steps to avoid or reduce pain. These are the most important home treatments for the first few days of back pain. Also see Home Treatment on page 114.

First Aid #1: Relax

Lie down in a comfortable position. This will allow your spinal muscles to relax.

First Aid #2: Ice

As soon as possible, apply ice or a cold pack to your injured back (10 to 15 minutes every hour). Cold applied for the first 3 days reduces pain and speeds healing.

First Aid #3: Pelvic tilts

This exercise gently moves the spine and stretches the lower back.

• Lie on your back with knees bent and feet flat on the floor.

• Slowly tighten your stomach muscles and press your lower back against the floor. Hold for 10 seconds (do not hold your breath). Slowly relax.

First Aid #4: Walk

Take a short walk (3 to 5 minutes) on a level surface (no slopes) every 3 hours. Walk only distances you can manage without pain, especially leg pain.

Any of these injuries can result in 2 to 3 days of acute pain and swelling in the injured tissue, followed by slow healing and a gradual reduction in pain. The pain may be felt in the low back, in the buttock, or down the leg. The goals of self-care are to relieve pain, promote healing, and avoid reinjury.

Back pain can also be caused by conditions that affect the bones and joints of the spine. Arthritis pain may be a steady ache, unlike the sharp, acute pain of strains, sprains, and disc injuries. If you think your back pain may be caused by arthritis, combine the self-care guidelines for back pain with those for arthritis on page 122.

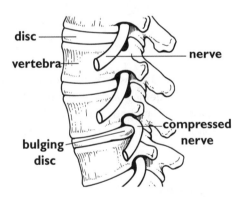

disc

vertebra

nerve

bulging disc

compressed nerve

A spinal disc that bulges or ruptures can put pressure on a nerve, causing pain.

Osteoporosis weakens all bones, including the spine, which can lead to broken bones and compression fractures. Compression fractures cause vertebrae to collapse. This can cause misalignment of the spine and lead to varying degrees of pain. See page 135 for more information about osteoporosis.

Sciatica

Sciatica is an irritation of the sciatic nerve, which is formed by the nerve roots coming out of the spinal cord into the lower back. The sciatic nerve extends down through the buttocks, branches, and extends to the feet. Sciatica can occur when an injured disc presses against the spinal nerve roots. Its main symptom is radiating pain, numbness, or weakness that is usually worse in the leg than in the back. In addition to the home treatment for back pain on page 114, the following may help:

- Avoid sitting if possible, unless it is more comfortable than standing.

- Alternate lying down with short walks. Increase your walking distance as you are able to do so without pain.

- Apply ice or a cold pack to the middle of your lower back. See page 108.

Prevention

The keys to preventing back pain are to use good body mechanics and to practice good health habits, such as getting regular exercise, maintaining a healthy body weight, and avoiding tobacco (nicotine weakens the discs in your back). Some of the tips presented in this chapter are things you will want to do every day, not only because they are good for your back, but because they are good for your overall health. The rest will come in handy if you are ever suffering from acute back pain.

Body Mechanics

Good body mechanics will reduce the stress on your back. Use good body mechanics all the time, not just when you have back pain.

Sitting

- Avoid sitting in one position for more than an hour at a time. Get up or change positions often.

- If you must sit a lot, the exercises on pages 111 to 114 are particularly important.

- If your chair doesn't give enough support, use a small pillow or rolled towel to support your lower back.

- When driving, pull your seat forward so that the pedals and steering wheel are within comfortable reach. Stop often to stretch and walk around. Consider placing a small pillow or towel roll behind your lower back.

Lifting

- Keep your upper back straight. Do not bend forward from the waist to lift.

- Bend your knees and let your arms and legs do the work. Tighten your buttocks and abdomen to further support your back.

- Keep the load as close to your body as possible, even if the load is light.

- While holding a heavy object, turn your feet, not your back. Try not to turn or twist your body.

- If possible, don't lift heavy objects above shoulder level.

- Use a hand truck or ask someone to help you carry heavy or awkward objects.

Avoid back strain when lifting heavy objects by keeping your upper back straight, bending your knees, and keeping the load close to your body.

Lying Down

If you have back pain at night, your mattress may be the problem. Try sleeping on a firmer mattress. Or, if you think your mattress is too firm, try one that's a little softer. Try these additional tips for more comfortable sleep:

- If you sleep on your back, you may want to use a towel roll to support your lower back or put a pillow under your knees.

- If you sleep on your side, try placing a pillow between your knees.

- Sleeping on your stomach is fine if it doesn't increase your back or neck pain.

Try placing pillows between or under your knees to relieve back pain while lying in bed.

Exercise

Regular exercise (stretching, strengthening, and aerobic exercise) helps you maintain your overall fitness and flexibility and strengthens the muscles that support your spine. Exercising also helps you maintain a healthy body weight, which reduces the load on your lower back. If you are interested in creating a personalized fitness plan, see Fitness starting on page 285.

Although there is no clear evidence that specific exercises can help prevent back pain, the exercises presented here are a common, practical approach to helping you maintain strength and flexibility. You may choose to make the exercises a part of your regular fitness routine.

Do not do these exercises if you have just injured your back. Instead, see "First Aid for Back Pain" on page 108.

Extension exercises strengthen your lower back muscles and stretch the stomach muscles and ligaments. Flexion exercises stretch the lower back muscles and strengthen the stomach muscles.

- You do not need to do every exercise. Do the ones that help you the most.

- If any exercise causes increasing or continuing back pain, stop the exercise and try something else. Stop any exercise that causes the pain to radiate away from your spine into your buttocks or legs, either during or after the exercise.

- Start with 5 repetitions, 3 to 4 times a day, and gradually increase to 10 repetitions. Do all exercises slowly.

Extension Exercises
Press-Ups

Begin and end every set of exercises with a few press-ups.

- Lie facedown with your arms bent, palms flat on the floor.

- Lift yourself up on your elbows, keeping the lower half of your body relaxed. If it's comfortable, press your chest forward.

Press-ups

• Keep your hips pressed to the floor. Feel the stretch in your lower back.

• Lower your upper body to the floor. Repeat this exercise slowly.

Shoulder Lifts

Shoulder lifts will strengthen the back muscles that support the spine.

• Lie facedown with your arms beside your body.

• Lift your shoulders straight up from the floor as high as you can without pain. Keep your chin down and your eyes facing the floor. Keep your torso and hips pressed to the floor.

Backward bend
(keep neck straight and chin down)

Shoulder lifts
(keep neck straight and chin down)

Backward Bend

Practice the backward bend at least once a day and whenever you work in a bent-forward position.

• Stand upright with your feet slightly apart. Back up to a countertop for greater support and stability.

• Place your hands in the small of your back and gently bend backward. Keep your knees straight (not locked) and bend only at the waist. See illustration. Hold the backward stretch for 1 to 2 seconds.

Flexion Exercises

Curl-Ups

Curl-ups strengthen your abdominal muscles, which work with your back muscles to support your spine.

• Lie on your back with knees bent (60° angle) and feet flat on the floor, arms crossed on your chest. Do not hook your feet under anything.

• Slowly curl your head and shoulders up until your shoulder blades barely rise from the floor. Keep your lower back pressed to the floor. To avoid neck problems, remember to lift your shoulders, and do not force your head up or forward. Hold for 5 to 10 seconds (do not hold your breath), and then curl down very slowly.

Curl-ups
(keep neck straight and chin tucked in)

Knee-to-Chest Stretch

The knee-to-chest exercise stretches the lower back muscles and relieves pressure on the joints where the vertebrae come together.

• Lie on your back with knees bent and feet close to your buttocks.

• Bring one knee to your chest, keeping the other foot flat on the floor (or the other leg straight, if that feels better on your lower back). Keep your lower back pressed to the floor. Hold for 5 to 10 seconds.

• Relax and lower your knee to the starting position. Repeat with the other leg.

Knee-to-chest stretch

Additional Strengthening and Stretching Exercises

Prone Buttocks Squeeze

This exercise strengthens the buttocks muscles, which support the back and help you lift with your legs. You may need to place a small pillow under your stomach for comfort.

• Lie flat on your stomach with your arms at your sides.

• Slowly tighten your buttocks muscles and hold for 5 to 10 seconds (don't hold your breath). Relax slowly.

Pelvic Tilts

See instructions on page 108.

Hamstring Stretch

This exercise stretches the muscles in the back of your thigh, which will allow you to bend your legs without putting stress on your back.

• Lie on your back in a doorway with one leg through the doorway on the floor. Put the leg you want to stretch straight up with the heel resting on the wall next to the doorway.

• Keep the leg straight and slowly move your heel up the wall until you feel a gentle pull in the back of your thigh. Do not overstretch.

• Relax in this position for 30 seconds; then bend the knee to relieve the stretch. Repeat with the other leg.

Hamstring stretch
(shading shows where stretch is felt)

Hip Flexor Stretch

This exercise stretches the muscles in the front of your hip.

• Kneel on one knee with your other leg bent in front of you.

• Slowly sink your hips so your weight shifts onto your front foot. The knee of your forward leg should be aligned over the ankle. Hold for 10 seconds. You should feel a stretch in the groin of the leg you are kneeling on. Repeat with the other leg.

Hip flexor stretch
(shading shows where stretch is felt)

Exercises to Avoid

Many common exercises actually increase the risk of low back pain. Avoid the following:

• Straight-leg sit-ups.

• Bent-leg sit-ups when you have acute back pain. (These may be safe to do if you make sure to keep your lower back pressed against the floor.)

• Leg lifts (lifting both legs while lying on your back).

• Lifting heavy weights above the waist (military press, biceps curls while standing).

• Any stretching done while sitting with the legs in a V.

• Toe touches while standing.

Home Treatment

Immediately after an injury and for the next few days, the most important home treatment includes the following:

• Follow the "First Aid for Back Pain" guidelines on page 108.

• Sit or lie in positions that are most comfortable and reduce your pain, especially any leg pain.

• Do not sit up in bed, and avoid soft couches and twisted positions. Avoid sitting for long periods of time. Follow the body mechanics guidelines discussed earlier.

• Bed rest can help relieve back pain but may not speed healing. Unless you have severe leg pain, 1 to 3 days of bed rest should relieve pain. More than 3 days of bed rest is not recommended and could actually delay healing.

- For bed rest, try one of the following positions (see illustrations on page 111):

  - Lie on your back with your knees bent and supported by large pillows, or lie on the floor with your legs on the seat of a sofa or chair.

  - Lie on your side with your knees and hips bent and a pillow between your legs.

  - If it doesn't increase your pain, lie on your stomach.

- Take aspirin or ibuprofen regularly as directed. Do not give aspirin to anyone younger than 20. Call your doctor if you've been told to avoid anti-inflammatory medications. Acetaminophen may also be used. Take these medications sensibly; the maximum recommended dose will reduce the pain. Masking the pain completely might allow movement that could lead to reinjury.

- Relax your muscles. See page 324 for progressive muscle relaxation.

You can try the following home treatment 2 to 3 days after the injury occurs:

- Apply heat to your sore back for 20-minute periods. Moist heat (hot packs, baths, showers) works better than dry heat. Some people find comfort in alternating between heat and ice packs, or using ice only.

- Continue daily walks (increase to 5 to 10 minutes, 3 to 4 times a day).

- Try swimming, which is good for your back. It may be painful immediately after a back injury, but lap swimming or kicking with swim fins often helps prevent back pain from recurring.

- When your pain has improved, begin easy exercises that do not increase your pain. One or two of the exercises described on pages 111 to 114 may be helpful. Start with 5 repetitions 3 to 4 times a day and increase to 10 repetitions as you are able.

When to Call a Health Professional

- If back pain occurs with chest pain or other symptoms of a heart attack (see page 55).

- If you lose bowel or bladder control.

- If you cannot walk or stand.

- If you have new numbness in the buttocks, genital or rectal area, or legs.

- If you have leg weakness that is not solely due to pain. Many people with low back pain say their legs feel weak. However, if leg weakness is so severe that you are unable to bend your foot upward, get up out of a chair, or climb stairs, you should see a doctor.

• If you have new or increased back pain with unexplained fever, painful urination, or other signs of a urinary tract infection. See page 103.

• If you have a dramatic increase in your chronic back pain, especially if it is unrelated to a new or changed physical activity.

• If you have a history of cancer or HIV infection and you develop new or increased back pain.

• If you have severe back pain that does not improve after a few days of home treatment.

• If you develop a new, severe pain in your lower back that does not change with movement and is not related to stress, muscle tension, or a known injury.

• If back pain does not improve after 2 weeks of home treatment.

Medical Doctors

In addition to diagnosing the cause of back pain and evaluating back injuries, a doctor (MD or DO) may also:

• Help you develop an individualized exercise and home care plan or modified work plan if needed.

• Prescribe muscle relaxants, anti-inflammatory drugs, and pain relievers. Note: If you do get a strong painkiller or muscle relaxer, it is especially important to avoid postures and activities that could cause you to reinjure your back.

• Suggest physical therapy.

• Recommend back surgery.

Physical Therapists

After the initial first aid treatments, a physical therapist with training in orthopedic treatment can:

• Identify specific muscle or disc problems.

• Provide or recommend other therapies, such as massage, acupuncture, or manual therapy, if you aren't improving.

• Develop a customized exercise program for your recovery and long-term protection.

Other Health Professionals

Chiropractors and osteopaths can provide relief from some types of back pain through spinal manipulation. (If you have a herniated disc, forceful spinal manipulation may make your condition worse.) Spinal manipulation usually works best if you have had symptoms for fewer than 4 weeks. If your symptoms don't improve after 1 month of spinal manipulation treatment, stop the treatment and have your pain reevaluated.

Acupuncturists, massage therapists, and others can also provide treatments that may give short-term relief. For more information, see Complementary Medicine starting on page 327.

Back Surgery

Rest, pain relievers, and exercise can relieve almost all back problems, including most disc problems.

 MORE INFO Most back surgeries are done to treat <u>disc</u> problems that have not improved with time and exercise. Surgery may also be appropriate in cases of spinal fracture, spinal infection, and other conditions. If you are considering surgery to treat your back pain, getting all the facts and thinking about your own needs and values will help you make a wise decision about treatment.

If you do plan to have surgery, the body mechanics guidelines and exercises in this chapter are still important. A strong, flexible back will help you recover more quickly after surgery.

Neck Pain

Most people occasionally feel pain, stiffness, or a "kink" in the neck. Neck pain may spread to the shoulders, upper back, or upper arms, and it may also cause headache. Pain may limit neck movement. This usually affects one side of the neck more than the other.

Neck pain is most often caused by tension, strain, or spasm in the neck muscles or inflammation of the ligaments, tendons, or joints in the neck. These problems typically result from prolonged or repeated activities or movements that stress the neck. Postures that put your neck in awkward positions—cradling the telephone between your ear and shoulder, sleeping on your stomach or with your neck twisted, or using a workstation that strains your neck—are also common causes.

Other causes of neck pain include:

• Injury resulting from a sudden movement of the head and neck (whiplash), a direct blow to the neck, or a fall.

• Arthritis or damage to the discs in the neck that results in a "pinched nerve." When this is the cause of neck pain, the pain usually spreads down the arm. Numbness, tingling, or weakness in the arm or hand may occur. When you have symptoms of a pinched nerve, a visit to a doctor is needed.

• Meningitis, a serious illness that requires emergency care. Meningitis causes a severe stiff neck with headache and fever (see page 162).

Prevention

Most neck pain can be prevented by using good posture, getting regular exercise, and avoiding prolonged periods in positions that stress the neck. You can also strengthen and protect your neck by doing neck exercises once a day. See page 118. If stress may be the cause of your neck pain, practice the progressive muscle relaxation exercises on page 324.

Neck Exercises

You do not need to do every exercise. Stick with the ones that help you the most. Do each exercise slowly. Stop any exercise that increases pain. Start by doing the exercises twice a day.

Dorsal glide: Sit or stand tall, looking straight ahead (a "palace guard" posture). Slowly tuck your chin as you glide your head backwards over your body. Hold for a count of 5; then relax. Repeat 6 to 10 times. This stretches the back of the neck. If you feel pain, do not glide so far back. You may find this exercise easier to do while lying on your back with ice on your neck.

Chest and shoulder stretch: Sit or stand tall and glide your head backward as in the dorsal glide exercise. Raise both arms so that your hands are next to your ears. As you exhale, lower your elbows down and back. Feel your shoulder blades slide down and together. Hold for a few seconds. Relax and repeat 6 to 10 times.

Shoulder lifts: Lie facedown with your arms beside your body. Lift your shoulders straight up from the floor as high as you can without pain. Keep your chin down and your eyes facing the floor. Keep your torso and hips pressed to the floor. Repeat 6 to 10 times.

Hands on head: Move your head backward, forward, and side to side against gentle pressure from your hands, holding each position for several seconds. Repeat 6 to 10 times.

Chest and shoulder stretch

Dorsal glide

Shoulder lifts

If your pain is **worse at the end of the day**, evaluate your posture and body mechanics during the day.

• Sit straight in your chair with your lower back supported. Avoid sitting for long periods without getting up or changing positions. Take mini-breaks several times each hour to stretch your neck muscles.

• If you work at a computer, adjust the monitor so that the top of the screen is at eye level. Use a document holder that puts the copy at the same level as the screen.

• If you use the telephone a lot, consider using a headset or speakerphone.

If your neck stiffness is **worse in the morning**, you may need better neck support when you sleep.

• Try folding a towel lengthwise into a 4-inch-wide pad and wrapping it around your neck. Pin it for good support.

• You may need a special neck support pillow. Look for a pillow that supports your neck comfortably when you lie on your back and on your side (try before buying). Avoid pillows that force your head forward when you are on your back.

• Avoid sleeping on your stomach with your neck twisted or bent.

• Morning neck pain may also be the result of activities done the day before.

Home Treatment

Much of the home treatment for back pain is also helpful for neck pain. See page 114.

• If you have recently been in an accident involving your neck, see Spinal Injuries on page 71.

• See the icing guidelines on page 108. If the problem is near your shoulder or upper back, it will usually help more to ice the back of your neck.

• After the first 72 hours (or if you have chronic pain), you may apply heat to the sore area for 20-minute periods.

• Use aspirin, ibuprofen, or acetaminophen to help relieve pain. Do not give aspirin to anyone younger than 20.

• Walking also helps relieve and prevent neck pain. The gentle swinging motion of your arms often relieves pain. Start with short walks of 5 to 10 minutes, 3 to 4 times a day.

• If neck pain occurs with headache, see Tension Headaches on page 191.

• Once the pain starts to get better, do the exercises on page 118.

When to Call a Health Professional

• If neck pain occurs with chest pain or other symptoms of a heart attack (see page 55). **Call 911 or other emergency services immediately**.

• If a stiff neck occurs with headache and fever. See "Encephalitis and Meningitis" on page 162.

• If you have severe neck pain after an injury or fall. See Spinal Injuries on page 71.

• If you develop new weakness or continuous numbness in your arms or legs.

• If pain extends or shoots down one arm, or you have numbness or tingling in your hands.

• If a blow or injury to your neck (whiplash) is causing new pain.

• If you are unable to manage your pain with home treatment.

• If the pain has lasted 2 weeks or longer without improvement despite home treatment.

I don't deserve this award, but then I have
arthritis and I don't deserve that either.
Jack Benny

6

Bone, Muscle, and Joint Problems

Our aches and pains remind us that life isn't always easy. But pain can be managed. This chapter covers pain from arthritis to plantar fasciitis. As with most chapters in this book, we hope you rarely have to refer to these pages. But when you do, we hope these guidelines will make your life more comfortable.

In many cases, you can determine the cause of bone, muscle, or joint problems by thinking back to how or when the pain started.

- A single episode of overuse or repeated heavy use of a joint can cause bursitis or tendon injury. See page 124.

- Joint pain that comes on gradually and seems unrelated to any specific injury may be due to arthritis.

- Traumatic injuries (turning an ankle or twisting a knee) usually cause strains, sprains, fractures, or dislocations. See page 72.

Arthritis

Arthritis refers to a variety of joint problems that cause pain, swelling, and stiffness. Simply put, arthritis means inflammation of a joint. Arthritis can occur at any age, but it affects older people the most.

There are more than 100 different types of arthritis. The chart on page 122 describes three common kinds of arthritis. Osteoarthritis is the most common type and can usually be managed at home. Rheumatoid arthritis and gout can improve with a combination of self-care and professional care.

Little is known about what causes most types of arthritis. Some seem to run in families; others seem to be related to imbalances in body chemistry or immune system problems. Many arthritis problems are the result of injury or long-term "wear and tear" on the joints.

Common Types of Arthritis

Type	Cause	Symptoms	Comments
Osteoarthritis	Breakdown of joint cartilage.	Pain and stiffness; common in knees, fingers, hips, feet, and back.	Most common after age 50.
Rheumatoid Arthritis	Inflammation of the membrane (synovium) lining the joint.	Pain, stiffness, warmth, and swelling in joints on both sides of the body; common in hands, wrists, elbows, feet, knees, and neck.	Occurs most often around age 40; more common in women.
Gout	Buildup of uric acid crystals in the joint fluid.	Sudden onset of burning pain, stiffness, and swelling; common in big toe, ankle, knee, wrist, and elbow.	Most common in men ages 30 to 50; may be aggravated by alcohol and exposure to cold.

Prevention

It may not be possible to prevent arthritis, but you can prevent a lot of pain by being kind to your joints. This is especially important if you already have arthritis.

- If activities that jar your body (such as running) cause pain, try activities that involve less impact (such as swimming).

- Control your weight.

- Exercise regularly. Exercise nourishes joint cartilage and removes waste products from the joints. It also strengthens the muscles around the joints, providing support and reducing injuries caused by fatigue. Stretching maintains your range of pain-free motion.

Home Treatment

- A warm shower or bath may help relieve morning stiffness. Try to avoid sitting still afterwards.

- If the joint is not swollen, apply moist heat for 20 to 30 minutes, 2 to 3 times a day. Do not apply heat to a swollen, inflamed joint.

- If the joint is swollen, apply cold packs for 10 minutes, once an hour. Cold will help relieve pain and reduce inflammation.

- Rest sore joints. Avoid activities that put weight or strain on the joints for a few days. Take short rest breaks from your regular activities throughout the day.

- Put each of your joints gently through its full range of motion once or twice each day.

- Exercise regularly to help maintain strength and flexibility in your muscles and joints. Try low-impact activities, such as swimming, water aerobics, biking, or walking.

- Take acetaminophen to relieve pain caused by osteoarthritis. Anti-inflammatory medications, such as aspirin, ibuprofen, or naproxen sodium, may help ease pain but can cause stomach upset.

- Enroll in an arthritis self-management program. Participants in these programs usually have less pain and fewer limitations on their activities.

When to Call a Health Professional

- If you have fever or a skin rash along with severe joint pain.

- If the joint is so painful that you cannot use it.

- If there is sudden, unexplained swelling, redness, warmth, or pain in one or more joints.

- If sudden back pain occurs with weakness in the legs or loss of bowel or bladder control.

- If joint pain continues for more than 6 weeks and home treatment is not helping.

- If you experience side effects (stomach pain, nausea, persistent heartburn, or dark, tarry stools) from aspirin or other arthritis medications. Do not exceed recommended doses of nonprescription medications without your doctor's advice.

Bunions and Hammer Toes

A bunion is an enlargement of the joint at the base of the big toe. A bunion develops when the big toe bends toward and sometimes overlaps the second toe. A hammer toe is a toe that bends up permanently at the middle joint. These foot problems sometimes run in families. Tight or high-heeled shoes increase the risk of both conditions and may make an existing problem worse.

A bunion is an enlargement of the joint at the base of the big toe.

A hammer toe is a toe that bends up permanently at the middle joint.

Prevention

Wear shoes with low or flat heels and roomy toe areas. Tennis or basketball court shoes are often best. Make sure your shoes fit properly.

Home Treatment

Once you have a bunion or hammer toe, there is usually no way to completely get rid of it. Home treatment will help relieve discomfort and keep the problem from getting worse.

• Wear low-heeled shoes that have roomy toe areas.

• Cushion the joint with moleskin or doughnut-shaped pads to prevent rubbing and irritation.

• Cut out the area over the bunion or hammer toe from an old pair of shoes, and wear them around the house. Or wear comfortable sandals that don't press on the area.

• Try ibuprofen or acetaminophen to relieve pain. Ice or cold packs may also help.

When to Call a Health Professional

• If severe pain in the big toe comes on suddenly and you have not been diagnosed with gout.

• If your big toe starts to overlap your second toe.

• If you have diabetes, poor circulation, or peripheral vascular disease. In people with these conditions, irritated skin over a bunion or hammer toe can easily become infected.

• If you develop a sore over the bunion or hammer toe.

• If pain does not respond to home treatment in 2 to 3 weeks.

 If severe pain or joint deformity interferes with walking or daily activities, you may want to consider surgical treatment. Surgery may not cure the problem completely. The more information you gather about the risks and benefits of <u>surgery for bunions</u> and hammer toes, the easier it will be for you to make a wise health decision.

Bursitis and Tendon Injury

A bursa is a small sac of fluid that helps the tissues surrounding a joint slide over one another easily. Injury or overuse of a joint or tendon can result in pain, redness, heat, and inflammation of the bursa, a condition known as bursitis. Bursitis often develops quickly, over just a few days, often after a specific injury, overuse, or prolonged direct pressure on a joint.

Tendons are tough, ropelike fibers that connect muscles to bones. Injury or overuse can cause pain, tenderness, inflammation, and tissue breakdown in the tendons or the tissues surrounding them.

Both bursitis and tendon injury can be related to job, sports, or household activities that require repeated twisting or rapid joint movements. The same home treatment is good for both problems.

Prevention

Stretch and warm up well before exercising, and increase the intensity of the activity gradually. Cool down afterwards by doing gentle stretches. See pages 125 to 127 for additional, joint-specific prevention tips.

Home Treatment

Bursitis or mild tendon injury will usually improve in a few days or weeks if you avoid the activity that caused it.

The most common mistake in recovery is thinking that the problem is gone when the pain is gone. Chances are, the problem will recur if you do not take steps to strengthen and stretch the muscles around the joint and change the way you do some activities.

- Rest the affected area. Change the way you do the activity that causes pain so that you can do it without pain. See pages 125 to 127 for joint-specific guidelines. To maintain fitness, substitute activities that don't stress the affected area.

- As soon as you notice pain, apply ice or cold packs for 10-minute periods, once an hour or as often as you can for 48 hours. Continue applying ice (10 minutes, 3 times a day) as long as it relieves pain. See page 133. Although heating pads or hot baths may feel good, ice or cold packs will reduce inflammation and promote healing.

- Aspirin, ibuprofen, or naproxen sodium may help ease pain and inflammation, but don't use medication to relieve pain while you continue overusing a joint. Do not give aspirin to anyone younger than 20.

- To prevent stiffness, gently move the joint through as full a range of motion as you can without pain. As the pain subsides, continue range-of-motion exercises, and add exercises that strengthen the affected muscles.

- Gradually resume the activity at a lower intensity. Increase the intensity slowly and only if pain does not recur.

- Warm up before and stretch after the activity. Apply ice to the injured area after exercise to prevent pain and swelling.

In addition to the general prevention and home treatment information for bursitis and tendon injury above, the following tips will be useful if you have a specific joint problem.

Wrist pain may be caused by tendon injury. Though this is not the same as carpal tunnel syndrome, the same home care may help. See page 128.

Elbow pain is often caused by one of the following common types of injuries to the forearm tendons. (The inside or outside of the elbow is defined by holding your arm at your side with the palm of your hand facing forward. The inside is the side closest to your body.)

Elbow pain is often caused by injury to a tendon in the forearm.

- **Tennis elbow** causes pain on the outside of the elbow where the muscles that bend the wrist back are attached.

- **Golfer's elbow** causes pain on the inside of the elbow where the muscles that bend the wrist down are attached.

To relieve elbow pain and prevent further injury:

- Rest the elbow and give it time to heal.

- Wear a brace or elbow sleeve.

- Support a sore elbow with a sling for 1 to 2 days. Do range-of-motion exercises daily.

- Strengthen the wrist, arm, shoulder, and back muscles to help protect the elbow.

- Avoid activities that require repetitive use of the wrist.

- Change activities that irritate the tendon:

  - Use tools with larger handles.

  - Use a two-handed tennis backhand stroke and a more flexible, midsize racquet.

  - Try to avoid hitting divots when playing golf.

  - Try to avoid sidearm pitching and throwing curve balls.

Shoulder pain that occurs on the outside of the upper arm is often caused by bursitis or tendon injury in the shoulder joint. Pain on the top of the shoulder or in the neck may be caused by tension in the trapezius muscles, which run from the back of the head across the back of the shoulders. See Neck Pain on page 117.

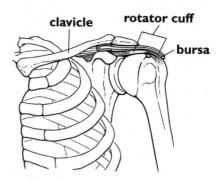

Bursitis, tendon injury, and muscle tension are common causes of shoulder pain.

Common symptoms of bursitis or tendon injury in the shoulder are pain, pinching, and stiffness when you raise your arm. The symptoms are often brought on by doing repeated overhead movements. Problems develop when you continue to use your shoulder without giving it time to rest. This leads to further swelling and pain.

For home treatment of shoulder pain, see page 125. Also keep the following in mind:

- Avoid activities that involve overhead reaching, but continue to use your shoulder.

- Practice the pendulum exercise to prevent stiffness: Bend forward and grasp the back of a chair with the hand of your "good" arm. Let the other arm dangle straight down from the shoulder. Move the dangling arm in clockwise circles; start with small circles and gradually make them bigger. Then make counterclockwise circles (small to large). Next, swing the arm forward and backward, then from side to side. Do this exercise 10 times a day.

- Use proper throwing techniques for baseball and football.

- Use a different swim stroke: breast stroke or sidestroke instead of the crawl or butterfly.

- Put your shoulder through its full range of motion every day to prevent stiffness.

Hip pain caused by tendon injury or bursitis may be felt at the side of the hip when you rise from a chair and take the first few steps, while you climb stairs, or while you drive. If pain is severe, sleeping on your side may also be painful. Pain in the front of the hip may also be caused by arthritis. See page 121. Hip pain can also cause knee or thigh pain. This is known as referred pain.

- Wear well-cushioned shoes and avoid high heels.

- Avoid activities that force one side of your pelvis higher than the other, such as running in only one direction on a track or working sideways on a slope.

- Sleep on your uninjured side with a pillow between your knees, or on your back with pillows beneath your knees.

- See the hip stretches on pages 114 and 288. Stretch after activity, when your muscles are warm.

Knee pain may be caused by bursitis or tendon injury. See Knee Problems on page 131.

Heel or foot pain may be caused by plantar fasciitis or Achilles tendon injury. See page 130. Pain in the front of the lower leg may be due to shin-splints. See page 133.

When to Call a Health Professional

- If there is fever, rapid swelling, or redness, or if you are unable to use a joint.

- If severe pain continues when the joint is at rest and you have applied ice.

- If the pain is severe.

- If the pain persists for 2 weeks or longer despite home treatment. Your doctor or a physical therapist can help you develop a specific exercise and home treatment plan.

Carpal Tunnel Syndrome

The carpal tunnel is a narrow passageway between the bones and ligaments in your wrist. The median nerve, which controls sensation in the fingers and some muscles in the hand, passes through this tunnel along with some of the finger tendons. Carpal tunnel syndrome (CTS) develops when there is pressure on the median nerve where it goes through the carpal tunnel.

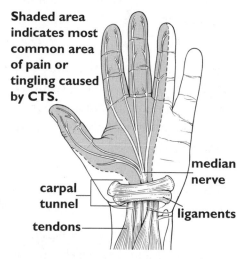

Shaded area indicates most common area of pain or tingling caused by CTS.

median nerve

carpal tunnel

ligaments

tendons

Pain and tingling in the hand may be caused by pressure on a nerve in the wrist.

Doing activities that use the same finger or hand movements over and over again can cause CTS. We do these activities in every part of our lives, including work, home, hobbies, and sports. Other causes include being overweight, a cyst (ganglion) on the tendon sheath in the wrist, or rheumatoid arthritis. Previous wrist injuries, pregnancy, diabetes, thyroid disease, and taking birth control pills also may increase your risk for CTS.

Pressure on the median nerve causes the following symptoms of CTS:

- Numbness or pain in your hand or wrist that wakes you up at night.

- Numbness or tingling in the fingers of one or both hands, except for the little finger.

- Numbness or pain that gets worse when you use your hand or wrist, especially when you grip an object or bend your wrist.

- Occasional aching pain in your arm from your hand to your elbow.

- A weak grip.

Prevention

- Stop any activity that you think may be causing finger, hand, or wrist numbness or pain. If your symptoms improve when you stop an activity, resume that activity gradually and with greater efforts to keep your wrist straight or only slightly bent.

- Use your whole hand (not just your fingers and thumb) to grasp objects.

- Reduce the speed and force of repetitive hand movements such as typing.

- Switch hands and change positions often when you are doing repeated motions.

- Take frequent breaks and rest your hands.

- If you are not able to change positions or equipment at work often enough to prevent numbness or pain, wear a wrist splint that will reduce the stress on your fingers, hand, or wrist.

- Pay attention to your posture. When you are typing, make sure your fingers are lower than your wrists (using a keyboard wrist support may help). When your forearms are hanging by your sides, keep your shoulders relaxed.

- Keep your arm, hand, and finger muscles strong and flexible and maintain good overall fitness.

- Avoid using too much salt if you tend to retain fluid.

Home Treatment

- Follow the prevention tips above.

- Use ibuprofen or naproxen sodium to relieve pain and reduce swelling.

- Apply ice or a cold pack to the palm side of the wrist. See "Ice and Cold Packs" on page 133.

- Avoid sleeping on your hands. Wear a wrist splint at night to relieve pressure on your wrist.

- Do simple range-of-motion exercises with your fingers and wrist to prevent stiffening. Stop if it hurts.

- Other lifestyle changes such as losing weight, quitting smoking, reducing the amount of alcohol you drink, and controlling diabetes may help relieve symptoms of CTS that are related to swelling.

- Vitamin B_6 has not been shown to be an effective treatment for CTS.

When to Call a Health Professional

- If tingling, numbness, weakness, or pain in your fingers and hand has not gone away after 2 weeks of home treatment.

- If you have little or no feeling in your fingers or hand.

- If you cannot do simple hand movements, or you accidentally drop things.

- If you cannot pinch your thumb and first finger together or you have no thumb strength.

- If you have problems at work because of pain in your fingers or hand.

 Most cases of carpal tunnel syndrome are treated without surgery. If you are considering surgery to treat CTS, gather as much information as possible about the risks and benefits of surgical treatment. Getting all the facts and thinking about your own needs and values will help you work with your doctor to make a wise health decision.

Heel Pain and Plantar Fasciitis

Plantar fasciitis is a condition that occurs when the thick, fibrous tissue that covers the bottom of your foot (plantar fascia) becomes inflamed and painful. Athletes, middle-aged people, and those who are overweight tend to develop plantar fasciitis. Prolonged standing and repetitive movements such as running and jumping can lead to heel pain and plantar fasciitis.

An excessive inward rolling of the foot (called pronation) during walking or running can also cause heel pain and plantar fasciitis. Pronation can be caused by wearing shoes that are worn out or have poor arch support, having tight calf muscles, or running downhill or on uneven surfaces.

Achilles tendon

plantar fascia

Foot or heel pain is often caused by inflammation of the plantar fascia or injury to the Achilles tendon.

Achilles tendon injury can cause pain in the back of the heel.

A **heel spur** is a calcium buildup that most often develops where the plantar fascia attaches to the heel bone. Heel spurs usually do not cause pain and do not need to be treated. (Rarely, a painful heel spur may need to be surgically removed.) The pain many people attribute to heel spurs is in most cases caused by plantar fasciitis, rather than by the heel spur itself.

Prevention

- Stretch your Achilles tendon and calf muscles several times a day (see page 288). Stretching is important for both athletes and nonathletes.

- Maintain a reasonable weight for your height.

- Always wear shoes with well-cushioned soles and good arch supports. Replace running shoes every 300 to 500 miles.

- Establish good exercise habits. If you are a runner, increase mileage slowly, limit your training on hilly terrain, and run on softer surfaces (grass or dirt) rather than concrete. Cross-train by alternating running with different sports.

Home Treatment

Treat heel pain when it first appears to keep plantar fasciitis or other problems from becoming chronic.

- Reduce all weight-bearing activities to a pain-free level. Try low-impact activities such as cycling or swimming to speed healing. You may need to check with your doctor about when you can gradually resume high-impact activities.

- Apply ice to your heel. See "Ice and Cold Packs" on page 133.

- You may wish to put nonprescription arch supports in your shoes.

- Do not go barefoot until the pain is completely gone. Wear shoes or arch-supporting sandals during all weight-bearing activities, even going to the bathroom during the night.

- Take aspirin, ibuprofen, or naproxen sodium to relieve pain. Do not give aspirin to anyone younger than 20.

- Stretch your calf muscles. See page 288.

- For Achilles tendon problems or plantar fasciitis, try putting heel lifts or heel cups in both shoes. Use them only until the pain is gone (continue other home treatment).

When to Call a Health Professional

- If heel pain occurs with fever, redness, or heat in your heel, or if there is numbness or tingling in your heel or foot.

- If a heel injury results in pain when you put weight on your heel.

- If pain continues when you are not standing or bearing any weight on your heel.

- If heel pain persists for 1 to 2 weeks despite home treatment.

 Your doctor may recommend other treatments for plantar fasciitis, such as taping, exercises, shoe inserts, or in some cases steroid injections. Surgery is usually done only as a last resort when other treatments fail to relieve pain.

Knee Problems

The knee is a vulnerable joint. It is basically just two long leg bones held together with ligaments and muscles. Problems develop when you put too much stress on the joint. The following are the three most common knee problems:

- Strained or sprained knee ligaments (such as the anterior cruciate ligament) usually occur when the knee is twisted in a direction that it does not normally go. Sometimes knee ligaments are torn, and when this happens knee cartilage (such as a meniscus) may also be damaged.

- Kneecap pain, also known as patellofemoral pain, occurs around or behind the kneecap (patella) when you run downhill, go up or down stairs, or after you sit for long periods of time.

- Patellar tendinitis, also known as jumper's knee, is an inflammation of the tendon that attaches the kneecap to the shinbone (tibia). It is common among basketball and volleyball players.

thigh bone (femur)

kneecap (patella)

ligaments

ligaments

meniscus

fibula

shinbone (tibia)

Knee problems can develop when the structures that support the joint are injured or become inflamed.

Prevention

• The best way to prevent knee problems is to strengthen and stretch the leg muscles evenly, especially those in the front and back of the thigh (quadriceps and hamstrings). See page 288.

• Avoid deep knee bends.

• Avoid running downhill unless you are fully conditioned.

• Avoid wearing shoes with cleats when playing contact sports.

• Wear shoes with good arch supports. Replace running shoes every 300 to 500 miles.

• Avoid wearing high-heeled shoes.

Home Treatment

• Apply ice to your knee. See "Ice and Cold Packs" on page 133.

• Rest your knee, and reduce by at least 50 percent the activities that cause pain.

• Wear a brace, an elastic or neoprene sleeve, or a band with a hole for the kneecap that holds the kneecap in place to help ease pain during activity. You can buy one at a pharmacy or sporting goods store.

• Stretch the front and back of your thigh muscles (quadriceps and hamstrings) after exercise, when they are warm. See pages 114 and 288.

• Also see Strains, Sprains, Fractures, and Dislocations on page 72 and Bursitis and Tendon Injury on page 124.

• If knee pain is not related to exercise or due to a recent or past injury, see Arthritis on page 121.

When to Call a Health Professional

• If the knee "gives out" or won't bear weight.

• If you felt or heard a "pop" in your knee at the time of an injury.

• If the knee begins to swell within 30 minutes of an injury.

• If you have signs of damage to the nerves or blood vessels, such as numbness, tingling, a "pins-and-needles" sensation below the injury, or pale or bluish skin.

• If the knee looks deformed.

• If you are unable to straighten or bend the knee, or if the joint "locks."

- If the knee is red, hot, swollen, or painful to touch.

- If pain is severe enough that you are limping, or if it does not improve within 2 days.

Muscle Cramps and Leg Pain

Leg pain and muscle cramps ("charley horse" or "stitch") are common. They often occur during exercise, especially during hot weather, or at night. Dehydration, low levels of potassium in the body, or using a muscle that is not stretched well may cause cramps.

Shinsplints cause pain in the front of the lower leg. Their cause is unclear, but they tend to develop when the legs are overused in high-impact activities.

Arthritis can also cause leg pain (see page 121). Leg pain that runs from the buttocks down the back of the leg and into the foot may be caused by sciatica. See page 109.

Phlebitis, an inflammation of a vein, also causes leg pain, usually in the calf of one leg. This condition can be serious if blood clots form in a deep vein, break loose, and lodge in the lungs. Phlebitis is most common after surgery or prolonged bed rest.

Decreased blood flow to the leg muscles caused by hardening of the arteries (called **intermittent claudication**) is another possible cause of leg cramps. Symptoms may

Ice and Cold Packs

Ice can relieve pain, swelling, and inflammation from injuries and other conditions such as arthritis. Apply ice consistently as long as you have symptoms. Use either a commercial cold pack or one of the following:

- Ice towel: Wet a towel with cold water and squeeze it until it is just damp. Fold the towel, place it in a plastic bag, and freeze it for 15 minutes. Remove the towel from the bag and place it on the affected area.

- Ice pack: Put about a pound of ice in a plastic bag. Add water to barely cover the ice. Squeeze the air out of the bag and seal it. Wrap the bag in a wet towel and apply it to the affected area.

- Homemade cold pack: See instructions on page 337.

Ice the area at least 3 times a day. For the first 48 hours, ice for 10 minutes once an hour. After that, a good pattern is to ice for 10 minutes 3 times a day: in the morning, in the late afternoon after work or school, and about half an hour before bedtime. Also ice after any prolonged activity or vigorous exercise.

Always keep a damp cloth between your skin and the cold pack, and press firmly against all the curves of the affected area. Do not apply ice for longer than 10 minutes at a time, and do not fall asleep with the ice on your skin.

include cramping pain in the calf that comes on with activity or exertion and is relieved by rest. Symptoms often occur after you walk a certain distance.

Fibromyalgia

Fibromyalgia is a condition that causes chronic muscle and soft tissue pain and tenderness on both sides of the body, above and below the waist. Fibromyalgia does not damage the body, destroy the joints, or cause any internal organ problems, but the pain may be severe enough to interfere with work and other activities.

The cause of fibromyalgia is not known. People who have fibromyalgia have many tender spots in specific areas of their bodies (trigger points). They often have trouble sleeping. There may also be stiffness, weakness, and fatigue. Fibromyalgia is more common in women than in men.

 Regular exercise, such as walking, biking, or swimming, is the cornerstone of treatment for fibromyalgia. Doctors sometimes prescribe medications to help treat the symptoms. If stress makes your symptoms worse, see page 323.

Prevention

- Warm up well and stretch before any activity. Also stretch after exercise to keep hot muscles from shortening and cramping.

- Drink extra fluids before and during exercise, especially during hot or humid weather.

- Include plenty of potassium in your diet. Bananas, orange juice, and potatoes are good sources.

- To avoid stomach muscle cramps ("stitches") during exercise, do side stretches before exercising and learn to breathe with your lower lungs. See Roll Breathing on page 323.

- If leg cramps wake you at night, take a warm bath and do some stretching exercises before going to bed. Keep your legs warm while sleeping.

Home Treatment

- If there is pain, swelling, or heaviness in the calf of only one of your legs, or if you have other symptoms that cause you to suspect phlebitis (see When to Call a Health Professional), call your doctor before you try home treatment.

- Gently stretch and massage the cramping muscle.

- Drink more fluids. Cramps are often related to dehydration.

MORE INFO **For more information, see the back cover.**

- The best treatment for shinsplints is ice, pain relievers (ibuprofen or acetaminophen), and 1 to 2 weeks of rest followed by a gradual return to exercise.

When to Call a Health Professional

- If you have any of the following symptoms of phlebitis:
  - Continuous leg or calf pain
  - Swelling of one leg
  - Any redness that is tender to the touch
  - Fever
- If you have signs of impaired blood flow such as:
  - Pain that comes on after you walk a certain distance and that goes away with rest.
  - Sudden onset of moderate to severe pain with coldness or pale skin in the lower part of the leg.
  - Pale or blue-black color to the skin of one or both legs, feet, or toes.
- If muscle cramps are not relieved by home treatment.

Growing Pains

Children age 6 to 12 often develop harmless "growing pains" in their legs at night. Other than growth itself, the cause is unknown. A heating pad, acetaminophen, or gentle massage of the legs may help.

Osteoporosis

Osteoporosis is a disease that causes a person's bones to become so weak that they can break during normal daily activities. Osteoporosis affects 20 million older Americans. Women are four times more likely to develop osteoporosis than men are.

Osteoporosis is more common after menopause, when estrogen levels decline. Risk factors for osteoporosis include family history of osteoporosis, lack of weight-bearing exercise, slender body frame, and Asian or European heritage. Women who smoke or drink are also at greater risk. Elevated thyroid hormone (hyper-thyroidism) may also cause osteoporosis.

Osteoporosis usually develops over many years without symptoms. The first signs of osteoporosis include loss of height, developing a curved upper back (dowager's hump), back pain, or broken bones.

Prevention

Weakening bones are a natural part of growing older. But if you start healthy habits early in life, you may be able to delay the development of osteoporosis.

- Get regular weight-bearing exercise, such as walking, jogging, climbing stairs, dancing, or weight lifting. Weight-bearing exercise helps keep bones strong.

• Eat a healthy diet that includes plenty of calcium and vitamin D. Both are needed for building healthy, strong bones. See page 299 for tips on getting more calcium in your diet. You can get a boost of vitamin D by drinking fortified milk or by spending 10 to 15 minutes in the sun each day. (If you have dark skin, you will need more time in the sun.) Take supplements of calcium and vitamin D if you think you are not getting enough in your diet.

• Don't smoke.

• Limit your alcohol intake to 1 drink per day or less.

• Cut down on caffeine. Caffeine increases calcium loss from your body and puts you at risk for osteoporosis.

• During menopause, estrogen therapy helps prevent osteoporosis. See "Hormone Therapy" on page 256.

If you already have osteoporosis, these healthy habits can help slow the disease process and possibly reduce your risk of broken bones.

When to Call a Health Professional

• If you think you have a broken bone; if you notice swelling; or if you cannot move a part of your body normally.

• If you have sudden, severe pain or problems bearing weight on the injured part of your body.

• If you notice that one of your arms or legs is misshapen. This may mean you have a broken bone.

• If you want to discuss your risk for developing osteoporosis.

 If you are at risk for osteoporosis and are nearing menopause, talk with your doctor about estrogen or hormone therapy. It is the most effective way to prevent osteoporosis. See pages 256 and 257.

Sports Injuries

Injuries are common among physically active people. Muscle aches and pains are likely to develop when you start a new activity (or resume an activity after taking a break from it), because the muscles used for the activity need time to build strength and endurance. Most sports injuries are caused by either accidents or overuse. Overuse injuries can be avoided if you train properly for activities and use appropriate equipment.

Prevention

• Warm up before exercising. Cold, stiff muscles and ligaments are more prone to injury. Cool down and stretch after activities. See page 289.

• Increase the intensity and duration of activities gradually. As your fitness level improves, you will be able to do increasingly strenuous exercise without injury.

• Use proper sports techniques and equipment. For example, wear supportive, well-cushioned shoes for running, aerobics, and walking; use a two-handed tennis backhand stroke; wear protective pads for in-line skating. Make sure that your bicycle is adjusted properly for your body. Wear a sport-specific helmet for your activity.

• Alternate hard workouts with easier ones to let your body rest. For example, if you run, alternate long or hard runs with shorter or easier ones. If you lift weights, don't work the same muscles 2 days in a row.

• Cross-train (do several activities regularly) to rest your muscles. Alternate days of walking or running with biking or swimming.

• Don't ignore aches and pains. When you feel the first twinge of pain, rest or reduce your activity for a few days. Apply ice and other home treatment, and you may avoid more serious problems.

Home Treatment

The biggest home treatment challenge for most people with sports injuries is to get enough rest to allow healing without losing overall conditioning.

• Maintain your fitness level by cross-training with activities that don't stress the injured area: swimming for sore ankles or feet; walking or biking for sore shoulders or elbows. Don't return to the activity that caused the injury too quickly.

• Resume your regular activity gradually. Start with a slow, easy pace, less weight (if you're lifting weights), fewer repetitions, or a shorter duration of activity, and increase only if you have no pain.

• Break your sport down into components. If you can throw a ball a short distance without pain, try increasing the distance. If you can walk comfortably, try jogging. If you can jog without pain, try running.

When to Call a Health Professional

Information on specific injuries can be found on the following pages:

• Bursitis and Tendon Injury, page 124.

• Tennis or golfer's elbow, page 126.

• Patellar tendinitis, page 131.

• Achilles tendon injury and plantar fasciitis, page 130.

• Strains, Sprains, Fractures, and Dislocations, page 72.

Temporomandibular (TM) Disorder

The temporomandibular joint (TMJ) is the joint in front of the ear that connects the lower jawbone (mandible) to the skull. Pain and discomfort in the jaw muscles and temporomandibular joint is called temporomandibular disorder (TM disorder).

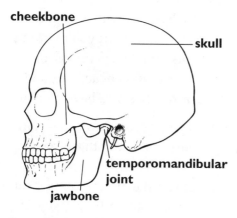

Pain and discomfort in the jaw muscles and jaw joint is called temporomandibular disorder.

The symptoms of TM disorder can include:

• Pain in one or both jaws when chewing or yawning.

• Painful clicking, popping, or grating in the jaw joint.

• Locking of the jaw in an open or closed position, or inability to "open wide."

• Headache, neck pain, facial pain, or shoulder pain.

The most common cause of TM disorder is tension in the jaw, neck, and shoulder muscles. This can be brought on by stress or by habits such as clenching or grinding your teeth. TM disorder can also occur when there is a problem, such as arthritis, in the joint itself.

 Home treatment and **MORE INFO** nonsurgical treatments will successfully relieve most symptoms of TM disorder.

Your doctor may recommend use of a plastic mouth plate (splint), physical therapy, or prescription pain relievers. Surgery is rarely needed and may cause further problems.

Prevention

The key to preventing TM disorder is reducing muscle tension in your jaw.

• Relax. If you have a lot of stress and anxiety in your life, try relaxation techniques (see page 323).

• Do not bite your nails or cradle the telephone receiver between your shoulder and jaw.

• Stop chewing gum or tough foods at the first sign of pain or discomfort in your jaw muscles.

• Change your diet. Eat softer foods, and use both sides of your mouth to chew your food.

• Maintain good posture. Poor posture may disturb the natural alignment between your facial bones and muscles and cause pain.

• Get regular dental checkups.

Home Treatment

• Continue the prevention tips.

• Avoid opening your mouth too wide.

• Rest your jaw, keeping your teeth apart and your lips closed. (Keep your tongue on the roof of your mouth, not between your teeth.)

• Put an ice pack on the joint for 8 minutes, 3 times a day. Gently open and close your mouth while the ice pack is on. If the jaw muscle is swollen, apply ice 6 times a day.

• Take ibuprofen or acetaminophen to reduce swelling and pain.

• If there is no swelling, apply moist heat to your jaw for 10 to 15 minutes 3 times a day. Gently open and close your mouth while the heat is on. Alternate with the cold pack treatments.

• If you are under severe stress or suffer from anxiety or depression, see Mental Health and Mind-Body Wellness starting on page 303.

When to Call a Health Professional

• If the pain is severe.

• If TM symptoms occur after an injury to the jaw.

• If your jaw locks in certain positions.

• If any jaw problem or pain lasts longer than 2 weeks without improvement.

• If you have noticed a change in the way your teeth fit together when you close your mouth.

Weakness and Fatigue

Weakness is a lack of physical or muscle strength and a feeling that extra effort is required to move your arms, legs, or other muscles.

Fatigue is a feeling of tiredness, exhaustion, or lack of energy.

Unexplained muscle weakness is usually more serious than fatigue. It may be caused by diabetes (see page 237), thyroid problems, stroke, or other problems related to the brain and spinal cord. Call your doctor immediately if you have sudden, unexplained muscle weakness.

Fatigue, on the other hand, can usually be treated with self-care. Most fatigue is caused by lack of exercise, stress or overwork, lack of sleep, depression, worry, or boredom. Colds and flu may cause fatigue and weakness, but the symptoms disappear as the illness runs its course.

Prevention

• Regular exercise is your best defense against fatigue. If you feel too tired to exercise vigorously, try a short walk.

• Eat a well-balanced diet.

• Make sure you are getting enough sleep. See page 314.

• Deal with emotional problems instead of ignoring or denying them. See page 303.

• Take steps to control your stress and workload. See page 321.

Home Treatment

• Follow the prevention guidelines and be patient. It may take a while before you feel energetic again.

• Listen to your body. Alternate rest with exercise.

- Limit medications that might contribute to fatigue. Tranquilizers and cold and allergy medications are particularly suspect.

- Reduce your use of caffeine, nicotine, and alcohol.

- Cut back on watching television. Spend that time with friends, try new activities, or travel to break the fatigue cycle.

When to Call a Health Professional

- If you have unexplained muscle weakness in one area of your body.

- If severe or persistent fatigue causes you to limit your usual activities for longer than 2 weeks despite home treatment.

- If you experience sudden, unexplained weight loss or gain.

- If you do not feel more energetic after 4 weeks of home treatment.

- If fatigue gets worse despite home treatment.

Chronic Fatigue Syndrome

Chronic fatigue syndrome (CFS) is a flulike illness that causes severe fatigue lasting longer than 6 months. The fatigue does not improve with rest. Other symptoms may include memory problems, headaches, sore throat, painful lymph glands, muscle and joint pain, and sleep problems.

CFS is difficult to diagnose. There are no definitive lab tests. Many other illnesses, such as depression, thyroid disorders, or mononucleosis, cause similar symptoms. A CFS diagnosis is made only after fatigue and other symptoms continue for at least 6 months and other possible causes have been ruled out.

 Treatment is focused on adequate rest, balanced diet, and gentle exercise. No medications are known to cure <u>chronic fatigue syndrome</u>, but many people may improve on their own over time. Treatment of the individual symptoms can be effective. For treatment of depression, which is common in people with CFS, see page 309.

Call your doctor if unexplained fatigue is severe, persistent, and interferes with your activities for more than 2 weeks despite home treatment and rest.

Life is made up of sobs, sniffles, and smiles,
with sniffles predominating.
O. Henry

7

Chest and Respiratory Problems

Chest and respiratory problems can be as simple as a minor cold or as life-threatening as a heart attack. For most respiratory problems, including allergies, colds, sore throats, sinusitis, and tonsillitis, this chapter will help you decide what to do at home and when to call your doctor.

Start this chapter with a look at the chart on the next page. If you don't find what you're looking for, please check the index.

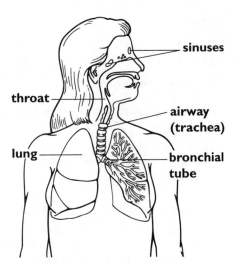

Respiratory problems can occur in the upper respiratory tract (nose, sinuses, throat, or trachea) or in the lower respiratory tract (bronchial tubes or lungs).

Allergies

Allergies come in many forms. The most common causes of allergies are particles in the air. Hay fever is the most common allergic disease. Allergy symptoms include itchy, watery eyes; sneezing; runny, stuffy, or itchy nose; and fatigue. The symptoms are a lot like cold symptoms, but they usually last longer. Dark circles under the eyes (allergic shiners) or postnasal drip may also accompany hay fever.

Chest, Respiratory, Nose, and Throat Problems

Symptoms	Possible Causes
Chest and Respiratory	
Wheezing or difficult (rapid, shallow, labored) breathing	Allergies, p. 141; Asthma, p. 146; Bronchitis, p. 149.
Cough, fever, yellow-green or rust-colored sputum, and difficulty breathing (possibly with chest-wall pain)	Bronchitis, p. 149; Pneumonia, p. 149.
Chest pain or discomfort with sweating or rapid pulse	Possible heart attack. Call for help. See p. 55. Chest Pain, p. 152.
Burning, pain, or discomfort behind or below the breastbone	Heartburn, p. 87; Chest Pain, p. 152.
Coughing	Coughs, p. 157.
Pounding or racing heartbeat; heart skipping or missing a beat	Heart Palpitations, p. 160.
Nose and Throat	
Stuffy or runny nose with watery eyes, sneezing	Allergies, p. 141; Colds, p. 155.
Cold symptoms with fever, headache, severe body aches, fatigue	Influenza, p. 161.
Thick green, yellow, or gray nasal discharge with fever and facial pain	Sinusitis, p. 164.
Foul odor from nose; swollen, inflamed nasal tissue	Objects in the Nose, p. 64; Sinusitis, p. 164.
Sore throat	Sore Throat, p. 165; Tonsillitis, p. 165.
Sore throat with white spots on tonsils, swollen glands, fever of 101° or higher	Strep Throat, p. 165.
Swollen tonsils, sore throat, fever	Tonsillitis, p. 165.
Swollen lymph nodes in the neck	Swollen Lymph Nodes, p. 169; Tonsillitis, p. 165.
Hoarseness, loss of voice	Laryngitis, p. 163.

You can often discover the cause of an allergy by noting when symptoms occur. Symptoms that occur at the same time each year (especially during spring, early summer, or early fall) are often caused by tree, grass, or weed pollen. Allergies that persist all year long may be due to dust, mites in household dust, cockroaches, mold spores, or animal dander. An animal allergy is often easy to detect: symptoms clear up when you stay away from the animal or its bedding.

Allergies seem to run in families. Parents with hay fever often have children with allergies. Hay fever may develop in children but is more common in teens and adults.

Life-Threatening Allergic Reactions

A few people have severe allergies to insect stings or to certain foods or drugs, especially antibiotics such as penicillin. For these people, the allergic reaction is sudden and severe and may cause breathing difficulty and a drop in blood pressure (anaphylactic shock).

An anaphylactic reaction is a medical emergency, and prompt care is needed. If you have ever had a severe allergic reaction, your doctor may suggest that you carry an epinephrine syringe (such as EpiPen or Ana-Kit) designed for giving yourself a shot that will decrease the severity of the reaction. If you have

What About Allergy Shots?

Allergy shots (immunotherapy) are a series of shots given to desensitize your body to substances that trigger allergic reactions (allergens). You may need to receive shots for 3 to 5 years before you stop having allergic reactions.

Immunotherapy is effective only if skin sensitivity testing has identified the specific allergy trigger. It is very effective against allergies to bee stings and other insect venom. For most people, immunotherapy is effective against grass, tree, and weed pollens, as well as house dust and house dust mites.

 Because of the time and expense involved, you need a realistic idea of the benefits before you agree to immunotherapy. Discuss these with your doctor. Allergy shots may be worthwhile for you if:

• You cannot avoid allergy triggers, or avoiding them has not helped.

• Your symptoms have bothered you a lot for at least 2 years.

• Home treatment has not been successful.

• Neither prescription nor nonprescription medications bring you relief.

• Immunotherapy has been shown to be effective for the allergens identified by your skin tests.

had an allergic reaction to a drug, wear a medical identification bracelet that will tell health professionals about your allergy in case you cannot.

Prevention

- If practical, avoid the substance that causes allergy attacks. See page 144 for more information about food allergies.

- Allergy shots (immunotherapy) may help control symptoms of allergies and asthma or may reduce the risk of having an anaphylactic reaction. See page 143.

Home Treatment

If you can discover the source of your allergies, avoiding that substance may be the best treatment. Keep a record of your symptoms and the plants, animals, foods, or chemicals that seem to trigger them.

General information about avoiding irritants:

- Avoid yardwork (raking, mowing), which stirs up both pollen and mold. If you must do yard work, wear a mask and take an antihistamine beforehand.

- Don't smoke, and avoid inhaling other people's smoke.

- Eliminate aerosol sprays, perfumes, room deodorizers, cleaning products, and other substances that may trigger allergy symptoms.

Food Allergies

Less than 1 percent of adults have true food allergies. Most adverse reactions to foods are due to food intolerances, reactions to food additives, or food poisoning. Most true food allergies are to nuts, shellfish, eggs, chocolate, wheat, and milk. An allergic reaction to a food can result in anaphylactic shock. See When to Call a Health Professional on page 145.

By gradually introducing simple solid foods into your child's diet, you will be able to identify possible food allergies. Children often outgrow food allergies by age 6. If your child was allergic to a food when younger, you may be able to reintroduce it as he or she gets older. If the reaction was severe, talk to a health professional before trying to reintroduce the food.

If your symptoms are seasonal and seem to be related to pollen:

- Keep your house and car windows closed. Keep bedroom windows closed at night.

- Limit the time you spend outside when pollen counts are high. Dogs and other pets may bring large amounts of pollen into your house.

If your symptoms are year-round and seem to be related to dust:

- Keep your bedroom and other places where you spend a lot of time as dust-free as possible.

- Avoid carpeting, upholstered furniture, and heavy draperies that collect dust. Vacuuming doesn't pick up house dust mites.

- Cover your mattress and box spring with dustproof cases and wipe them clean weekly. Avoid wool or down blankets and feather pillows. Wash all bedding in hot water once a week.

- Consider using an air conditioner or air purifier with a special HEPA filter. Rent one before buying to see if it helps.

If your symptoms are year-round and are worse during damp weather, they may be related to mold or mildew:

- Keep your home well ventilated and dry. Keep the humidity below 50 percent. Use a dehumidifier during humid weather.

- Use an air conditioner, which removes mold spores from the air. Change or clean heating and cooling system filters regularly.

- Clean bathroom and kitchen surfaces often with bleach to reduce mold growth.

If you are allergic to a pet:

- Keep the animal outside, or at least out of your bedroom.

- If your symptoms are severe, the best solution may be to find a new home for the pet.

Antihistamines and decongestants may relieve some allergy symptoms. Use caution when taking these drugs. See pages 344 and 345.

For more information about allergies, including immunotherapy, call LungLine, a service of the National Jewish Medical and Research Center at 1-800-222-LUNG (5864).

When to Call a Health Professional

Call 911 or other emergency services immediately if you develop signs of a severe allergic reaction (anaphylaxis). The following severe symptoms may occur soon after you take a drug, eat a certain food, or are stung by an insect:

- Lightheadedness (feeling like you might pass out) or confusion.

- Swelling around the lips, tongue, or face that is interfering with breathing or is getting worse.

- Wheezing or difficulty breathing.

Call a health professional:

- If your lips, tongue, or face are swollen, even if you are not having difficulty breathing and the swelling is not getting worse.

- If there is significant swelling around the site of an insect sting (e.g., the entire arm or leg is swollen).

- If you develop a skin rash, itching, feeling of warmth, or hives.

Call your doctor if allergy symptoms worsen over time and home treatment doesn't help. Your doctor may recommend stronger medication or allergy shots (immunotherapy). See page 143.

Asthma

Asthma is a condition that causes long-term inflammation of the airways. The inflammation makes the airways overreact to certain particles in the air. During an asthma episode, the muscles surrounding the tubes that carry air into the lungs (bronchial tubes) go into spasm; the mucous lining of the lungs swells; and secretions build up in the lungs, suddenly making breathing difficult.

A person who is having an asthma episode (attack) may make a wheezing or whistling sound while breathing. The person usually coughs a great deal and may spit up mucus. Sometimes a chronic, dry cough, especially at night or early in the morning, is the only symptom of mild asthma.

Many things can trigger asthma, including allergens such as dust mites, dust, pollen, cockroaches, and animal dander. In general, viral respiratory infections, such as colds, are the most common triggers of asthma. Other triggers include exercise, cold air, cigarette or wood smoke, chemical vapors, pain relievers (especially aspirin), food preservatives and dyes, and emotional stress.

Asthma usually develops during childhood but may also begin later in life. The first episode often follows a cold or the flu. Asthma is more common in children who are exposed to cigarette smoke in the home. Many children outgrow asthma symptoms as they get older, but the symptoms may return later in life.

 Most children and adults can control their asthma by avoiding triggers that cause attacks and using medications to manage symptoms. Severe attacks can usually be treated with inhaled or injected medications. Asthma attacks are rarely fatal if they are treated promptly and appropriately.

Prevention

There is no way to prevent asthma. However, you may be able to limit the length and severity of asthma episodes if you can avoid or control your exposure to things that trigger asthma symptoms.

- Review home treatment for allergies on page 144.

- Control cockroaches. Do not leave food or garbage in open containers. Use poison bait and traps to kill cockroaches. Avoid chemical sprays, which can trigger an asthma attack.

- Avoid smoke of all kinds. If you smoke cigarettes, stop. See page 26 for tips on quitting. Avoid places where other people may be smoking, and make sure your home is a smoke-free environment. Don't use wood-burning stoves.

- Avoid irritants in the air. Stay indoors when the air pollution or pollen count is high. Try to avoid strong odors, fumes, and perfume.

- Avoid breathing cold air. In cold weather, breathe through your nose, and cover your nose and mouth with a scarf or a cold weather mask.

- Aspirin, ibuprofen, and similar pain medications can cause severe asthma attacks in some people. Discuss the use of these medications with your doctor, and use them with caution. If these medications bother you, don't use them. Try acetaminophen instead.

- Do not use nonprescription cold and cough medications unless your doctor tells you to do so.

- Stress may be a factor in triggering asthma attacks. Practice the relaxation exercises on page 323.

- Reduce your risk of colds and flu by washing your hands often and getting a flu shot each year.

- If you use a humidifier, clean it thoroughly once a week.

- Build up the strength of your lungs and airways:

  - Get regular exercise. Swimming or water aerobics may be good choices because you are less likely to have an asthma attack when you breathe moist air. If vigorous exercise triggers asthma attacks, talk with your doctor. Adjusting your medication and your exercise routine may help.

  - Practice roll breathing as described on page 323.

Asthma Action Plan

An asthma action plan is a written plan that tells you how to manage your asthma symptoms at home. It helps take the guesswork out of treating your asthma. The plan will outline the medication you will take for your asthma symptoms and when to take it, depending on the zone you are in (green, yellow, or red). In order to determine what zone you are in, you will have to know how to measure your ability to exhale using a peak flow meter. The plan may also tell you when to talk to your health professional about your asthma symptoms.

The asthma action plan zones include:

- Green zone plan: Routine care to keep asthma symptoms from starting.

- Yellow zone plan: How to stop asthma symptoms and keep an asthma episode (attack) from getting worse. This may involve taking other medications in addition to the ones you usually take to control your asthma.

- Red zone plan: What to do for a severe asthma episode. This is a medical emergency.

• Work with your doctor to develop an asthma action plan so you can manage your symptoms at home. Make sure family members and friends know about your plan so they can help you during an asthma episode. See page 147.

• When you aren't having symptoms, follow your plan to treat ongoing airway inflammation. Get regular checkups to make sure your asthma action plan is working well for you.

• Learn to use a peak flow meter to monitor your ability to exhale. Used regularly, this device will give you an idea of how your lungs normally function. It also helps you tell when an asthma attack may be coming so you can take steps to prevent or treat it.

Since triggers for asthma attacks are often not known, you need to monitor your symptoms so you can prevent or treat asthma attacks before they become severe. Using an asthma action plan developed by a doctor to guide your home treatment, you may be able to prevent emergency room visits or admissions to the hospital for asthma symptoms.

Home Treatment

Once an asthma attack begins, prompt home treatment can provide relief.

• Learn to use a metered-dose inhaler. Inhalers help get the right amount of medication to your airways. A device called a spacer is now recommended for use with an inhaler. Ask your doctor to watch you use your inhaler and spacer to make sure you are doing it right. With practice, most people can use an inhaler and spacer correctly.

• Drink extra fluids to thin the mucus in the bronchial tubes. Try to drink at least 2 quarts of water per day.

• Be confident that your home treatment will control the severity of the attack.

• Keep a diary outlining your asthma attack. After you've had an attack, write down what triggered it, what helped end it, and any concerns you have about your asthma action plan. Take your diary when you see your doctor for your regular checkups. Ask questions you may have about your plan or medication.

When to Call a Health Professional

Always follow your asthma action plan if you have one. **Call 911 or other emergency services** if you are having severe asthma symptoms and:

• You are having severe difficulty breathing.

• Your medications have not helped after 20 minutes.

Call a health professional:

• If you have symptoms that may indicate heart problems, such as chest pain or shortness of breath. See page 152.

- If you are having a severe asthma attack (peak flow is less than 50 percent of your best), even if your medications have relieved some symptoms.

- If your asthma symptoms don't get better after you follow your asthma action plan.

- If you are coughing up yellow, dark brown, or bloody mucus.

- If acute asthma symptoms (wheezing, coughing, difficulty breathing) have happened for the first time.

- To discuss exactly what to do when an attack begins. Once you understand and have confidence in your asthma medication, you can often handle mild attacks without professional help.

- If you begin to use your asthma medication more often than usual. This may be a sign that your asthma is getting worse.

- If you or the people who live with you have not been educated about immediate treatment for asthma attacks.

- If the medication required to treat an asthma attack is not available.

- To talk about adjusting your medication. Your doctor needs your feedback to figure out the best medicine and the right dosage for you.

- To assess allergies, which may worsen asthma attacks.

- To get a referral to a support group. Talking with others who have asthma can give you information and boost your confidence in dealing with prevention and treatment.

Bronchitis and Pneumonia

Bronchitis is an inflammation and irritation of the airways that lead to the lungs. Viruses are the usual cause of bronchitis, but it can also be caused by bacteria or by exposure to cigarette smoke or air pollution. The inflammation caused by acute bronchitis is not permanent. It goes away when the infection or irritation goes away.

Symptoms of bronchitis usually begin 3 to 4 days after an upper respiratory infection, such as a cold, goes away. Symptoms often include a dry cough that may become productive (produce sputum), mild fever, fatigue, discomfort or tightness in the chest, and wheezing.

 MORE INFO Frequent lung infections, especially in a person who smokes, may lead to the development of chronic bronchitis. Tobacco smokers are also at high risk for developing emphysema. Chronic bronchitis, emphysema, and other lung conditions, such as asthma, are known as chronic obstructive pulmonary disease (COPD).

Tuberculosis (TB)

Tuberculosis is a contagious disease caused by organisms that usually infect the lungs (pulmonary TB). When a person who has pulmonary TB coughs, sneezes, or laughs, TB-causing organisms are released into the air where other people can inhale them. This is how TB is spread. Children and people with weak immune systems are particularly prone to TB.

Most people who are exposed to TB never develop symptoms because their immune systems are able to stop the disease. People who develop symptoms of TB, such as persistent cough, weight loss, fatigue, night sweats, and fever, need drug treatment to stop the disease from progressing and to reduce the risk of spreading TB to others. Treatment, which consists of several medications, may last from 6 months to 2 years.

People who have weak immune systems due to AIDS or other diseases, who abuse alcohol and drugs, or who have a chronic lung disease called silicosis are at high risk for developing progressive TB, which can damage the lungs or spread to other parts of the body.

To prevent TB infection, avoid close contact with people who have TB if possible. If you live with someone who has TB, ask your doctor what you can do to protect yourself from TB infection and whether you need to be tested for TB.

Pneumonia is an infection or inflammation that affects the bronchial tubes and lungs. Pneumonia is usually caused by bacteria, but viruses and other organisms can cause it as well. It may also develop as a complication of another viral illness, such as measles or chickenpox.

Pneumonia sometimes follows a viral respiratory infection, such as a cold or bronchitis. Having bronchitis and another lung disease, such as asthma, may increase your risk for pneumonia.

A person who has bacterial pneumonia is usually very sick. Symptoms may include:

- Productive cough with yellow, green, rust-colored, or bloody sputum (mucus coughed up from the lungs).
- Fever and shaking chills.
- Rapid, shallow breathing.
- Chest-wall pain that is often made worse by coughing or taking a deep breath.
- Rapid heartbeat.
- Fatigue that is worse than you would expect from a cold.

Prevention

- Get a pneumococcal vaccination if you are over 65, or if you are younger than 65 and have a chronic lung disease such as emphysema. (If you are younger than 65 and you have asthma, talk to your doctor about whether you should receive the pneumococcal vaccine). See page 19.

- Get a yearly flu shot. See page 161.

- Give proper home care to minor respiratory problems such as colds and flu. See pages 155 and 161.

- Stop smoking. People who smoke or are around smokers have more frequent bouts of bronchitis.

- Avoid polluted air and don't exercise outdoors when the ozone concentration is high.

- Keep up your resistance to infection by eating a healthy diet, getting plenty of rest, and exercising regularly.

Home Treatment

Here is what you can do at home to prevent complications from bronchitis or pneumonia and feel better.

- Take the entire course of all prescribed medications. Although most cases of bronchitis can be managed with home treatment, severe or persistent symptoms may require prescription medication. Treatment for pneumonia almost always involves antibiotics.

- Drink 8 to 12 glasses of water per day. Extra fluids help thin the mucus in the lungs so it can be coughed out.

- Get some extra rest. Let your energy go to healing.

- Take aspirin, ibuprofen, or acetaminophen to reduce fever and relieve body aches. Do not give aspirin to anyone younger than 20.

- Use a nonprescription cough suppressant that contains dextromethorphan to help quiet a dry, hacking cough so you can sleep. Avoid cough preparations that contain more than one active ingredient. See Cough Preparations on page 345.

- Breathe moist air from a humidifier, hot shower, or a sink filled with hot water. The heat and moisture will thin mucus so it can be coughed out.

- If you have classic flu symptoms, try home treatment and reassess your symptoms in 48 hours. See Influenza (Flu) on page 161.

When to Call a Health Professional

Call if you develop any of the following symptoms. They may mean that your lung infection is getting worse or that you are developing a bacterial lung infection.

- A cough that:
  - Occurs with wheezing or difficulty breathing that is new or different.
  - Brings up bloody sputum.
  - Frequently produces yellow, green, or rust-colored sputum from the lungs (not postnasal drainage), lasts longer than 2 days, and occurs along with a fever of 101° or higher.

- Lingers more than 7 to 10 days after other symptoms have cleared, especially if it is productive (brings up sputum). A dry, hacking cough may last several weeks after a viral illness such as a cold.

• A fever of 105° or higher that does not go down after 30 to 60 minutes of home treatment.

• A fever of 104° or higher that does not go down after 2 hours of home treatment.

• A fever higher than 101° with shaking chills and a productive cough.

• A fever that persists despite home treatment. Many viral illnesses cause fevers of 102° or higher for short periods of time (up to 12 to 24 hours). Call a doctor if the fever stays high:

- 102° or higher for 2 full days

- 101° or higher for 3 full days

- 100.4° or higher for 4 full days

• Labored, shallow, or rapid breathing with shortness of breath.

• Significant chest-wall pain (pain in the muscles of the chest) when you cough or breathe.

• Fatigue that is worse than what you would expect from a cold.

Also call:

• If you are unable to drink enough fluids to avoid becoming dehydrated or if you are unable to eat.

• If the sick person is an infant, an older adult, or someone who is chronically ill, especially with lung problems.

• If any cough lasts longer than 2 weeks.

Chest Pain

Call 911 or other emergency services immediately if you think you may be having a heart attack. See "Am I Having a Heart Attack?" on page 153.

Call your doctor if you have continuous chest discomfort or pain and there is no obvious cause.

If the person who is having heart attack symptoms loses consciousness, follow the Rescue Breathing and CPR guidelines on page 40.

Angina is pain, pressure, heaviness, or numbness behind the breastbone or across the chest. It occurs when there is not enough oxygen reaching the heart muscle. It is a symptom of coronary artery disease. The pain caused by angina may radiate to the upper back, neck, jaws, shoulders, or arms. Angina may be brought on by stress or exertion and is relieved by rest and use of prescribed medication.

A **heart attack** (myocardial infarction) is caused by blocked blood flow to the heart muscle. The pain of a heart attack is usually more severe than angina, lasts longer, and does not go away with rest or by taking medication that was previously effective for angina. Other symptoms that may be present include sweating, nausea, shortness of breath, weakness, or indigestion.

Am I Having a Heart Attack?

You may be having a heart attack if you have chest discomfort or pain that:

❑ Lasts longer than 20 minutes and is not relieved by rest or nitroglycerin.

❑ Feels like pressure, tightness, squeezing, crushing, intense burning, or aching in your chest.

In addition to chest pain, you may also have:

❑ Pain spreading to your back, shoulder, neck, jaw or teeth, arm, or wrist.

❑ Sweating.

❑ Shortness of breath.

❑ Dizziness.

❑ Fainting.

❑ Nausea or vomiting.

❑ Unusual weakness.

❑ Fast and irregular heartbeat.

❑ Sense of doom.

The more boxes you check, the more likely it is that you are having a heart attack. There may be other explanations for chest pain, but you need to **call 911 or other emergency services immediately** if you think you could be having a heart attack.

Factors that may increase your risk of a heart attack include:

• Smoking.

• Family history of heart disease.

• Diabetes.

• High blood pressure.

• High cholesterol.

• Inactive lifestyle.

• High stress levels.

Chest pain is a key warning sign of a heart attack, but it may also be caused by other problems.

If chest pain increases when you press your finger on the painful site, or if you can pinpoint the spot that hurts, it is probably chest-wall pain, which may be caused by strained muscles or ligaments or by a fractured rib. An inflammation of the cartilage in the chest wall (called costochondritis) can also cause chest-wall pain. Chest-wall pain usually lasts only a few days. Aspirin or ibuprofen may help. Do not give aspirin to anyone younger than 20.

A shooting pain that lasts a few seconds, or a quick pain at the end of a deep breath, is usually not a cause for concern. Hyperventilation (see page 57) can also cause chest pain.

Chest pain caused by pleurisy (inflammation of the membrane that surrounds the lungs) or pneumonia (see page 149) will get worse when you take a deep breath or cough. An ulcer (see page 100) can cause chest pain, usually below the breastbone, that is worse when your stomach is empty. Gallstones (see page 92) may cause pain in the right side of the chest or around the shoulder blade. The pain may worsen after a meal or in the middle of the night. Heartburn (see page 87) can also cause chest pain. Shingles (page 205) may cause a sharp, burning, or tingling pain that feels like a tight band around one side of the chest.

Home Treatment

For chest-wall pain caused by strained muscles or ligaments or a fractured rib:

• Use pain relievers such as aspirin, ibuprofen, or acetaminophen. Do not give aspirin to anyone younger than 20.

• Use an ice pack to help relieve pain the first few days after an injury.

• After applying ice during the first 72 hours (or until the swelling has gone down), apply heat (a hot water bottle, warm towel, or heating pad) to help relieve pain. Use heat that is no warmer than bath water or the low setting on a heating pad. To prevent burns, do not go to sleep with a heating pad turned on.

• Use products such as Ben-Gay or Icy-Hot to help soothe sore muscles.

• Avoid any activity that strains the chest area. As your pain gets better, slowly return to your normal activities.

When to Call a Health Professional

Call 911 or other emergency services immediately if symptoms of a heart attack are present (see page 152).

If a doctor has diagnosed the cause of your chest pain and prescribed a home treatment plan, follow it. **Call 911 or other emergency services** if the pain worsens and may be caused by a heart problem, or if you develop any of the heart attack symptoms listed on page 152.

Call a health professional:

• If you suspect that you have angina and your symptoms have not been diagnosed.

• If symptoms of angina do not respond to your prescribed treatment, or if the pattern of your angina changes.

• If minor chest pain occurs without the symptoms of a heart attack and any of the following apply:

  - You have a history of heart disease or blood clots in the lungs.

  - Chest pain is constant, nagging, and not relieved by rest.

  - Chest pain occurs with symptoms of pneumonia. See page 149.

  - Mild chest pain lasts longer than 2 days without improvement.

Colds

The common cold is brought to you by any one of 200 viruses. The symptoms of a cold include runny nose, red eyes, sneezing, sore throat, dry cough, headache, and general body aches. There is a gradual 1- or 2-day onset. As a cold progresses, the nasal mucus may thicken. This is the stage just before a cold completes its course. A cold usually lasts a week or two.

Colds occur throughout the year but are most common in late winter and early spring. The average child has six colds a year; adults have fewer.

Using a mouthwash will not prevent a cold, and antibiotics will not cure a cold. There is no cure for the common cold. If you catch a cold, treat the symptoms.

Sometimes a cold will lead to a bacterial infection (see page 156) such as bronchitis or pneumonia. Good home treatment of colds can help prevent complications.

If a person seems to have a cold all the time, or if cold symptoms last 2 weeks or longer, suspect allergies (see page 141) or sinusitis (see page 164).

Prevention

- Eat well and get plenty of sleep and exercise to keep up your resistance.

- Try to avoid people who have colds.

- Keep your hands away from your nose, eyes, and mouth, but cover your mouth when you cough or sneeze.

- Wash your hands often, particularly when you are around people who have colds.

- Humidify your bedrooms or your whole house if possible.

- Don't smoke.

Home Treatment

Home treatment for a cold will help relieve symptoms and prevent complications.

- Get extra rest. Slow down just a little from your usual routine. It isn't necessary to stay home in bed, but take care not to expose others to your cold.

- Drink plenty of liquids. Hot water, herbal tea, or chicken soup will help relieve congestion.

- Take aspirin, ibuprofen, or acetaminophen to relieve aches. Do not give aspirin to anyone younger than 20 because of the risk of Reye syndrome (see page 221).

- Humidify your bedroom and take hot showers to relieve nasal stuffiness.

- Check the back of your throat for postnasal drip. If you see streaks of mucus, gargle with warm water to prevent a sore throat.

Viral or Bacterial?

Viral infections

- Usually produce symptoms in several parts of the body at once: sore throat, runny nose, headache, muscle aches. In the digestive system, viruses cause nausea, vomiting, or diarrhea.

- Typically include colds, flu, bronchitis, and stomach flu.

- Cannot be cured by antibiotics.

Bacterial infections

- Sometimes follow viral infections.

- Usually affect one area of the body: sinuses, lungs, an ear.

- May be cured by antibiotics.

Call a health professional if you develop any of the following symptoms of a bacterial infection:

- Fever of 104° or higher that does not go down after 2 hours of home treatment.

- Fever higher than 101° with shaking chills and productive cough (brings up sputum).

- Fever that persists despite home treatment. Many viral illnesses cause fevers of 102° or higher for short periods of time (up to 12 to 24 hours). Call a doctor if the fever stays high:

  - 102° or higher for 2 full days
  - 101° or higher for 3 full days
  - 100.4° or higher for 4 full days

- Labored, shallow, rapid breathing with shortness of breath.

- Sputum is yellow, green, rust-colored, or bloody, and other symptoms (fever, productive cough, fatigue) are worse. Sputum that is coughed up from the lungs is more significant than mucus that has drained down the back of the throat (postnasal drip).

- Nasal discharge changes from clear to colored (yellow or green) after 5 to 7 days of a cold, and other symptoms (sinus pain, fever) are worse. If nasal discharge is colored from the start of a cold, call if it lasts longer than 7 to 10 days.

- Cough that lingers more than 7 to 10 days after other symptoms have cleared, especially if it is productive (brings up sputum). A dry, hacking cough may last several weeks after a viral illness such as a cold.

- Use disposable tissues, not handkerchiefs, to reduce the chance of spreading the cold virus to others.

- If your nose is red and raw from rubbing it with tissues, put a dab of petroleum jelly on the sore area.

- Avoid cold remedies that contain a combination of drugs to treat many different symptoms. Treat each symptom separately. Take a decongestant for stuffiness, a cough medicine for a cough. See Home Treatment for coughs on page 157.

- Do not use nasal decongestant sprays for more than 3 days in a row. Continued use may lead to a "rebound" effect, causing the mucous membranes to become more swollen than they were before you used the spray. See page 344 to learn how to make nose drops at home.

- Avoid antihistamines. They are not an effective treatment for colds.

- If you have classic flu symptoms, try home treatment and reassess your symptoms in 48 hours. See Influenza (Flu) on page 161.

When to Call a Health Professional

- If you develop signs of a bacterial infection (see "Viral or Bacterial?" on page 156).

- If you develop facial pain, fever, and other signs of sinusitis (see page 164).

Coughs

Coughing is the body's way of removing foreign material or mucus from the lungs. Coughs have distinctive traits that you can learn to recognize.

Productive coughs produce phlegm or mucus (sputum) that comes up from the lungs. This kind of cough generally should not be suppressed. It is needed to clear mucus from the lungs.

Nonproductive coughs are dry coughs that do not produce sputum. A dry, hacking cough may develop toward the end of a cold or after exposure to an irritant, such as dust or smoke. Dry coughs that follow viral illnesses may last up to several weeks and often get worse at night.

A chronic, dry cough, especially at night or early in the morning, may be the only sign of mild asthma. See page 146.

Long-term (chronic) coughs are often caused by the backflow (reflux) of stomach acid into the lungs and throat. If you suspect that problems with stomach acid reflux may be causing your cough, see Heartburn on page 87.

Prevention

- Don't smoke. See page 26 for tips on quitting. Avoid other people's smoke. A dry, hacking "smoker's cough" means your lungs are constantly irritated.

- Drink 8 to 10 glasses of water every day. You are drinking enough if you are urinating more often than usual.

Home Treatment

- Drink lots of water. Water helps loosen phlegm and soothe an irritated throat. Also try drinking hot tea or hot water with honey or lemon juice in it. Do not give honey to children younger than 1 year of age.

Description and Treatment of Coughs

Type of Cough	Possible Causes
Loud cough like a seal's bark	Croup, p. 223.
Dry cough in the morning that gets better as the day goes on	Dry air; cigarette smoking. Increase fluids. Humidify the bedroom. Stop smoking. Also see Coughs, p. 157.
Hacking, dry, nonproductive cough; may be worse at night	Common for several weeks following a viral illness. May be due to postnasal drip, smoking, or mild asthma. Increase fluids. Try a decongestant. Stop smoking. Also see Coughs, p. 157; Asthma, p. 146.
Productive cough following a cold or flu	Bronchitis, p. 149; Pneumonia, p. 149; Sinusitis, p. 164.
Dry, sudden-onset cough after a choking episode, most often in an infant or toddler	Foreign object in the throat. See "Preventing Choking," p. 40.

- Cough drops can soothe an irritated throat. Expensive, medicine-flavored cough drops are not any better than inexpensive, candy-flavored ones or hard candy.

- Elevate your head with extra pillows at night to ease a dry cough.

- Use cough suppressants wisely. Avoid cold remedies that combine drugs to treat many symptoms. It is generally better to treat each symptom separately. See Cough Preparations on page 345.

- Coughing is useful because it brings up mucus from the lungs and helps prevent bacterial infections. People with asthma and other lung diseases need to cough. If you have a dry, hacking cough that does not bring anything up, ask your health professional about an effective cough suppressant medication.

- Do not take anyone else's prescription cough medication.

- Avoid exposure to dust, smoke, and other irritants, or wear an appropriate mask to protect yourself from the irritant.

- If you have classic flu symptoms, try home treatment and reassess your symptoms in 48 hours. See Influenza (Flu) on page 161.

When to Call a Health Professional

- If you develop signs of a bacterial infection (see "Viral or Bacterial?" on page 156).

- If a cough lingers more than 7 to 10 days after other symptoms have cleared, especially if the cough is productive (brings up sputum). A dry, hacking cough may last several weeks after a viral illness such as a cold.

- If any cough lasts longer than 2 weeks.

Fever

A fever is a high body temperature. It is a symptom, not a disease. A fever is one way your body fights illness. A temperature of up to 102° can be helpful because it helps the body respond to infection. Most healthy adults can tolerate a fever as high as 103° to 104° for short periods of time without problems.

For specific fever guidelines for children younger than 4 years of age, see page 228.

Home Treatment

- Drink 8 to 12 glasses of water a day. You are drinking enough if you are urinating more often than usual.

- Take acetaminophen, aspirin, or ibuprofen to lower fever. Do not give aspirin to anyone younger than 20 because of the risk of Reye syndrome (see page 221).

- Take and record your temperature every 2 hours and whenever symptoms change.

- Take a sponge bath with lukewarm water if a fever causes discomfort.

- Watch for signs of dehydration. See page 84.

- Dress lightly.

- Eat light, easily digested foods, such as soup.

- If you have classic flu symptoms, try home treatment and reassess your symptoms in 48 hours. See Influenza (Flu) on page 161.

When to Call a Health Professional

- If a fever higher than 104° to 105° does not come down after 2 hours of home treatment.

- If a fever higher than 103° to 104° does not come down after 12 hours of home treatment.

- If you have a persistent fever. Many viral illnesses cause fevers of 102° or higher for short periods of time (up to 12 to 24 hours). Call a doctor if the fever stays high:

  - 102° or higher for 2 full days

  - 101° or higher for 3 full days

  - 100.4° or higher for 4 full days

- If body temperature rises to 103° or higher, all sweating stops, and the skin becomes hot, dry, and flushed (possible heat stroke, see page 56).

- If a fever occurs with other signs of a bacterial infection (see page 156).

- If fever occurs with any of the following symptoms:

  - Very stiff neck and headache (see "Encephalitis and Meningitis" on page 162).

  - Shortness of breath and cough (see Bronchitis and Pneumonia on page 149).

  - Pain above the eyes or the cheekbones (see Sinusitis on page 164).

  - Pain or burning when urinating (see Urinary Tract Infections on page 103).

  - Abdominal pain, nausea, and vomiting (see Stomach Flu and Food Poisoning on page 98, or Appendicitis on page 81).

- If a fever is accompanied by disturbing symptoms, such as confusion, decreased alertness, or unusual behavior.

- If you develop a fever after you start taking a new medication.

Heart Palpitations

Heart palpitations are an uncomfortable sensation that your heart is beating rapidly or irregularly. Heart palpitations can feel like:

- A pounding or fluttering feeling in your chest.

- A feeling that your heart is doing a "flip-flop," or that it is skipping or missing a beat.

- Your heart is racing, or there is an extra heartbeat.

- Your heart is beating in your neck.

Although palpitations may be caused by a heart problem, they often occur because of stress, fatigue, or overuse of alcohol or stimulants (caffeine, nicotine). People who experience severe anxiety may have heart palpitations. See Anxiety on page 308. Many medications, including diet pills, antihistamines, decongestants, and some herbal products, can cause heart palpitations.

 Nearly everyone has heart palpitations from time to time. There is usually no cause for concern. However, if you have heartbeat changes that are new and different or that occur with chest pain, shortness of breath, or lightheadedness, or if you have risk factors for heart disease (smoking, high blood pressure, high cholesterol, inactive lifestyle, or high stress levels), see your doctor to have your condition evaluated.

Prevention

- Stop smoking.

- Avoid caffeine and alcohol or limit your intake.

- If you take prescription or non-prescription medications regularly, ask your pharmacist if the drugs you take can cause heart palpitations.

- If anxiety or stress may be causing heart palpitations, see Anxiety on page 308 and try the relaxation exercises on page 323.

- Make physical activity a daily habit. (If you frequently have heart palpitations, talk to your doctor before starting an exercise program.)

- See your doctor for regular check-ups if you have risk factors for heart attack (see page 153). Early detection and management of heart problems is the best way to prevent serious illness.

Home Treatment

- Take deep breaths and try to relax. This may slow a racing heart.

- If you start to feel lightheaded (like you might pass out), lie down to avoid injuries that might result if you pass out and fall down.

- Keep a record of the date and time; your activities when the irregular heartbeat happened; how long the irregular beats lasted; how many "skipped" beats there were; and any other symptoms.

- Follow the prevention guidelines.

When to Call a Health Professional

Call 911 or other emergency services immediately if symptoms of a heart attack are present (see page 152).

Call a health professional:

- If heart palpitations occur with any of the following symptoms:

  - Weakness or fatigue.

  - Lightheadedness (feeling like you might pass out).

  - Confusion.

  - Feeling as if something bad is going to happen.

  - Feeling like your heart beats irregularly all the time.

- If heart palpitations are new or different than before and are not relieved by home treatment.

Influenza (Flu)

Influenza, or flu, is a viral illness that commonly occurs in the winter and affects many people at once. Flu is not the same as the common cold—the symptoms of flu are usually more severe and come on quite suddenly. Symptoms include fever (100° to 104°), shaking chills, body aches, muscle pain, headache, pain when you move your eyes, fatigue, weakness, and runny nose. Symptoms may last up to 10 days. Most other viral illnesses have milder symptoms that don't last as long.

Although a person with the flu feels very sick, the illness seldom leads to more serious complications. However, flu can be dangerous for babies, older adults, and people with some chronic conditions.

Antiviral medications are recommended for people at high risk for complications from the flu. These drugs can reduce the severity and duration of some types of influenza if they are taken before or soon after symptoms develop. People at low risk for complications may choose to take medication for the flu so that they feel better faster. These medications work best if taken no more than 48 hours after symptoms first appear.

Prevention

- Get a flu shot each autumn if you are over 50; if you have a chronic illness, such as asthma, heart disease, or diabetes; or if you live in a nursing home.

- Consider annual flu shots if you or your family members are likely to be exposed to the disease through work or by being around other children, or if you just want to reduce the chance that you and your family will catch the disease. The vaccine can be given to anyone over 6 months of age.

- Keep up your resistance to infection by eating a healthy diet, getting plenty of rest, and exercising regularly.

- Avoid exposure to the flu virus. Wash your hands often and keep your hands away from your nose, eyes, and mouth.

- Stop smoking.

Encephalitis and Meningitis

Encephalitis is an inflammation of the brain that may occur after a viral infection, such as chickenpox, flu, measles, mumps, mononucleosis, cold sores, or genital herpes. Mosquitoes and ticks spread encephalitis in some parts of the world, including the U.S.

Meningitis is a viral or bacterial illness that causes inflammation in the tissues that surround the brain and spinal cord. It may follow an infection, such as an ear or sinus infection, or a viral illness.

Encephalitis and meningitis are serious illnesses that have similar symptoms. Call a health professional immediately if the following symptoms develop, especially after a viral illness or after you are bitten by mosquitoes:

- Severe headache with stiff neck, fever, nausea, and vomiting

- Drowsiness, lack of energy, confusion, memory problems, or unusual behavior

Home Treatment

- Get plenty of rest.

- Drink extra fluids to replace fluids lost from fever, to ease a scratchy throat, and to keep nasal mucus thin. Hot tea with lemon, plain water, fruit juice, and soup are all good choices.

• Take acetaminophen, aspirin, or ibuprofen to relieve fever, headache, and muscle aches. Do not give aspirin to anyone younger than 20 because of the risk of Reye syndrome (see page 221).

When to Call a Health Professional

It is common for adults with influenza to have high fevers (up to 104°) for 3 to 4 days. When trying to decide if you need to see a health professional, consider the likelihood that you have the flu versus a possible bacterial infection. If it is the flu season and many people in your community have similar symptoms, it is likely that you have the flu. Call a health professional:

• If you want to take antiviral medication to reduce the severity of the flu. Medication is recommended for babies, older adults, and people with chronic health problems.

• If you develop signs of a bacterial infection (see page 156).

• If you seem to get better, then get worse again.

Laryngitis

Laryngitis is an infection or irritation of the voice box (larynx). The most common cause is a viral infection such as a cold. Other causes include allergies; excessive talking, singing, or yelling; cigarette smoke; and the backflow (reflux) of stomach acid into the throat. Heavy drinking or smoking can lead to chronic laryngitis.

Symptoms include hoarseness or loss of voice, the urge to clear your throat, fever, tiredness, throat pain, and cough.

Prevention

To prevent hoarseness, lower your voice as soon as you feel minor pain. Give your vocal cords a rest.

Home Treatment

• Your voice box will usually heal in 5 to 10 days. Medication does little to speed recovery.

• If hoarseness is caused by a cold, treat the cold (see page 155). Hoarseness may last up to 1 week after a cold goes away.

• Rest your voice. Talk as little as possible. Don't shout or whisper, and avoid clearing your throat.

• Stop smoking and avoid other people's smoke. See page 26 for tips on quitting.

• Humidify your bedrooms or your whole house if possible.

• Drink 8 to 12 glasses of water a day. You are drinking enough if you are urinating more often than usual.

• To soothe the throat, gargle with warm salt water (1 teaspoon of salt in 8 ounces of water), or drink weak tea or hot water with honey or lemon juice in it. Do not give honey to children younger than 1 year of age.

• If you suspect that problems with stomach acid reflux may be contributing to your laryngitis, see Heartburn on page 87.

When to Call a Health Professional

• If you develop signs of a bacterial infection (see page 156).

• If hoarseness persists for 3 to 4 weeks.

Sinusitis

Sinusitis is an inflammation or infection of the mucous membranes lining the sinuses and nasal passages. The sinuses are hollow spaces in the head. Sinusitis causes the sinuses to become blocked, leading to pain and pressure in the face.

Sinusitis most often follows a cold and may also be associated with allergies, an infected tooth (dental abscess), air pollution, and other factors. Sinusitis can occur in infants and children as well as adults.

The key symptom of sinusitis is pain over the cheekbones and upper teeth, in the forehead over the eyebrows, or around and behind the eyes. There may also be headache, swelling around the eyes, fever, stuffy nose, coughing, or mucus draining down the back of the throat (postnasal drip). In children, coughing and nasal discharge that last more than 7 to 10 days along with complaints of headache and facial pain are signs that the problem may be sinusitis, not just a cold.

If your symptoms are severe or continue for more than 10 to 14 days, you may need to take antibiotics. A sinus infection can lead to chronic sinusitis if it does not respond to home treatment or antibiotics, or if it is not treated at all.

Prevention

• Treat nasal congestion caused by colds promptly. See page 155.

• Avoid cigarette, cigar, and pipe smoke in your home and workplace. Smoke irritates inflamed membranes in your nose and sinuses.

• If you have allergies, avoid the things that trigger your allergy attacks.

Home Treatment

Home treatment can often relieve early symptoms of sinusitis, such as facial pressure and stuffiness, and get your sinuses draining normally again so that you may not need antibiotic treatment.

• Drink extra fluids to keep mucus thin. Drink at least 8 to 10 glasses of water or juice per day.

• Apply moist heat (a warm towel or gel pack) to your face several times a day for 5 to 10 minutes at a time.

• Breathe warm, moist air from a steamy shower, a hot bath, or sink filled with hot water.

• Increase the humidity in your home, especially in the bedrooms. Avoid cold, dry air.

- Take an oral decongestant, use a decongestant nasal spray, or use a mucus-thinning agent (see page 344). Do not use a nasal decongestant spray for more than 3 days in a row. Avoid products that contain antihistamines unless your symptoms may also be related to allergies.

- Take aspirin, acetaminophen, or ibuprofen to relieve facial pain and headache. Do not give aspirin to anyone younger than 20 because of the risk of Reye syndrome (see page 221).

- Check the back of your throat for postnasal drip. If you see streaks of mucus, gargle with warm water to prevent a sore throat.

- Blow your nose gently. Do not close one nostril when blowing your nose.

- Salt water (saline) irrigation helps wash mucus and bacteria out of the nasal passages. Use nonprescription saline nose drops or a homemade solution (see page 344):

  - Use a bulb syringe and gently squirt the solution into your nose, or snuff the solution from the palm of your hand, one nostril at a time.

  - The salt water should go in through your nose and come out your mouth.

  - Blow your nose gently afterward. Repeat the salt water wash 2 to 4 times a day.

When to Call a Health Professional

- If cold symptoms last longer than 10 to 14 days or worsen after the first 7 days.

- If you have a severe headache that is different from a "normal" headache and is not relieved by acetaminophen, aspirin, or ibuprofen.

- If you have facial swelling, or if your vision changes or gets blurry.

- If nasal discharge changes from clear to colored (yellow or green) after 5 to 7 days of a cold, and other symptoms (sinus pain, fever) worsen. If nasal discharge is colored from the start of a cold, call if it lasts longer than 7 to 10 days.

- If facial pain (especially in one sinus area or along the ridge between the nose and lower eyelid) persists after 2 days of home treatment.

- If sinusitis symptoms persist after you have taken a full course of antibiotics.

Sore Throat, Strep Throat, and Tonsillitis

Most sore throats are caused by viruses and may occur with a cold or may follow a cold. A mild sore throat may be caused by dry air, smoking, air pollution, or yelling. People who have allergies or stuffy noses may breathe through their mouths while sleeping, which can cause a mild sore throat.

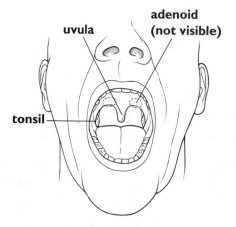

uvula

adenoid (not visible)

tonsil

Location of tonsils and adenoids

Sore throats can also be caused by inflammation of the tonsils (tonsillitis) or adenoids (adenoiditis). This is common in children. Tonsillitis and adenoiditis are usually caused by a virus. In addition to sore throat, symptoms of tonsillitis or adenoiditis include fever, swollen lymph nodes, and tiredness along with cold symptoms, such as runny nose and a cough. It may be painful to swallow, and the tonsils are often bright red, spotted with pus, and swollen. Adenoiditis can also cause headache and vomiting. Chronically inflamed adenoids may block the passageway between the ears and the throat (eustachian tubes), contributing to ear infections. See page 179.

Strep throat is a sore throat caused by streptococcal bacteria. It is more common in children from 3 to

15 years of age. A person can get strep throat even if his or her tonsils have been removed.

In general, the more coldlike your symptoms are, the less likely it is that you have strep throat or another bacterial infection. Strep throat causes some or all of these symptoms:

• Severe and sudden sore throat

• Fever of 101° or higher

• Swollen lymph nodes in the neck

• White or yellow coating on the tonsils

Strep throat is treated with antibiotics to prevent rheumatic fever. Antibiotics are effective in preventing rheumatic fever if started within 9 days of the onset of the sore throat.

Another cause of persistent sore throat is mononucleosis (mono, or "the kissing disease"), which is caused by the Epstein-Barr virus. Mono is most common in older teens and young adults. In addition to a severe sore throat, fever, and fatigue, mono symptoms often include weakness, body aches, and swollen lymph nodes in the neck. Another less common symptom is pain in the upper left part of the abdomen caused by enlargement of the spleen. Mono is diagnosed with a blood test called the monospot test.

Most people recover from mono after several weeks. However, for some people it may take several months to get their normal energy level back, and it is normal for the lymph nodes to remain enlarged for up to 1 month (see Swollen Lymph Nodes on page 169). There is no specific treatment for mono except rest, plenty of fluids, salt water gargles for throat pain, and aspirin or acetaminophen for body aches. Do not give aspirin to anyone younger than 20.

A less common cause of sore throat is the backflow (reflux) of stomach acid into the throat. Although reflux is often associated with heartburn or an "acid" taste in the mouth, sometimes a sore throat is the only symptom. If you think stomach acid reflux may be causing your throat pain, see Heartburn on page 87.

Prevention

- Drink 8 to 12 glasses of water a day.

- Identify and avoid irritants that cause sore throat (such as smoke, fumes, or yelling). For tips on quitting smoking, see page 26.

- Avoid contact with people who have strep throat. People who have strep throat should stay home from work, school, or day care until 24 hours after starting antibiotic treatment.

- If you have mono, try to keep from spreading the virus: don't share eating or drinking utensils; avoid kissing; and do not donate blood until your symptoms are gone and you are feeling better.

Tonsillectomy and Adenoidectomy

 It was once common to remove children's tonsils and adenoids. Today, in recognition of the risks, costs, and limited benefits, tonsillectomy and adenoidectomy are done less often, and only when the benefits greatly outweigh the risk, inconvenience, and pain.

Tonsillectomy may be recommended if at least one of the following criteria is met:

- There have been at least 4 to 6 severe tonsillitis infections caused by strep bacteria in the past year despite treatment with at least 2 different antibiotics.

- The enlarged tonsils cause severe breathing difficulty or sleep disturbance.

- There are deep pockets of infection in the tonsils that haven't responded to drug treatment.

Adenoidectomy may be recommended if at least one of the following criteria is met:

- The enlarged adenoids are blocking the airway, causing breathing difficulty and sleep disturbance.

- The adenoids are believed to cause persistent ear infections, despite antibiotic treatment.

If your doctor recommends surgery but none of the above criteria are met, it may be wise to get a second opinion. See page 14.

Home Treatment

Home care is usually all that is needed for viral sore throats and tonsillitis. If you are taking antibiotics for strep throat, these tips will also help you feel better.

• Gargle with warm salt water (1 teaspoon of salt in 8 ounces of water). The salt reduces swelling and discomfort.

• If you have postnasal drip, gargle often to prevent more throat irritation.

• Drink more fluids to soothe your sore throat. Honey and lemon in hot water or in weak tea may help. Do not give honey to children younger than 1 year of age.

• Stop smoking, and avoid other people's smoke.

• Acetaminophen, aspirin, or ibuprofen will relieve pain and reduce fever. Do not give aspirin to anyone younger than 20 because of the risk of Reye syndrome (see page 221).

• Some nonprescription throat lozenges (such as Sucrets Maximum Strength, Spec-T, and Tyrobenz) are safe, effective, and have a local anesthetic to soothe pain. Regular cough drops or hard candy may also help.

When to Call a Health Professional

• If any one of the following symptoms develops:

  - Difficulty swallowing

  - Excessive drooling caused by inability to swallow

  - Labored or difficult breathing

• If you develop a severe sore throat after being exposed to strep throat.

• If a sore throat occurs with 2 of these 3 symptoms of strep throat:

  - Fever of 101° or higher

  - White or yellow coating on the tonsils

  - Swollen lymph nodes in the neck

• If a rash occurs with sore throat. **Scarlet fever** is a rash that may occur when there is a strep throat infection. Like strep throat, scarlet fever is treated with antibiotics.

• If you cannot trace the cause of a sore throat to a cold, allergy, smoking, overuse of your voice, or other irritation.

• If a mild sore throat lasts longer than 2 weeks.

• If a child has at least 4 to 6 episodes of tonsillitis in 1 year despite antibiotic treatment.

• If a child persistently breathes through his or her mouth, snores, or has a very nasal- or muffled-sounding voice. These are signs of chronic adenoid inflammation.

Swollen Lymph Nodes

The lymph nodes are small glands located throughout the body. The most noticeable lymph nodes are those in the neck. The lymph nodes swell as the body fights minor infections from colds, insect bites, or small cuts. More serious infections can cause the lymph nodes to greatly enlarge and become very firm and tender.

Swelling in the lymph nodes on either side of the neck is common with a cold or sore throat. The lymph nodes in the groin may swell if there is a vaginal or other pelvic infection, or if there is a cut or sore on the leg or foot.

Swollen lymph nodes may be felt in the areas shown.

Lymph nodes may remain hard long after the initial infection goes away. This is especially true in children, whose lymph nodes may get smaller but remain hard and visible for several weeks.

Home Treatment

• There is no specific home treatment for swollen lymph nodes. Continue treating the cold or other infection that is causing the lymph nodes to swell.

• Your child may develop hard, swollen lymph nodes following a cold or minor infection. If the lymph nodes near the site of the infection are not tender and are not getting larger, you can monitor them at home and report them at the child's next regular doctor visit.

When to Call a Health Professional

• If the lymph nodes are large, very firm, red, and very tender.

• If swollen lymph nodes are associated with other signs of infection in a nearby cut or sore. See page 67.

• If you develop swollen lymph nodes after traveling outside the U.S. or in wilderness areas.

• If swollen lymph nodes continue to get bigger, or appear without apparent cause and persist for 2 weeks or longer.

• If swollen lymph nodes appear in areas other than the ones shown on page 169.

Snoring

Up to 50 percent of all adults snore occasionally, and about 25 percent of all adults are habitual snorers. Snoring is caused by blockage of the airways in the back of the mouth and nose. These airways can be blocked for many reasons, such as excess neck tissue caused by being overweight or a stuffy nose caused by allergies or a cold. Some people who snore have sleep apnea. Sleep apnea is present when a person repeatedly stops breathing for 10 to 15 seconds or longer during sleep.

Snoring can disrupt a person's sleep patterns, so he or she may be sleepy and less alert during the day. A person's snoring can also disrupt the sleep of other family members or roommates. Here are some tips for people who snore:

• Exercise daily to maintain a healthy body weight and improve muscle tone. Avoid exercise within 2 hours of bedtime, because exercise may make it harder to fall asleep.

• Avoid heavy meals, alcohol, sleeping pills, and antihistamines before bedtime.

• Sleep on your side rather than your back. (Sew a pocket onto the back of your pajama top, and put a tennis ball inside the pocket. This will keep you from sleeping on your back.)

• Establish regular sleeping patterns. Go to bed at the same time every night, even on weekends.

• Let the person who doesn't snore fall asleep first.

 If snoring becomes a problem for you and affects your family life, see a health professional. An examination of the nose, mouth, and neck may be needed. A doctor may also want to do a sleep study to see if sleep apnea is one of the reasons why you snore. Treatment will depend on what is causing you to snore.

You can observe a lot just by watching.
Yogi Berra (naturally)

8

Eye and Ear Problems

From dry eyes to pinkeye and earaches to earwax, your eyes and ears can cause you trouble. With home care and patience, most of these problems will clear up. This chapter will explain what you can do at home and when to get professional help.

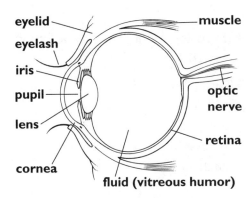

The structures at the front of the eye (lens, pupil, cornea, iris) let light into the eye. Light hits the back of the eye (retina) and is changed into nerve signals that are carried to the brain by the optic nerve. The brain reads the signals from the optic nerve as images that you "see."

Blood in the Eye

Sometimes blood vessels in the whites of the eyes break and cause a red spot or speck. This is called a subconjunctival hemorrhage. The blood may look alarming, especially if the spot is large, but it is usually not a cause for concern. The red spot will go away in 2 to 3 weeks.

However, call a health professional immediately if your eye is bloody and painful; if there is blood in the colored part of the eye; or if the bleeding followed a blow or injury to the eye. Also call if bleeding in the eye occurs often; occurs after you begin taking blood thinners (anticoagulants); or covers more than one-fourth of the white of the eye.

Eye Problems

Symptoms	Possible Causes
Red, itchy, watery eyes	Allergies, p. 141. Think about allergy to eye care products, makeup, or smoke. Possible contact lens problem, p. 174.
Excessive discharge from eye; red, swollen eyelids; sandy feeling	Eye Infections, p. 173. Possible contact lens problem, p. 174.
Pimple or swelling on eyelid	Styes, p. 175.
Pain in the eye	Chemical Burns, p. 47; Migraine Headaches, p. 190; Cluster Headaches, p. 192; Objects in the Eye, p. 63; Possible contact lens problem, p. 174; Eye Infections, p. 173.
Severe eye pain, blurred vision, reddened eyeball	**See a doctor now!**
Red spot on white of eye	Blood in the Eye, p. 171.
Black eye	Bruises (black eye), p. 44.
Dry, scratchy eyes	Dry Eyes, p. 172.

Dry Eyes

Eyes that don't have enough moisture in them may feel dry, hot, sandy, or gritty. Low humidity, smoke, the natural aging process, certain diseases, and certain medications (such as antihistamines, decongestants, some antidepressants, or birth control pills) can cause dry eyes.

Home Treatment

• Give your eyes a rest. While reading, watching television, or using a computer, take frequent breaks and close your eyes. If you can, blink your eyes more often.

• If possible, avoid smoke and other eye irritants.

• Try a nonprescription artificial tear solution, such as Akwa Tears, Duratears, or HypoTears. Do not use eyedrops for reducing redness (such as Visine) to treat dry eyes.

When to Call a Health Professional

Call a health professional if your eyes are persistently dry and artificial tears do not help.

Floaters and Flashes

Floaters are spots, specks, and lines that "float" across your field of vision. They are caused by stray cells or strands of tissue that float in the vitreous humor, the gel-like substance that fills the eyeball. Floaters can be annoying but are not usually serious. However, if you see floaters or flashes of light for the first time, or if you have a sudden increase in floaters or flashes, call your eye doctor or family doctor. If you have had floaters for some time, or if you have occasional flashes, mention it at your next routine eye exam.

Eye Infections

Conjunctivitis, or pinkeye, is an inflammation of the membrane (conjunctiva) that lines the eyelid and the surface of the eye. Bacteria and viruses (which can be very contagious), allergies, dry air, and irritants in the air such as smoke, fumes, or chemicals can cause pinkeye.

The symptoms of pinkeye may include redness in the whites of the eyes, red and swollen eyelids, lots of tears, itching or burning, a sandy feeling in the eyes, and sensitivity to light. There may be a discharge that causes the eyelids to stick together during sleep. Antibiotic ointment may be needed if the discharge is yellow or green.

Prevention

• Do not share towels, handkerchiefs, pillows, eye makeup, or contact lens equipment or solutions.

• Wash your hands before and after treating pinkeye in your own eyes or someone else's.

• Wear safety glasses when working with chemicals. If a chemical gets into your eye, immediately flush the eye with water. See page 47 or page 63.

Home Treatment

Although most cases of pinkeye will clear up on their own in 5 to 7 days, viral pinkeye can last many weeks. Pinkeye caused by allergies or pollution will last as long as you are exposed to the irritating substance. Good home care will speed healing and ease discomfort.

• Apply cold or warm compresses several times a day to relieve discomfort.

• Gently wipe the edge of the eyelid with moist cotton or a clean, wet washcloth to remove encrusted matter. Wipe from the inside corner (next to the nose) to the outside. Use a clean surface for each wipe.

• Don't wear contact lenses or eye makeup until the inflammation is gone. Discard eye makeup after an eye infection, and clean your contacts and storage case.

Contact Lenses

If you wear contact lenses, these tips will help you avoid problems.

Follow the cleaning instructions for your lenses. Keep your lenses and anything that touches them (hands, storage containers, solution bottles, makeup) very clean. Wash your hands before handling your contacts.

Use a commercial saline solution. (Generic brands are just as good as name brands.) Homemade solution is easily contaminated with bacteria. Never wet your lenses with saliva, which contains bacteria that may cause an eye infection.

Insert your contacts before applying eye makeup. Do not apply makeup to the inner rim of the eyelid. Replace eye makeup every 3 to 6 months to reduce the risk of contamination.

When worn for long periods of time, extended-wear lenses are more likely to cause severe eye infections. If you choose to wear them, follow the wearing and cleaning schedule your eye care professional recommends.

Symptoms of a possible problem with your contacts include unusual redness, pain, or burning in the eye; discharge; blurred vision; or extreme sensitivity to light. Remove your lenses and disinfect them. If symptoms last longer than 2 to 3 hours after you remove your contacts, call your eye care professional.

Visit your eye care professional once a year to check the condition of your lenses and the health of your eyes.

Inserting eyedrops

- If eyedrops are prescribed, insert them as follows:

  - For older children and adults: Pull the lower lid down with two fingers to create a little pouch. Put the drops there. Close the eye for several minutes to let the drops move around.

  - For younger children: Ask the child to lie down with eyes closed. Put a drop in the inner corner of the eye. When the child opens the eye, the drop will run in.

  - Be sure the dropper is clean and does not touch the eye, eyelid, or the eyelashes. If the dropper does touch the eye, do not put it back in the bottle. Throw it away and replace it.

- Putting antibiotic ointment in the eye can be tricky, especially with children. If you can get it on the eyelashes, it will melt and get into the eye.

- Make sure any nonprescription medicine you use is ophthalmic (for eyes), not otic (for ears).

- Wash your hands thoroughly before and after treating pinkeye.

Cataracts and Glaucoma

A cataract is a painless, cloudy area in the lens of the eye. Cataracts may cause vision problems such as cloudy, foggy, or filmy vision; glare from lamps, sunlight, or car headlights; and double vision. They are common in older adults.

Glaucoma is an eye disorder that damages the optic nerve at the back of the eye. The damage is often related to excess pressure in the eye. Glaucoma rarely has symptoms and develops slowly over several years. If it is not treated, however, it may lead to blindness.

Cataracts and glaucoma are easy to detect during routine eye exams. Both respond well to treatment. Talk with your doctor about the best schedule of eye exams for you, based on your age and risk factors for these eye problems.

Call your health professional immediately if you have sudden blurry vision, loss of vision, or pain in the eye.

 If you are considering cataract surgery, gather as much information as possible about the risks and benefits of surgery. Getting all the facts and thinking about your own needs and values will help you work with your doctor to make a wise health decision.

When to Call a Health Professional

- If there is pain in the eye (rather than irritation), blurring, or loss of vision that is not cleared even momentarily by blinking.

- If the eye is painfully sensitive to light.

- If the skin around the eye or the eyelid is red.

- If it feels like there is a foreign object in the eye.

- If the eye is red and there is a yellow, green, or bloody discharge that does not begin to go away in 24 hours.

- If there is an abnormal difference between the sizes of the pupils.

- If symptoms of an eye infection last longer than 7 days.

Styes

A sty is a noncontagious infection of the eyelash follicle. It looks like a small, red bump, much like a pimple, either in the eyelid or on the edge of the lid. It comes to a head and breaks open after a few days.

Styes are very common and are not a serious problem, although they can be painful. Most will go away on their own with home treatment and don't require removal.

Home Treatment

- Do not rub your eye, and do not squeeze or open the sty.

- Apply warm, moist compresses for 10 minutes, 3 to 6 times a day, until the sty comes to a head and drains.

- Do not wear eye makeup or contact lenses until the sty heals.

PRK and Lasik

PRK and LASIK are two different surgical procedures that can correct vision problems such as nearsightedness, farsightedness, and astigmatism. For each procedure, a surgeon uses laser instruments to reshape the cornea (the clear tissue that covers the iris and pupil) in a way that allows improved vision. These procedures take only a few minutes to complete. If both eyes need correction, they can be treated at the same time.

Some people may still need to wear glasses or contact lenses after the surgery, especially when light is dim and at night (usually the prescription is not as strong). A person may see halos around lights for up to 6 months after having corrective eye surgery.

PRK and LASIK cannot restore vision loss caused by cataracts or macular degeneration; nor can they prevent these age-related eye changes from happening.

When to Call a Health Professional

- If the sty is very painful, grows larger quickly, or continues to drain.

- If the sty interferes with your vision.

- If the sty gets worse despite home treatment or doesn't heal within 1 week.

- If the redness and swelling around the sty spread to involve the entire eyelid or the eyeball.

Dizziness and Vertigo

Dizziness is a word that is often used to describe two different sensations: lightheadedness and vertigo. Knowing the difference can help you and your health professional narrow down the list of possible problems.

Lightheadedness is a feeling that you are about to pass out (faint). Although you may feel unsteady, there is no sensation of movement. Lightheadedness usually goes away or improves when you lie down. If lightheadedness gets worse, it can lead to a fainting spell with nausea or vomiting.

Lightheadedness usually does not indicate a serious problem. It is common to feel lightheaded occasionally. Lightheadedness is often caused by a momentary drop in blood pressure and reduced blood flow to the brain when you get up too quickly from a seated or lying position. This is called **orthostatic hypotension**. It may be caused by dehydration or medications such as water pills (diuretics), high blood pressure medications, and certain heart medications.

Lightheadedness is common when you have flu, a cold, or allergies. Vomiting, diarrhea, and fever can cause dehydration and lightheadedness. Other common causes of lightheadedness include hyperventilation, stress, anxiety, drinking alcohol, or using illegal drugs. A more serious cause of lightheadedness is bleeding. If a person is bleeding internally, lightheadedness and fatigue may be the first noticeable symptoms of blood loss.

Eye Twitches

Eye twitches or muscle spasms around the eye are most often associated with fatigue or stress. Twitches will usually stop on their own in a short time, and they will improve with rest or reduced stress.

Call a health professional if twitches occur with redness, swelling, discharge from the eye, or fever, or if eye twitches last longer than 1 week.

An uncommon cause of lightheadedness is an abnormality in your heart rhythm that reduces blood flow. This can cause recurrent episodes of lightheadedness and can lead to fainting (cardiac syncope). Unexplained fainting needs to be evaluated by a health professional. See Fainting on page 78.

Vertigo is a sensation that you or your surroundings are spinning or moving when there is no actual movement. Vertigo is often related to inner ear problems. It may occur with nausea and vomiting. Standing or walking may be impossible when you have severe vertigo.

The most common form of vertigo is triggered by changes in the position of your head, such as when you move your head from side to side, bend your head back to look up, or lie down. This is called **benign positional vertigo**.

Vertigo also may be caused by labyrinthitis, an inflammation in the part of the inner ear that controls balance. Labyrinthitis is usually caused by a viral infection and sometimes follows a cold or the flu.

Other underlying problems that can contribute to vertigo are Meniere's disease (a balance problem believed to be caused by a buildup of fluid in the inner ear), migraine headaches, multiple sclerosis, stroke, and, in rare cases, a brain tumor.

Ear Problems

Symptoms	Possible Causes
Earache and fever; pulling at ears by infants and small children, especially with inconsolable crying	Ear Infections, p. 179.
Pain while chewing; headache	TM Disorder, p. 137.
Pain when ear is wiggled or while chewing; itching or burning in ear	Swimmer's Ear, p. 184.
Discharge from ear	Swimmer's Ear, p. 184; eardrum rupture, p. 179.
Feeling of fullness in ear, with runny or stuffy nose, cough, fever	Colds, p. 155; Ear Infections, p. 179.
Feeling of something moving or "bumping around" in ear	Objects in the Ear, p. 63.
Hearing loss; inattentiveness	Hearing Loss, p. 183; Earwax, p. 181; serous otitis, p. 180.
Ringing or noise in the ears	Tinnitus, p. 186.

Home Treatment

Lightheadedness is usually not a cause for concern unless it is severe, persistent, or occurs with other symptoms such as an irregular heartbeat or fainting. The greatest danger of lightheadedness or vertigo is the injuries that might result if you fall.

• When you feel lightheaded, lie down for a minute or two. This will allow more blood to flow to your brain. After lying down, sit up slowly and remain sitting for 1 to 2 minutes before slowly standing up.

• If you have a cold or the flu, rest and extra fluids will help prevent lightheadedness.

• Do not drive, operate machinery, or put yourself in any other potentially dangerous situation while you are having vertigo or feeling lightheaded.

• When you are having vertigo, avoid lying flat on your back, and keep your eyes open. Propping yourself up slightly may help relieve the spinning sensation.

When to Call a Health Professional

Call 911 or other emergency services immediately:

- If vertigo is accompanied by severe headache, confusion, loss of speech or sight, weakness in the arms or legs, or numbness in any part of the body.

- If lightheadedness occurs with chest pain that is squeezing or crushing, or occurs with any other symptoms of a heart attack (see page 55).

- If someone who is feeling dizzy loses consciousness and you are unable to arouse the person.

- If vertigo or loss of balance occurs with other signs of serious illness, such as headache with severe stiff neck, fever, irritability, confusion, or a seizure. (See "Encephalitis and Meningitis" on page 162.)

- If severe and persistent lightheadedness is accompanied by a sudden change in your normal heart rate.

Call a health professional:

- If lightheadedness or vertigo develops after an injury.

- If you have vertigo that is severe (may cause vomiting) or that occurs with hearing loss.

- If you suspect dizziness may be a side effect of a medication.

- If you experience vertigo that:
  - Occurs frequently and has not been diagnosed.
  - Lasts longer than 5 days.
  - Is significantly different from other episodes.

- If you have repeated spells of lightheadedness over a few days.

- If you feel lightheaded and your pulse is less than 50 or more than 150 beats per minute. See page 58 to learn how to take your pulse.

Ear Infections

Ear infections can occur in the middle ear or the ear canal. For information about infections in the ear canal, see Swimmer's Ear on page 184.

A middle ear infection (otitis media) often develops during a cold. Colds can cause the eustachian tube (which connects the middle ear to the throat) to swell and close. When the eustachian tube is closed, air cannot reach the middle ear. This creates a vacuum that draws fluid into the middle ear. Bacteria or viruses then grow in the fluid, causing a middle ear infection.

The infected fluid that is trapped in the middle ear puts pressure on the eardrum. In some cases, the pressure may continue to build until the eardrum ruptures. A single **eardrum rupture** usually is not serious and rarely causes hearing loss. However, repeated eardrum ruptures can lead to permanent hearing loss (see "Recurrent Ear Infections and Persistent Effusion" on page 182).

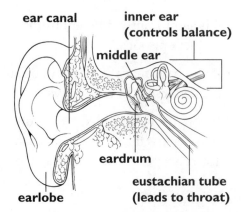

ear canal

inner ear
(controls balance)

middle ear

eardrum

eustachian tube
(leads to throat)

earlobe

Ear infections can occur in the ear canal or middle ear. Dizziness can be caused by an inflammation of the inner ear.

Symptoms of a middle ear infection include ear pain, dizziness, ringing or a feeling of fullness in the ear, hearing loss, fever, headache, and runny nose. Children who can't yet talk may tug on their painful ears. Drainage from the ear that is bloody or looks like pus may indicate a ruptured eardrum. Ear pain caused by a middle ear infection usually improves once an eardrum ruptures.

When a person has fluid buildup in the middle ear, it is called **otitis media with effusion**. Effusion generally occurs after a middle ear infection has cleared up. There may be no symptoms, or there may be a muffling of sound, minor hearing loss, and mild discomfort. Effusion that occurs after a middle ear infection is not a cause for concern and probably will not require treatment unless it lasts longer than 3 months and causes significant hearing loss. See "Recurrent Ear Infections and Persistent Effusion" on page 182.

Prevention

- Breast-feed your baby. Breast-fed babies have fewer ear infections. If you bottle-feed your baby, hold the baby in an upright position to prevent milk from getting into the eustachian tubes. Do not allow infants to fall asleep with a bottle (however, it is all right to let a nursing baby fall asleep at the breast).

- Avoid exposing children to cigarette smoke, which is associated with more frequent ear infections.

- If possible, limit your child's contact with other children who have colds.

- Wean your child from his or her pacifier at about 6 months of age. Babies who continue to use their pacifiers after 12 months of age are more likely to develop ear infections.

- Wash your hands often if you have a cold or other upper respiratory infection to prevent spreading the infection.

- Make sure your child is up to date with his or her immunizations.

Home Treatment

- Apply heat to the ear to ease the pain. Use a warm washcloth or a heating pad set on low. Don't use a heating pad on an infant or a child. Don't use a heating pad in bed; you may fall asleep and burn yourself.

- Acetaminophen, aspirin, or ibuprofen will help relieve earache. Do not give aspirin to anyone younger than 20.

• Drink more clear liquids.

• If dizziness occurs, see page 176.

• If an ear infection has caused the eardrum to rupture, avoid getting water in the ear until the eardrum heals (about 3 to 4 weeks).

When to Call a Health Professional

• If ear pain is severe or increases despite home treatment.

• If ear pain occurs with other signs of serious illness, such as headache with severe stiff neck, fever, irritability, or confusion. (See "Encephalitis and Meningitis" on page 162.)

• If your baby pulls or rubs his or her ear and appears to be in pain (crying, screaming).

• If your child has a fever over 102° with other signs of an ear infection.

• If an infant younger than 3 months has a fever of 100.4° or higher.

• If you suspect that the eardrum has ruptured or if there is drainage from the ear that looks like pus or contains blood.

• If symptoms do not improve after 48 hours of treatment with an antibiotic.

• If your child has ear tubes and develops an earache or has drainage from the ear.

• If mild ear pain continues for longer than 3 to 4 days.

• If there is redness or swelling behind the ear.

Earwax

Earwax is a protective secretion that filters dust, repels water, and keeps the ears clean. Normally, earwax is liquid, drains freely from the ears, and does not cause problems.

Occasionally, earwax will build up, harden, and cause some hearing loss or discomfort. Poking at the wax with cotton swabs, fingers, or other objects will only push the wax deeper into the ear canal and pack it against the eardrum. When wax is tightly packed, professional help is needed to remove it.

In general, it is best to leave earwax alone. You can handle most earwax problems that do occur by avoiding cotton swabs and following the home treatment tips.

Home Treatment

Do not use home treatment if you suspect that the eardrum is ruptured, if there is drainage from the ear that looks like pus or contains blood, or if the person has ear tubes.

To remove earwax safely:

• Soften and loosen the earwax with warm (body temperature) mineral oil. Place 2 drops of mineral oil in the ear twice a day for 1 or 2 days.

• Once the wax is loose and soft, all that is usually needed to remove it from the ear canal is the spray from a warm, gentle shower. Direct the water into the ear, and then tip the head to let the earwax drain out.

Recurrent Ear Infections and Persistent Effusion

If your child has at least 3 ear infections in a 6-month period, or 4 infections in a 1-year period, talk to your family doctor or pediatrician about preventive antibiotic treatment. This is a low dose of antibiotics given daily throughout the season when your child is prone to ear infections.

However, there is growing debate among health professionals about the use of preventive antibiotics for two reasons. First, the effectiveness of antibiotics in preventing ear infections is questionable. And second, there is growing concern that routine use of antibiotics may cause bacteria to change so that common antibiotics cannot kill them.

If your child has repeated ear infections (3 in 6 months, or 4 to 6 in a year), your doctor may suggest inserting ear tubes (tympanostomy tubes) through your child's eardrums to help prevent ear infections. The tubes remain in the child's eardrums for 6 to 12 months.

In some children, fluid remains in the middle ear more than 3 to 4 months after an ear infection clears up. If this occurs in your child, he or she should be given a hearing test because long-lasting effusion can cause hearing loss or speech delays. If your child has effusion and significant hearing loss in both ears at the same time for more than 3 to 4 months, your doctor may recommend ear tubes.

 The decision about whether to treat recurrent ear infections is made on a case-by-case basis. Ask your doctor about the long-term risks and benefits of all the available treatment options.

• Use a nonprescription wax softener (such as Debrox or Murine), followed by gentle flushing with warm water in a bulb ear syringe each night for 1 to 2 weeks. Putting cool or hot fluids in the ear may cause dizziness, so make sure the water is warm.

When to Call a Health Professional

• If the wax buildup remains hard, dry, and compacted after 1 week of home treatment.

• If earwax is causing ringing in your ears, a full feeling in your ears, or hearing loss.

• If earwax buildup occurs with other problems such as nausea or difficulty with balance.

• If an earwax problem develops in a person who has a ruptured eardrum or ear tubes or who has had previous ear surgery.

MORE INFO **For more information, see the back cover.**

Hearing Loss

More than 28 million Americans cope with some degree of hearing loss. Most hearing loss is caused by problems in the inner ear or in the acoustic nerve, which sends sound signals to the brain. This is called **sensorineural hearing loss**. The damage to the inner ear that causes sensorineural hearing loss can be the result of exposure to loud noise, certain medications (including high doses of aspirin), or changes that come with age. In some cases, children are born with this type of hearing loss. People with sensorineural hearing loss may have trouble understanding the speech of others yet be very sensitive to loud sounds. They may also hear ringing, hissing, or clicking noises.

Hearing loss that develops when something prevents sound from reaching the inner ear is called **conductive hearing loss**. The most common cause is packed earwax in the ear canal, which can be easily treated (see page 181). Infection, abnormal bone growth, and excess fluid in the ear are other causes of conductive hearing loss.

People who have conductive hearing loss often say that their own voice sounds loud while other voices sound muffled. There may be a low level of ringing in the ear (tinnitus).

Depending on the underlying problem, conductive hearing loss is usually treated by ear flushing, medication, or surgery.

A more unusual form of hearing loss is caused by damage to the hearing centers in the brain. This is called **central deafness**, and it can occur after a head injury or stroke. The person's ear works normally, but his or her brain has difficulty interpreting sounds.

Some hearing loss may be the result of decreased blood flow to the inner ear or parts of the brain that help process information from the ear. If you have circulatory problems caused by heart disease, high blood pressure, or diabetes, be sure to follow your care plan for keeping those conditions under control.

Prevention

- Avoid loud noise whenever possible. If you know you are going to be exposed to it at work, at home, at the shooting range, or in other settings, wear earplugs or protective earmuffs. The noise generated by snowmobiles, motorcycles, lawnmowers, power tools and appliances, high-volume music, and other sources can permanently damage your hearing.

- Never use cotton swabs, hairpins, or other objects to remove earwax or to scratch your ears. They can damage the ear canal or eardrum. See page 181.

- Ask your pharmacist if any medications you are taking can affect your hearing. For example, the use of certain antibiotics, blood pressure medications, ibuprofen, and large doses of aspirin (8 to 12 tablets per day) is linked to hearing loss.

• During air travel, swallow and yawn frequently when the plane is coming down to land. If you have a cold, the flu, or a sinus infection, take a decongestant a few hours before the plane is scheduled to land.

When to Call a Health Professional

• If hearing loss develops suddenly (within a matter of days or weeks).

• If you have hearing loss in one ear only.

• If you develop a hearing problem while taking medication, including aspirin or ibuprofen.

• If you are thinking about wearing hearing aids. Make an appointment with a hearing specialist (otolaryngologist) if:

- You often ask people to repeat themselves or have difficulty understanding words.

- You have difficulty hearing when someone speaks in a whisper.

- You cannot hear soft sounds, such as a dripping faucet, or high-pitched sounds.

- You continuously hear a ringing or hissing background noise.

- A hearing problem is interfering with your life.

Swimmer's Ear

Swimmer's ear (otitis externa) is inflammation or infection of the ear canal (the passage leading from the external ear to the eardrum). It often develops after water has gotten into the ear. Sand or other debris that gets into the ear canal may also cause swimmer's ear.

Other causes of inflammation in the ear canal include a cut inside the ear or injury from a cotton swab or other object; prolonged use of earplugs; soap or shampoo buildup; and chronic skin conditions such as eczema and psoriasis.

Symptoms include pain, itching, and a feeling of fullness in the ear. The ear canal may be swollen. A more severe infection can cause increased pain, discharge from the ear, and possibly some hearing loss. Unlike a middle ear infection, the pain of an ear canal infection is worse when you chew, press on the "tag" in front of the ear, or wiggle your earlobe.

Prevention

• Keep your ears dry. After swimming or showering, shake your head to remove water from the ear canals. Gently dry your ears with the corner of a tissue or towel, or use a blow dryer on its lowest setting, held several inches from your ear.

- Put a few drops of rubbing alcohol or alcohol mixed with an equal amount of white vinegar in the ear after swimming or showering. Pull your ear up and back to let the liquid go deep into the ear canal; then tilt your head and let it drain out. You can also use nonprescription drops (Star-Otic, Swim-Ear) to prevent swimmer's ear.

- Never use cotton swabs, hairpins, or other objects to clean wax out of your ears. This can damage the ear canal or eardrum. See page 181.

- Avoid prolonged use of earplugs.

- Avoid getting soap and shampoo in the ear canal. To remove dirt or sand that gets into the ear while swimming, direct a gentle stream of warm water from the shower or a bulb syringe into your ear; then tip your head to let the water drain out.

Home Treatment

- Make sure there isn't an object or insect in the ear. See Objects in the Ear on page 63.

- If the eardrum may be ruptured or there is drainage from the ear that looks like pus or contains blood, do not insert eardrops or anything else into the ear unless a health professional has told you to do so.

- Gently rinse the ear using a bulb syringe and a solution of equal parts white vinegar and rubbing alcohol. Make sure the solution is at body temperature. Putting cool or hot fluids in the ear may cause dizziness.

Never stick a dropper into the ear canal. Put drops on the outer ear near the opening of the ear canal, and gently wiggle the ear until the drops flow into the canal.

- Avoid getting water in the ear until the irritation clears up. Cotton lightly coated with petroleum jelly can be used as an earplug. Do not use plastic earplugs.

- If your ear is itchy, try nonprescription swimmer's eardrops before and after getting your ears wet.

- To insert eardrops, have the person lie down, ear facing up. Warm the drops first by rolling the container between your hands. Place drops on the wall of the ear canal in small quantities so air can escape and drops can get into the ear. Wiggling the outer ear or pulling the ear up and back will help. See illustration on page 185.

- To ease ear pain, apply a warm washcloth or a heating pad set on low. (Don't use a heating pad on an infant or a child. Never use a heating pad in bed; you may fall asleep and burn yourself.) There may be some drainage when the heat melts earwax. As long as the drainage does not contain pus or blood, it is not of concern.

• Acetaminophen or aspirin may also help relieve pain. Do not give aspirin to anyone younger than 20.

When to Call a Health Professional

• If symptoms persist or worsen after 3 days of home treatment.

• If the ear canal is swollen, red, and very painful.

• If redness extends to the outer ear.

• If there is redness or swelling around or behind the ear.

• If there is discharge from the ear that looks like pus or contains blood.

• If ear pain follows a cold. See page 155.

• If dizziness or unsteadiness develops.

Tinnitus

Most people experience occasional ringing (or roaring, hissing, buzzing, or tinkling) in their ears. The sound usually lasts only a few minutes. If it becomes persistent, you may have tinnitus.

Tinnitus is often the result of damage to the nerves in the inner ear caused by prolonged exposure to loud noise. Other causes include excess earwax, ear infection, dental problems, head or ear injuries, and medications, especially antibiotics and large amounts of aspirin. Excessive alcohol or caffeine intake can also cause tinnitus or make existing tinnitus worse. In rare cases, tinnitus can be caused by a brain tumor.

Most tinnitus that comes and goes does not require medical treatment. However, if tinnitus is accompanied by other symptoms, becomes persistent, or starts to localize to one ear, a visit to a health professional usually is needed. Often there is no cure for tinnitus, but your health professional can help you learn how to live with the problem.

Prevention

Follow the prevention tips for Hearing Loss on page 183.

Home Treatment

• Cut back on or eliminate alcohol and beverages containing caffeine.

• Limit your use of aspirin, ibuprofen, and naproxen sodium.

• If you think earwax may be the cause of tinnitus, see Earwax on page 181.

When to Call a Health Professional

• If tinnitus develops suddenly and affects only one ear.

• If you have new tinnitus with other symptoms such as significant hearing loss, vertigo (see page 176), loss of balance, nausea, or vomiting.

• If tinnitus develops after an injury to the head or ear.

• If tinnitus lasts longer than 2 weeks despite home treatment.

*I'm very brave generally, only today I happen to
have a headache.*
Tweedledum in Alice in Wonderland

9

Headaches

Headaches are one of the most common health complaints. Some possible causes include tension, eyestrain, infection, allergy, injury, hunger, changes in the flow of blood in the vessels of the head, or exposure to chemicals.

Most headaches that occur without other symptoms will respond well to self-care. The majority of headaches are caused by tension and respond well to prevention measures and home treatment. See page 192.

An unusual headache that is very different from any you have had before, or a change in the usual pattern of your headaches, is a cause for concern. See "Headache Emergencies" on page 190. However, if you have had similar headaches before and your doctor has recommended a treatment plan for them, emergency care may not be needed.

Headaches that routinely occur during or after physical exertion, sexual activity, coughing, or sneezing may be a sign of a more serious disease and should be discussed with a health professional.

Headaches in Children

Migraine headaches (see page 190) often begin during childhood or adolescence and are the most common form of headache in children.

Children's headaches can also be related to stress about school, sports, relationships, or peer pressure. Even fun activities can be overdone and cause fatigue and headaches. Many times, just talking about a problem with your child may help. Encourage your children to talk openly about problems and stress at school.

Possible Headache Causes

If headache occurs:	Possible causes include:
On awakening.	Tension Headaches, p. 191; Allergies, p. 141; Sinusitis, p. 164; Neck Pain, p. 117; TM Disorder, p. 137.
In jaw muscles or in both temples.	TM Disorder, p. 137; Tension Headaches, p. 191.
Each afternoon or evening; after hours of desk work; with sore neck and shoulders.	Tension Headaches, p. 191; Neck Pain, p. 117.
On one side of the head, with visual disturbances or runny nose.	Migraine Headaches, p. 190; Cluster Headaches, p. 192.
After a blow to the head.	Head Injuries, p. 53.
After exposure to chemicals (paint, varnish, insect spray, cigarette smoke).	Chemical headache. Get into fresh air. Drink water to flush poisons.
With fever, runny nose, or sore throat.	Flu, p. 161; Sore Throat, p. 165; Colds, p. 155; Sinusitis, p. 164.
With fever, stiff neck, nausea, and vomiting.	Encephalitis and Meningitis, p. 162.
With runny nose, watery eyes, and sneezing.	Allergies, p. 141.
With fever and pain in the cheekbones or over the eyes.	Sinusitis, p. 164.
On mornings when you drink less caffeine than usual.	Caffeine-withdrawal headache. Cut back slowly, p. 192.
Following a stressful event.	Tension Headaches, p. 191.
At the same time during the menstrual cycle.	Premenstrual Syndrome, p. 261.
With new medication.	Drug allergy. Contact your doctor.
With severe eye pain.	Possible acute glaucoma, p. 175. **See a doctor now!**

Hunger can also cause headaches in children. A daily breakfast and a nutritious after-school snack may prevent headaches. Eyestrain and lack of sleep are other possible headache causes. Children will often have headaches along with sore throats, colds, sinus problems, or other infections.

Treatment for headaches in children and teens is based on the same factors as adult headache treatment: how often the headaches occur; how severe the pain is and how long it lasts; and how much the headaches disrupt normal activities. However, in children there is an increased emphasis on nondrug treatments.

Although migraines in children can be managed in much the same way as migraines in adults, less is known about the long-term effects of migraine medications in children. Some medications are not recommended for young children.

Home Treatment

- If your child's doctor has prescribed a specific treatment for the child's headaches, begin treatment as soon as your child reports the headache.

- For headaches that are mild and occur only occasionally, let your child rest quietly in a darkened room with a cool compress on his or her forehead. If rest does not relieve your child's headache, try a nonprescription medication such as acetaminophen or ibuprofen.

Follow the dosage directions on the package for your child's age group. Do not give aspirin to anyone younger than 20 because of the risk of Reye syndrome (see page 221).

- If your child tends to have mild headaches that occur frequently, encourage him or her to go on with normal activities. Do not allow your child to avoid chores or other activities unless his or her headache pain is moderate or severe. It is useful to "practice what you preach" in this area. When you have a headache, deal with it in a matter-of-fact way. Try to maintain your own usual activities when you have a headache, and adopt a calm approach to managing the pain. If your children see you successfully managing your headaches, they will be likely to do the same for themselves.

- Talk to your child. Let him or her know you care. Extra attention and quiet time may be all that are needed to relieve the headache.

When to Call a Health Professional

- If a severe headache occurs with signs of encephalitis or meningitis (see page 162), especially if your child recently had a viral illness.

- If a headache is severe and is not relieved by relaxing or taking a nonprescription pain reliever.

- If a headache occurs with other symptoms, such as abdominal pain, nausea, or vomiting, and is not relieved by home treatment and taking a nonprescription pain reliever.

- If a child's headaches occur twice a week or more, or if you are using pain relievers to control a child's headaches more than once a week.

- If you cannot discover a reasonable cause for your child's headaches.

- If headaches awaken your child at night or are worse early in the morning.

- Also see "Headache Emergencies" on page 190.

Migraine Headaches

Migraine headaches are severe, usually one-sided headaches that often occur with nausea, vomiting, and extreme sensitivity to light or sound. People often describe migraine headaches as throbbing or piercing. The pain may range from mild to terribly severe.

Although the headaches are usually one-sided, there may be pain on both sides of the head. In some people, the pain may switch sides each time they have a migraine.

Migraine headaches sometimes occur with an aura, a collection of symptoms that usually develop 15 to 30 minutes before a migraine headache begins. Visual disturbances, such as flashing lights, distortion in the size or shape of objects, or blind or dark spots in the field of vision, are the most common symptoms of an aura. An aura may also include symptoms that affect the nervous system, such as numbness or tingling in the face or arm, strange smells or sounds, or weakness on one side of the body. Some people have more vague symptoms, such as hunger, excessive thirst, or changes in mood or energy level, that appear 1 to 2 days before the headache develops.

Migraines are more common in females than in males. The headaches may begin during childhood, but most begin during the teens and early 20s. In women, they are often associated with menstrual periods.

Headache Emergencies

Call your doctor now if you have:

- A very sudden "thunderclap" headache.

- A sudden, severe headache unlike any you have had before.

- Headache with stiff neck, fever, nausea, vomiting, drowsiness, or confusion.

- Headache with weakness, paralysis, numbness, visual disturbances, slurred speech, confusion, behavior changes, or seizures.

- Headaches following a recent fall or blow to the head. See page 53 for information on head injuries.

Prevention

- Keep a diary of your headache symptoms. See "Tracking Your Headaches" on page 193. Once you know what events, foods, medications, or activities bring on your headaches, you may be able to prevent or limit their recurrence.

- Do what you can to manage stress. See Stress and Distress on page 321 for tips.

Home Treatment

- At the first sign of a headache, try to go to a quiet, dark place and relax. Sleeping can relieve migraines.

- Some people find that taking a pain reliever such as acetaminophen or ibuprofen at the first sign of a headache brings relief. However, frequent use of pain relievers can cause rebound headaches (headaches that return as the effects of the pain relievers wear off).

- Apply a cold pack to the painful area or put a cool cloth on your forehead. Do not apply heat, since it may make a migraine worse.

- Have someone gently massage your neck and shoulder muscles, or give yourself a massage.

- Practice a relaxation exercise such as progressive muscle relaxation or roll breathing. See pages 323 and 324.

- If a doctor has prescribed medication for your migraines, take the recommended dose at the first sign that a migraine is starting.

When to Call a Health Professional

- If you suspect that your headaches are migraines.

- If headaches are becoming more frequent or more severe.

Also see "Headache Emergencies" on page 190.

 Professional diagnosis and treatment, combined with your self-care, can help decrease the impact of migraines on your life. Discuss relaxation and biofeedback techniques with your doctor. They help many people prevent migraines. If nondrug treatments are not effective, there are many new prescription drugs available that can help you cope with migraines.

Tension Headaches

More than 90 percent of headaches are tension headaches, which become more frequent and severe during times of emotional or physical stress. Tightness or pain in the muscles of the neck, back, and shoulders may accompany a tension headache. A previous neck injury or arthritis in the neck can also cause tension headaches.

A tension headache may cause pain all over your head, a pressure sensation, or a feeling like having a tight band around your head. Your head may feel like it is in a vise. Some people feel a dull, pressing, burning sensation above the eyes.

The pain may also affect the jaw, face, neck, and upper back. You can rarely pinpoint the center or source of pain.

Prevention

• Reduce emotional stress. Take time to relax before and after you do something that has caused a headache in the past. Try the progressive muscle relaxation or roll breathing exercises on pages 323 and 324.

• Reduce physical stress. When sitting at a desk, change positions often, and stretch for 30 seconds each hour. Make a conscious effort to relax your jaw, neck, shoulder, and upper back muscles.

• Evaluate your neck and shoulder posture at work and make adjustments if needed. See page 117.

• Exercise daily. It can help relieve muscle tension and reduce stress.

• Treat yourself to a massage. Some people find regular massages very helpful in relieving tension. See page 333.

• Limit your caffeine intake to 1 to 2 cups per day. People who drink a lot of caffeinated beverages often develop a headache several hours after they have their last caffeinated beverage or may wake with a headache that is relieved by drinking caffeine. Cut down slowly to avoid caffeine-withdrawal headaches.

Cluster Headaches

Cluster headaches are sudden, very severe, sharp, stabbing headaches that occur on one side of the head, usually in the temple or behind the eye. They are much more common in men than in women.

During a cluster headache, the eye and nostril on the affected side may be runny, and the eye may also be red. The pain often begins at night and may last from a few minutes to a few hours.

Cluster headaches occur in periods of time called cluster periods, which may last days or months and then disappear for months or even years. During a cluster period, a person may have headaches several times a day. To prevent headaches during a cluster period, avoid alcohol and tobacco products, maintain a regular sleep schedule, and try to reduce your overall stress level.

See your doctor if you think you have cluster headaches or if you have persistent, severe headaches with no apparent cause. Also see "Headache Emergencies" on page 190.

Home Treatment

- Stop whatever you are doing and sit quietly for a moment. Close your eyes and inhale and exhale slowly. Try to relax your head and neck muscles.

- Take a stretch break or try a relaxation exercise. See page 323.

- Gently and firmly massage your neck muscles. See page 118 for neck exercises.

- Apply heat to the painful area with a heating pad, hot water bottle, or a warm shower.

- Lie down in a dark room with a cool cloth on your forehead.

- Taking acetaminophen or ibuprofen often helps relieve a tension headache. However, using nonprescription or prescription headache medications too often may make headaches more frequent or severe.

When to Call a Health Professional

- If a headache is severe and cannot be relieved with home treatment.

- If unexplained headaches continue to occur more than 3 times a week.

- If headaches become more frequent and severe.

- If headaches occur during or after physical exertion, sexual activity, coughing, or sneezing.

- If headaches awaken you out of a sound sleep or are worse first thing in the morning.

- If you need help discovering or eliminating the source of your tension headaches.

- Also see "Headache Emergencies" on page 190.

Tracking Your Headaches

If you have recurring headaches, keep a record of your symptoms. This record will help your doctor if medical evaluation is needed. Write down:

1. The date and time each headache started and stopped.

2. Any factors that seemed to trigger the headache: food, smoke, bright light, stress, activity.

3. The location and nature of the pain: throbbing, aching, stabbing, dull.

4. The severity of the pain.

5. Other physical symptoms: nausea, vomiting, visual disturbances, sensitivity to light or noise.

6. If you are a woman, note any association between headaches and your menstrual cycle or your use of birth control pills or hormone replacement therapy.

*I have a simple philosophy...
scratch where it itches.*
Alice Roosevelt Longworth

10

Skin, Hair, and Nail Problems

Skin problems can be a nuisance, but they are rarely life-threatening. Diagnosing skin problems may require a doctor's help, especially the first time you have a particular ailment. Use the chart on the next page and the index to find the skin problem you're interested in. Also see "Childhood Rashes" on page 216.

Acne

Acne is the term for blemishes (pimples or blackheads) that commonly form on the face, chest, upper back, or shoulders. A pimple forms when an oil duct in the skin is blocked, and secretions and bacteria build up under the skin. Acne usually starts during the teen years and often persists into adulthood.

Many women get a few pimples just before their menstrual periods. Stress and some birth control pills may make acne worse. Fatty foods, such as chocolate and nuts, are not considered to be a cause of acne.

 Many cases of <u>acne</u> will respond to home treatment, especially if they are mild. For severe or persistent cases, your doctor can prescribe stronger topical medication, antibiotics, or other drugs.

Prevention

• Gently wash your face with a mild soap, such as Dove, or one that contains benzoyl peroxide, such as Oxy Sensitive. Wash as often as necessary to keep your face clean (at least once a day), but do not scrub or overdry.

• While foods are no longer considered a significant cause of acne, eat a healthy diet and avoid any food that seems to cause pimples.

Skin Problems

Symptoms	Possible Causes
Raised, red, itchy welts or fluid-filled bumps after an insect bite or taking a drug	Allergies, p. 141; Hives, p. 207; Insect and Spider Bites and Stings, p. 60.
Red, painful, swollen bump under the skin	Boils, p. 200.
Red, flaky, itchy skin	Dry Skin, p. 204; Atopic Dermatitis, p. 198; Fungal Infections, p. 205; Rashes, p. 209.
Crusty, honey-colored rash, most often between the nose and upper lip	Impetigo, p. 232.
Rash that develops after wearing new jewelry or clothing, being exposed to poisonous plants, eating a new food, or taking a new drug	Rashes, p. 209; Allergies, p. 141.
Red, itchy, blistered rash	Possible poison ivy, oak, sumac. See Rashes, p. 209; Chickenpox, p. 220.
Painful blisters in a band around one side of the body	Shingles, p. 205.
Change in the shape, size, or color of a mole, or a persistently irritated mole; a sore that does not heal	Skin Cancer, p. 210.
Cracked, blistered, itchy, peeling skin between the toes	Fungal Infections (athlete's foot), p. 205.
Red, itchy, weeping rash on the groin or thighs	Fungal Infections (jock itch), p. 205; Impetigo, p. 232.
Scaly, itchy, bald spots or sores on the scalp	Fungal Infections (ringworm), p. 205.
Flaky, silvery patches of skin, especially on the knees, elbows, or scalp	Psoriasis, p. 199.
Sandpapery skin rash with sore throat and a "raspberry" tongue	Scarlet Fever, p. 168.
Sores on the lip or in the mouth	Canker Sores, p. 201; Cold Sores (fever blisters), p. 202.

Home Treatment

- Cleanliness is essential. Wash your face, shoulders, chest, and back with lukewarm (not hot) water and a very gentle soap, such as Aveeno, Cetaphil, Neutrogena, or Basis. Avoid drying soaps, such as deodorant soaps. Always rinse well.

- Keep long hair off your face and shoulders, and wash it daily.

- Avoid touching your face or other areas that have acne.

- Don't squeeze pimples. This can cause infection and scarring.

- Nonprescription benzoyl peroxide gel or cream is one of the best treatments for acne. Start with the lowest strength, and increase the strength if your skin is able to tolerate it. Apply a very thin layer of the medication once a day, half an hour after washing. It may take up to 2 months to work and may cause mild redness and dryness. Never use more than 5% benzoyl peroxide unless a doctor recommends that you do so.

- Use only water-based lotions and cosmetics that do not clog skin pores (noncomedogenic), and only if they don't aggravate acne.

- Controlling stress may help reduce acne flare-ups. See page 321.

When to Call a Health Professional

- If acne gets worse despite 6 to 8 weeks of home treatment.

- If you have severe red or purple inflammation, cysts, or nodules under the skin.

- If scars develop as acne heals.

- If you develop acne after starting a new medication.

Rosacea

Rosacea causes the nose, cheeks, chin, and forehead to develop acne and become reddened and oily. Tiny blood vessels become visible on the skin's surface. The skin of the nose may become very red and bumpy if the condition is severe. Sometimes called "adult acne," rosacea most often affects young and middle-aged adults.

People who blush easily or whose facial flushing produces a redness that lasts longer than is typical may be more likely to develop rosacea. The condition tends to run in families.

Symptoms of rosacea may get worse in response to spicy foods; alcohol; exposure to sun, heat, or very cold temperatures; strenuous exercise; or certain skin care products, perfumes, or sunscreens.

If you have rosacea, try to identify and avoid things that trigger your symptoms and cause you to flush. Medications can help control pimples and redness. Laser treatment can be used to treat the blood vessels on the surface of the skin and reduce redness.

Atopic Dermatitis

Atopic dermatitis (AD) is a chronic skin disorder that often develops in people who have asthma, hay fever, and other allergies. It causes an itchy, red, raised rash that may weep or ooze clear fluid. The rash may develop tiny blisters, which break and crust over. The blisters are prone to infection, especially if scratching is not controlled.

In children, AD appears most often on the face, scalp, arms, thighs, and torso. AD is often worse during infancy. It improves in many children by age 5 or 6. Most children have outgrown it entirely by their early teens.

In adults, it usually appears on the neck and in the bend of the elbows and knees. Adults whose hands or feet are often exposed to irritating substances, such as chemicals, develop AD on those areas.

Home Treatment

Helping the skin retain moisture is important to successful treatment of AD.

- Take brief, daily baths or showers with lukewarm (not hot) water. Use a gentle soap (such as Dove, Oil of Olay, or Neutrogena) or nonsoap cleanser (such as Cetaphil or Aveeno). If possible, bathe without soap, or use soap in the armpits and groin area only.

- After bathing, pat skin dry and immediately apply a moisturizer (Lubriderm, Moisturel). The moisturizer may help keep your skin from drying out. Reapply it often.

- Use a humidifier in the bedroom.

- Taking an oral antihistamine (such as Benadryl) may help relieve itching and relax you enough to allow sleep. Avoid antiseptic and antihistamine creams and sprays, because they irritate the skin.

- Avoid contact with any irritants or allergens that cause problems. Wear gloves when working with irritating substances.

- Wash clothes and bedding in mild detergent and rinse at least twice. Do not use fabric softener if it irritates your skin. Avoid wools and scratchy fabrics.

- For more tips on relieving itching, see page 204.

When to Call a Health Professional

- If there are crusting or oozing sores, serious scratch marks, or skin discoloration. Also see "Signs of Infection" on page 67.

- If itching interferes with sleep, and home treatment is not working.

- If you cannot control atopic dermatitis with home treatment.

Psoriasis

Psoriasis is a chronic skin condition that causes raised red patches topped with silvery, scaling skin. These usually occur on the knees, elbows, scalp, and back. The fingernails, palms, and soles of the feet may also be affected. Psoriasis can also cause a form of arthritis.

The patches, called plaques, are made of dead skin cells that accumulate in thick layers. Normal skin cells are replaced every 30 days. In people who have psoriasis, skin cells are replaced every 3 to 6 days.

Psoriasis is not contagious. It may come and go. Small patches of psoriasis can often be treated with regular use of hydrocortisone creams. Tar products (lotions, gels, shampoos) may also be useful, although they may increase your skin's sensitivity to the sun. Limited exposure to the sun may also help (protect unaffected skin with sunscreen).

Stress may contribute to psoriasis. Stress reduction may help in some cases. See page 321.

Call your doctor if psoriasis covers much of your body or is very red. Extensive or severe cases often need professional care.

Blisters

Blisters are usually the result of persistent or repeated rubbing against the skin. Some illnesses, such as shingles, cause blisterlike rashes (see page 205). Burns can also blister the skin. See page 45.

Prevention

- Avoid shoes that are too tight or that rub your feet.
- Wear gloves to protect your hands when doing heavy chores.

Home Treatment

- If a blister is small and closed, leave it alone. Protect it from further rubbing by applying a loose bandage. Avoid the activity or shoes that caused the blister to form.
- If a small blister is in a weight-bearing area, protect it with a doughnut-shaped moleskin pad. Leave the area over the blister open.
- If a blister is larger than 1 inch across, it is usually best to drain it. The following is a safe method:
  - Wipe a needle with rubbing alcohol.
  - Gently puncture the edge of the blister.
  - Press the fluid in the blister toward the hole you have made so it can drain.

• Once you have opened a blister, or if it has torn open:

  - Wash the area with soap and water.

  - Do not remove the flap of skin covering a blister unless it is very dirty or torn, or if pus is forming under the skin flap. Gently smooth the skin flap flat over the tender skin underneath.

  - Apply an antibiotic ointment and a sterile bandage. Do not use alcohol or iodine on an open wound. They will delay healing.

  - Change the bandage once a day or anytime it gets wet or dirty to reduce the chance of infection.

  - Remove the bandage at night to let the area dry.

When to Call a Health Professional

• If blisters form often and you do not know the cause.

• If signs of infection develop. See page 67.

• If you have diabetes or peripheral vascular disease and blisters are forming on your hands, feet, or legs.

Boils

A boil is a red, swollen, painful bump under the skin, similar to an overgrown pimple. Boils are often caused by infected hair follicles.

Bacteria from the infection form an abscess or pocket of pus. The abscess can become large and cause severe pain.

Boils occur most often in areas where there is hair and chafing. The face, neck, armpits, breasts, groin, and buttocks are common sites.

Prevention

• Wash boil-prone areas with soapy water. An antibacterial soap may help. Dry thoroughly.

• Avoid clothing that is too tight.

Home Treatment

• Do not squeeze, scratch, drain, or open the boil. Squeezing can push the infection deeper into the skin. Scratching can spread the bacteria to other parts of the body.

• Wash yourself well with an anti-bacterial soap to keep the infection from spreading.

• Apply hot, wet washcloths to the boil for 20 to 30 minutes, 3 to 4 times a day. Do this as soon as you notice a boil. The heat and moisture can help bring the boil to a head, but it may take 5 to 7 days. Applying a hot water bottle or a waterproof heating pad over a damp towel may also help.

• Continue using warm compresses for 3 days after the boil opens. Apply a bandage to keep draining material from spreading, and change the bandage daily.

Calluses and Corns

Calluses and corns are hard, thickened skin that is exposed to friction and pressure. Calluses are common on the soles of the feet, the heels, and the hands. Corns usually form on the toes.

Soak your feet in warm water, and rub the callus or corn with a towel or pumice stone. You may need to do this for several days until the thickened skin is gone. Nonprescription products for removing calluses and corns are also available. If a callus or corn breaks open or becomes sore, see your doctor.

Do not try to cut or burn off corns or calluses. If you have diabetes or peripheral vascular disease, talk with your doctor before attempting to remove troublesome corns or calluses.

When to Call a Health Professional

If needed, your doctor can drain the boil and treat the infection. Call the doctor:

- If the boil is on your face, near your spine, or in the anal area.
- If signs of worsening infection develop. See page 67.
- If any other lumps, particularly painful ones, develop near the infected area.
- If the pain limits your normal activities.

- If you have diabetes.
- If the boil is as large as a Ping-Pong ball.
- If the boil has not improved after 5 to 7 days of home treatment.
- If many boils develop over several months.

Canker Sores

Canker sores are painful, open sores that form on the inside of the mouth. Possible causes of canker sores include injury to the inside of the mouth, infection, certain foods, stress, genetic tendency to get canker sores, and female hormones. The sores usually heal in 7 to 10 days.

Prevention

- Avoid injuring the inside of your mouth:
  - Chew food slowly and carefully.
  - Use a soft-bristle toothbrush, and brush your teeth thoroughly but gently.
  - Don't chew on toothpicks, plastic straws, or other objects.
- Avoid foods that seem to cause sores.
- Don't smoke or chew tobacco products.

Home Treatment

- Avoid coffee, spicy and salty foods, nuts, chocolate, and citrus fruits when you have open sores in your mouth.

- Apply a nonprescription canker sore medication to protect the sore, ease pain, and speed healing.

- Rinse your mouth with an antacid (such as Maalox or Mylanta) or with a mixture of 1 tablespoon of hydrogen peroxide in 8 ounces of water.

- Applying a thin paste of baking soda and water to the sore may relieve pain.

When to Call a Health Professional

- If mouth sores develop after you start taking a medication.

- If a canker sore, or any sore, does not heal in 14 days, or if multiple sores appear.

- If a sore is very painful or recurs frequently.

- If white spots that are not canker sores appear in the mouth and are not improving after 1 to 2 weeks.

Cold Sores

Cold sores (fever blisters) are small, red blisters that usually appear on the lip and outer edge of the mouth. They often weep a clear fluid and scab over after a few days. They are sometimes confused with impetigo (see page 232), which usually develops between the nose and upper lip. The fluid that weeps from impetigo is cloudy and honey-colored, not clear.

Cold sores are caused by a herpes virus. Herpes viruses (chickenpox is another kind) stay in the body after the first infection. Later, something triggers the virus to become active again. Cold sores may appear after colds, fevers, exposure to the sun, stressful times, or during menstruation. Sometimes they develop for no apparent reason.

Prevention

- Avoid kissing a person who has a cold sore. Also avoid direct skin contact with genital herpes sores (see page 279) or herpes sores elsewhere on the body.

- Use sunscreen on your lips and wear a hat if exposure to the sun seems to trigger cold sores.

- Reducing stress may help in some cases. Practice relaxation exercises often. See page 323.

Home Treatment

- Apply ice or a cool, wet towel to the area 3 times a day. This may help reduce redness and swelling.

- Apply petroleum jelly to ease cracking and dryness.

- Use a lip protector such as Blistex or Campho-Phenique to ease the pain. Don't share the product with anyone else.

- Apply vitamin E gel or a product containing aloe vera, goldenseal, or bee propolis to the sore.

- Be patient. Cold sores usually go away in 7 to 10 days.

When to Call a Health Professional

Call if sores last longer than 2 weeks or you have frequent outbreaks of cold sores. A prescription medication may reduce the frequency and severity of outbreaks.

Dandruff

Dandruff occurs when the skin cells of the scalp flake off. This flaking is natural and occurs all over your body. On the scalp, however, flakes can mix with oil and dust to form dandruff. Dandruff cannot be cured, but it can be controlled.

Home Treatment

• Try frequent and thorough shampooing with any shampoo. Wash hair daily if it controls dandruff.

• If dandruff is excessive and itchy, try a dandruff shampoo (such as Head & Shoulders, Sebulex, T-Gel, or Tegrin). Work the dandruff shampoo into your scalp and leave it on for several minutes before rinsing thoroughly.

When to Call a Health Professional

Call if frequent shampooing or shampooing with a dandruff shampoo doesn't control dandruff.

Birthmarks

Birthmarks are relatively common. Most are harmless. Over time they may fade, increase in size or thickness, or stay the same.

Macular stains (sometimes called salmon patches, angel kisses, or stork bites) are light pink birthmarks that appear on the upper lip, eyelids, forehead, and back of the neck. They usually fade within a few months.

Hemangiomas are soft, red, or blue lumps formed by clusters of blood vessels. They may be present at birth or appear during the first few months. They may grow for up to 6 months, stabilize for a short time, and then usually begin to recede and fade. Nearly all disappear by age 9.

Port-wine stains are pink or wine-colored birthmarks that appear most often on the head and face. They are permanent, become darker as the child grows, and may need to be treated by a dermatologist or plastic surgeon to stop them from expanding.

Report any changes in birthmarks to your health professional. Birthmarks need to be removed if they interfere with breathing or vision or disfigure the face. If surgery is desired for cosmetic reasons, it is best to talk with your health professional about the best timing for surgery.

Dry Skin

Dry, itchy, flaky skin is the most common skin problem, especially in the winter. It develops when the skin loses water (not oil) to the air. Dry indoor air is a common cause, as is excessive bathing in hot water.

Prevention

• Avoid showers. They strip the skin's natural oil, which helps hold in moisture. Baths are much kinder to the skin than showers are.

• Use bath oils in the bathwater. Be careful not to slip.

• Use mild soaps (such as Dove or Cetaphil), especially under the arms and in the groin area.

• Use a moisturizing lotion immediately after your bath.

Home Treatment

• Follow the prevention guidelines above.

• For very dry hands, try this for a night: Apply a thin layer of petroleum jelly and wear thin cotton gloves to bed. (Dry feet may benefit from similar treatment.)

• Avoid scratching, which damages the skin. If itching is a problem, see "Relief From Itching" on page 204.

When to Call a Health Professional

• If you itch all over your body but there is no obvious cause or rash.

• If itching is so bad that you cannot sleep, and home treatment is not helping.

• If you have open sores from scratching.

Relief From Itching

• Keep the itchy area well moisturized. Dry skin may make itching worse.

• Take an oatmeal bath to help relieve itching: Wrap 1 cup of oatmeal in a cotton cloth, and boil as you would to cook it. Use this as a sponge and bathe in tepid water without soap. Or try an Aveeno colloidal oatmeal bath.

• Calamine lotion is helpful for poison ivy or poison oak rashes.

• Try a nonprescription 1% hydrocortisone cream for small itchy areas. Use very sparingly on the face or genitals. If itching is severe, your doctor may prescribe a stronger steroid cream or ointment.

• Try a nonprescription oral antihistamine such as Benadryl or Chlor-Trimeton.

• Cut nails short or wear gloves at night to prevent scratching.

• Wear cotton or silk clothing. Avoid wool and acrylic fabrics next to the skin.

Fungal Infections

Fungal infections of the skin most commonly affect the feet, groin, scalp, or nails. Fungi grow best in warm, moist areas of the skin, such as between the toes, in the groin, and in the area beneath the breasts.

Athlete's foot is the most common fungal skin infection. Symptoms include cracked, blistered, and peeling areas between the toes and on the soles of the feet and itching. Athlete's foot often recurs and must be treated each time.

Jock itch causes severe itching and moistness on the skin of the groin and upper thighs. There may be red, scaly, raised areas on the skin that weep or ooze pus or clear fluid.

Ringworm is a fungal infection that grows on the outer layer of skin, hair, or nails.

On the skin, ringworm appears as patches that are clear in the center and have edges that are red, peeling, or have blisterlike bumps. The skin is often very itchy. The rash can spread quickly.

On the scalp and beard, ringworm appears as round or oval patches of baldness, which may be scaly, red, crusty, or swollen with little blisterlike bumps. The hair on the scalp and beard may have flakes that look like dandruff.

Fungal infections of the **fingernails** and **toenails** cause discoloration, cracking, thickening, and often softening of the nails. They are difficult to treat and often cause permanent damage to the nails.

Shingles

Shingles (herpes zoster) is caused by the reactivation of the chickenpox virus in the body years after the initial illness. The virus usually affects one or two of the large nerves that spread outward from the spine, causing pain and a rash in a band around one side of the chest, abdomen, or face. The rash will blister and scab, then clear up over the course of a few weeks.

No one knows what makes the virus active again. Shingles can affect anyone who has had chickenpox. However, older adults and people with weakened immune systems are more likely to get shingles. People with weakened immune systems include those who have had a bone marrow or an organ transplant; have cancer, especially of the lymph system; or are infected with HIV.

Exposure to the shingles rash can cause chickenpox in a person who has not had chickenpox before.

If you suspect shingles, call your doctor or advice nurse to discuss medication that can limit the pain and rash. If possible, call as soon as you notice the rash. Medication works best when it is started immediately.

Thrush is a yeast infection that occurs in the mouth, especially in babies. It causes a white coating inside the mouth, often on the inside of the cheeks, that may look like milk but is hard to remove. Thrush may develop after taking antibiotics. (Yeast infections also develop in the vagina. See page 265.)

Prevention

• Keep your feet clean, cool, and dry. Dry well between the toes after swimming or bathing. Use antifungal powder to prevent infection or reinfection.

• Wear leather shoes or sandals that allow your feet to "breathe," and wear cotton socks to absorb sweat. Use powder on your feet and in your shoes. Give shoes 24 hours to dry between wearings.

• Wear thongs or shower sandals in public pools and showers.

• Keep your groin area clean and dry. Wash and dry well, especially after exercising. Wear cotton underclothes and avoid tight pants and panty hose.

• Teach children not to play with dogs or cats that have bald or mangy spots on their coats.

• Don't share hats, combs, brushes, or towels.

Home Treatment

• Follow the prevention guidelines.

• For athlete's foot and jock itch, use a nonprescription antifungal powder or lotion, such as Micatin, Lamasil, or Lotrimin AF. Always wash the affected area before applying the powder or lotion. Use the medication for 1 to 2 weeks after the symptoms clear up to prevent recurrence. Do not use hydrocortisone cream on a fungal infection.

• Ringworm on the body can be treated with one of the antifungals listed above.

When to Call a Health Professional

• If signs of infection are present. See page 67.

• If you have diabetes and develop athlete's foot. People with diabetes are at increased risk for infection and may need professional care.

• If you experience a sudden loss of patches of hair associated with flaking, broken hairs, and inflammation of the scalp; or if several members of your household are experiencing hair loss.

• If ringworm is severe and spreading or is present on the scalp. Prescription medicine may be needed.

 If a fungal infection does not improve after 2 weeks or clear up after 1 month despite home treatment, you may want to consider prescription medication. Discuss the options with your doctor.

Hives

Hives are raised, red, itchy, often fluid-filled patches of skin (wheals or welts) that may appear and disappear at random. They range in size from less than ¼ inch to 3 inches or more, and they may last a few minutes or a few days.

A single hive commonly develops after an insect sting. Multiple hives often develop in response to a drug, food, or infection. Other possible causes of hives include plant allergies, inhaled allergens, stress, cosmetics, and exposure to heat, cold, sunlight, or natural rubber latex. Often a cause cannot be found.

Home Treatment

- Avoid the substance that causes hives.

- Apply cool water compresses to help relieve itching. Also see page 204.

- Take an oral antihistamine (such as Benadryl or Chlor-Trimeton) to treat the hives and relieve itching. Once the hives have disappeared, decrease the dose of the medication slowly over 5 to 7 days.

When to Call a Health Professional

Call 911 or other emergency services if spreading hives occur with dizziness, wheezing, difficulty breathing, tightness in the chest, or swelling of the tongue, lips, or face.

Call a health professional:

- If hives develop soon after you start taking a new drug.

- If hives cover all or most of your body.

- If hives persist for 24 hours despite home treatment.

Ingrown Toenails

Ingrown toenails usually develop when an improperly trimmed toenail cuts into the skin at the edge of the nail or when you wear shoes that are too tight. Because the cut can easily become infected, prompt care is needed.

Prevention

- Cut toenails straight across and leave the nails a little longer at the corners so that the sharp ends don't cut into the skin.

- Wear roomy shoes, and keep your feet clean and dry.

Home Treatment

- Soak your foot in warm water for 15 minutes to soften the skin around the nail.

- Wedge a small piece of wet cotton under the corner of the nail to cushion the nail and lift it slightly to keep it from cutting the skin. Repeat daily until the nail has grown out and can be trimmed.

- Daily foot soaks in warm water will help relieve swelling or tenderness while toenails grow out.

Cut toenails straight across.

When to Call a Health Professional

• If signs of infection develop. See page 67.

• If you have diabetes or circulatory problems and develop an ingrown toenail.

Lice and Scabies

Lice are tiny, white, wingless insects that may live on the skin, hair, or clothing. They feed by biting the skin and sucking blood. The bites itch and may cause an allergic rash. Head lice live in the hair on the head; body lice live on clothing; and pubic lice (also called crabs) live in the groin, underarms, and eyelashes.

Lice are spread by close physical contact or contact with the clothing, bedding, brushes, or combs of an infected person. Pubic lice can be spread through sexual contact.

Scabies are tiny mites that burrow under the skin and lay eggs. This burrowing causes an allergic rash that may itch intensely. Scabies are often found between folds of skin on the fingers and toes, wrists, underarms, and groin. The scabies mites

are spread through close contact with an infested person or the person's bedding, clothing, or towels. Scabies are usually treated with a prescription medication that is applied over the entire body and left on overnight. Itching may last for several weeks after treatment.

Prevention

Be alert for signs of lice: itching and lice or tiny eggs (nits) attached to the hair shafts of the head. Prompt treatment can help prevent spreading lice to others.

People who have lice or scabies should avoid close contact with others to prevent spreading the insects or mites that cause these conditions.

Home Treatment

• Nix and RID are nonprescription medications for lice. Follow the manufacturer's directions for use exactly. For head lice, comb the hair well with a fine-toothed comb after treatment to remove all nits.

• On the day you start treatment, wash all dirty clothing, bedding, and towels in hot water to help get rid of lice, nits, and mites. Iron or dry clean things that cannot be washed, or freeze them for 24 hours.

• Some schools have a "no nits" policy stating that children may not return to school until they are free of lice nits. Children who have been treated for scabies can return to school after treatment is completed.

• Contact your pharmacist or health department for more information about treatment and preventing reinfestation.

When to Call a Health Professional

Call if treatment with nonprescription medication is not successful. Stronger prescription drugs are available.

Rashes

A rash (dermatitis) is any irritation or inflammation of the skin. Rashes can be caused by illness, allergy, or heat, and sometimes by emotional stress. For rashes related to childhood illnesses, see page 216. If the rash developed after you were bitten by a tick, see page 76.

Poison ivy and other plant rashes are often red, blistered, and itchy and appear in lines where the leaves brushed against the skin.

When you first get a rash, ask yourself these questions to help determine the cause (also see pages 196 and 216):

• Did a rash that is contained to a specific area (localized) develop after you came in contact with anything new that could have irritated your skin: poison ivy, oak, or sumac; soaps, detergents, shampoos, perfumes, cosmetics, or lotions; jewelry or fabrics; new tools, appliances, latex gloves, or other objects? The location of the rash is often a clue to the cause.

• Have you eaten anything new that you may be allergic to?

• Are you taking any new medications, either prescription or nonprescription?

• Have you been unusually stressed or upset recently?

• Is there joint pain or fever with the rash?

• Is the rash spreading?

• Does the rash itch?

poison ivy

poison oak

poison sumac

The oil on the leaves of these plants can cause an uncomfortable, itchy, red skin rash with blisters or hives.

Prevention

• If you are exposed to poison ivy, oak, or sumac, wash your skin with rubbing alcohol or plenty of water within 10 to 15 minutes to get the allergy-causing oil off your skin. This may help prevent or reduce the rash. Use soap only after using plenty of water. Also wash your clothes, your dog, and anything else that may have come in contact with the plant.

• Avoid products that have caused a rash in the past: detergents, cosmetics, lotions, clothing, jewelry, etc.

• Use fragrance- and preservative-free or hypoallergenic detergents, lotions, and cosmetics if you have frequent rashes.

Home Treatment

• Wash affected areas with water. Soap can be irritating. Pat dry thoroughly.

• Apply cold, wet compresses to reduce itching. Repeat frequently. Also see page 204.

• Keep cool, and stay out of the sun.

• Leave the rash exposed to the air. Baby powder can help keep it dry. Avoid lotions and ointments until the rash heals. However, calamine lotion is helpful for plant rashes. Use it 3 to 4 times a day.

• Use hydrocortisone cream to provide temporary relief of itching. Use very sparingly on the face and the genital area.

When to Call a Health Professional

• If signs of infection develop. See page 67.

• If you suspect a medication reaction caused the rash.

• If a rash occurs with fever and joint pain.

• If a rash occurs with a sore throat. See scarlet fever on page 168.

• If a rash appears and you aren't sure what is causing it.

• If a rash does not clear up after 2 to 3 weeks of home treatment.

Skin Cancer

Skin cancer is the most common type of cancer. Most skin cancer is caused by sun damage and occurs on the face, neck, and arms, where sun exposure is greatest. Light-skinned, blue-eyed people are more likely to develop skin cancer. Dark-skinned people have less risk.

Most skin cancers are nonmelanoma skin cancer, which includes basal cell and squamous cell carcinoma. Nonmelanoma skin cancer is rarely life-threatening. Melanoma is a more serious type of skin cancer. It may affect only the skin, or it may spread (metastasize) to other organs and bones. Melanoma can be life-threatening.

 Most nonmelanoma skin cancers are easy to treat if they are caught early. Early surgical removal of thin melanomas can cure the disease in most cases.

Skin cancers differ from noncancerous growths in the following ways:

• They tend to bleed more than noncancerous growths do and are often open sores that do not heal.

• They tend to be slow-growing. However, melanoma may appear suddenly and grow quickly.

Prevention

Most skin cancers can be prevented by avoiding excessive exposure to the sun (including sunlamps). Most damaging sun exposure has occurred by age 20, so keep your children protected (see page 212). Repeated sun exposure and severe sunburns are major factors in some types of skin cancer.

Home Treatment

Examine all areas of your skin with a mirror or with another person's help. Look for unusual moles, spots, bumps, or sores that won't heal. Pay special attention to areas that get a lot of sun exposure: hands, arms, back, chest, neck (especially the back of the neck), face, ears, etc. Report any changes to your doctor.

When to Call a Health Professional

Call your doctor if you notice any unusual skin changes or growths, especially if they bleed and continue to change.

If your moles do not change over time, there is little cause for concern. If you have a family history of malignant melanoma, let your doctor

know because you may be at higher risk for malignant melanoma. Call your doctor if you notice any of the following "ABCD" changes in a mole or other skin growth:

• **A**symmetrical shape: One half does not match the other half.

• **B**order irregularity: The edges are ragged, notched, or blurred.

• **C**olor not uniform: Watch for shades of red and black, or a red, white, and blue mottled appearance.

• **D**iameter: A mole is larger than a pencil eraser. (Harmless moles are usually smaller than this.)

Also call if you notice:

• Scaliness, oozing, bleeding, or spreading of pigment into surrounding skin.

• Appearance of a bump or nodule on the mole, or any change in the appearance of the mole.

• Itching, tenderness, or pain.

Asymmetrical shape

Border irregular

Color varied

Diameter larger than a pencil eraser

Watch for these "ABCD" mole changes.

Sunburn

A sunburn is usually a first-degree burn that involves the outer surface of the skin. Sunburns are painful but can usually be treated at home unless they are extensive. Severe sunburns can be serious in infants, small children, and older adults.

Repeated sun exposure and sunburns increase the risk of skin cancer.

Prevention

If you are going to be outdoors for more than 15 minutes, take the following precautions:

- Wear light-colored, loose-fitting, long-sleeved clothes and a broad-brimmed hat to shade your face. Wear sunglasses that provide ultraviolet (UV) protection.

- Use a sunscreen that has a sun protection factor (SPF) of 15 or higher. Sunscreens labeled "broad spectrum" can protect the skin from the two types of harmful sun rays (UVA and UVB).

- Apply the sunscreen at least 30 minutes before you will be exposed to the sun.

- Apply sunscreen to all the skin that will be exposed to the sun, including the nose, ears, neck, scalp, and lips. It needs to be applied evenly over the skin.

- Reapply sunscreen every 2 to 3 hours while in the sun and more often if you are swimming or sweating a lot.

- Older adults have sensitive skin and should always use a sunscreen with an SPF of 30 or higher.

- Drink lots of water. Sweating helps cool the skin.

- Avoid the sun between 10 a.m. and 4 p.m., when the burning rays are strongest. Seek shade whenever possible.

- Don't forget the kids. Sun exposure may be very hard on their tender skin. Teach your young children safe sun habits—hats and sunscreen—early. Babies should not be exposed to direct sunlight. Do not use sunscreens on babies younger than 6 months.

Home Treatment

- Drink plenty of water and watch for signs of dehydration (especially in infants or children). See page 84. Also watch for signs of heat exhaustion. See page 56.

- Cool baths or compresses can be very soothing. Take acetaminophen or aspirin for pain. Don't give aspirin to anyone younger than 20.

- A mild fever and headache can accompany a sunburn. Lie down in a cool, quiet room to relieve headache.

- There is nothing you can do to prevent peeling; it is part of the healing process. Lotion can help relieve itching.

When to Call a Health Professional

• If you develop signs of heat stroke (red, hot, dry skin; confusion). See page 56.

• If symptoms of heat exhaustion (dizziness, nausea, headache) persist after you have cooled off.

• If you develop signs of severe dehydration. See page 84.

• If you have severe blistering (over 50 percent of the affected body part) or severe pain with fever or if you feel very ill.

• If you have a fever of 102° or higher.

Warts

Warts are skin growths that are caused by a virus. They can appear anywhere on the body. Warts are not dangerous, but they can be bothersome.

Little is known about warts. Most types are only slightly contagious. They can spread to other areas on the same person but rarely to other people. Genital and anal warts are an exception; they are easily transmitted through sexual contact and may increase a woman's risk for cervical cancer. See page 279.

Plantar warts appear on the soles of the feet. Most of the wart lies under the skin surface and may make you feel like you are walking on a pebble.

Warts appear and disappear spontaneously. They can last a week, a month, or even years. Because warts seem to come and go for little reason, it's possible that they are sensitive to slight changes in the immune system. Although there is no scientific explanation for why it works, in some cases you can "think" warts away.

When necessary, your doctor can remove warts. Unfortunately, they often come back.

Home Treatment

• Try the least expensive method of treating warts first. You may save a trip to your doctor. If you find a treatment that works for you, stick with it.

• If the wart bleeds a little, cover it with a bandage and apply light pressure to stop the bleeding.

• If the wart is in the way, rub it with a pumice stone or a file or apply a nonprescription product containing salicylic acid. (If you have diabetes or peripheral vascular disease, do not irritate the wart or use salicylic acid on it without first discussing these treatments with a health professional.)

• If treatment with salicylic acid causes the area to become tender, taking a 2- to 3-day break from treatment may help relieve pain.

• If you use a pumice stone or file, both the debris from the wart and the area of the pumice stone or file that touched the wart can be infectious. Don't use these items for any other purpose or you may spread the wart-causing virus. Wash your hands with soap after you touch the debris from the wart or the pumice stone or file.

• For plantar warts, apply a doughnut-shaped pad to cushion the wart and relieve pain. Before you go to bed, apply salicylic acid to the wart, and cover the wart with a bandage (or wear a sock). Wash the medication off in the morning.

• Don't cut or burn off a wart.

When to Call a Health Professional

• If a wart looks infected after being irritated or knocked off.

• If a plantar wart is painful when you walk, and foam pads do not help.

• If you have warts in the anal or genital area. See page 279.

• If a wart develops on your face and is a cosmetic concern.

 If a wart causes continual discomfort, or if warts are numerous enough to be a problem, they may need to be surgically removed. Talk with your doctor about the risks and benefits of removing warts surgically.

Hair Loss

Many people lose hair as they grow older. Such hair loss is natural and is largely the result of heredity. Balding poses no health risks other than sunburn, which you can prevent by wearing a hat and using sunscreen when outdoors. While men tend to lose hair from the hairline and crown of the head, women's hair becomes thinner all over.

 If you are thinking about medication (such as minoxidil) or surgical treatment for hair loss, make sure you understand the risks of treatment, how many treatments you will need, and how long the results will last.

Bald spots are not the same as baldness. Wearing tight braids or habitually tugging or twisting your hair may cause bald spots. Ringworm is a fungal infection that causes scaly bald spots. See page 205. A condition called alopecia areata causes patchy hair loss that may require treatment with prescription medications.

Thinning hair can signal problems such as thyroid disease or lupus. Emotional or physical stress can cause short-term hair loss, as can changes in hormone levels during pregnancy and menopause.

If hair loss is sudden, or if it develops after you start taking a new medication, call your doctor.

MORE INFO **For more information, see the back cover.**

My mother had a great deal of trouble with me,
but I think she enjoyed it.
Mark Twain

11

Infant and Child Health

When your children get sick or hurt, you are usually the first person to provide care. Your calmness, confidence, and competence in caring for your children's health problems will help them enjoy good health and learn the importance of self-care for their own use as they mature.

Virtually every health problem in this book can affect children. However, a few are almost exclusively childhood concerns. For convenience, we have grouped these problems into this chapter. If the problem you are looking for is not in this chapter, please look for it in the index.

Facts About Infants and Young Children

The following brief notes are of particular concern to parents. This information may help dispel some unnecessary fears and give you some guidance.

Umbilical Cords and Bellybuttons

Clean the bellybutton (navel) 3 to 4 times a day with a bit of cotton moistened with a little rubbing alcohol. Pull the cord up gently but firmly to clean the base. Try not to get alcohol on the skin around the navel.

Keep the cord dry and do not give your baby a tub or pan bath until the cord has fallen off and the navel is healed. Fold diapers below and shirts above the cord to promote drying.

The cord will drop off and the navel will heal in 1 to 3 weeks. After the cord comes off, there may be a moist or bloody oozing for a few days. This does not need special treatment.

Call your doctor if there is redness or swelling around the navel or a large amount of foul-smelling discharge from the navel.

The appearance of the bellybutton is not affected by the way the cord is tied off. A small lump of tissue sometimes remains after the cord falls off.

If the lump is small, treatment is usually not needed. If it is larger and does not fall off after 2 weeks, call your doctor.

Childhood Rashes

Rashes that come with childhood illnesses are hard to tell apart. Review all symptoms before deciding what to do.

Description	Possible Illness
Red, pimplelike spots that turn to blisters; fever	Chickenpox, p. 220.
Rash in diaper area only	Diaper Rash, p. 224.
Red rash on face that looks like slapped cheeks; pink rash that comes and goes on torso; possible fever	Fifth Disease, p. 235.
Red or pink dots on head, neck, shoulders; more common in infants	Prickly Heat, p. 234.
Sudden high fever for 2 to 3 days followed by rose-pink rash on torso, arms, and neck after fever goes down	Roseola, p. 236.
Fine pink rash that starts on face and covers whole body; swollen glands behind ears	Rubella (rare), p. 17.
Fever, runny nose, hacking cough; red eyes 2 to 3 days before spotty red rash covers whole body	Measles (rare), p. 17.
High fever, sore throat, sandpapery rash, and raspberry-textured tongue	Scarlet fever, p. 168.
Blisters on mouth and tongue appearing 1 to 2 days after onset of fever and sore mouth or throat; painless, blistering rash on fingers, hands, feet	Hand-Foot-Mouth Disease, p. 233.

Breast-Feeding

Breast milk is the ideal food for babies younger than 4 to 6 months. The American Academy of Pediatrics recommends that babies be breast-fed for at least the first year of life. However, the length of time that breast-feeding should continue differs for each mother and her child. Although breast-feeding is best, babies can also get good nutrition from formula.

Breast milk contains substances that help your baby resist infections and other diseases. Breast-fed babies have fewer colds and ear infections, less diarrhea, and less vomiting. Breast milk is easier to digest than formula.

Getting some instruction helps ensure that you can breast-feed successfully. If possible, take a breast-feeding class. The La Leche League and the Nursing Mothers Counsel are other good sources of breast-feeding information, advice, and support.

Circumcision

 MORE INFO Circumcision is surgery to remove the foreskin of a newborn boy's penis. There are both benefits and risks associated with circumcision. Discuss them with your doctor. The decision is entirely up to you.

A major benefit is that circumcision makes it easier to keep the penis clean, which reduces your baby's risk for urinary tract infections. Circumcision also reduces the already low risk of penile cancer

The risks of circumcision are slight. Complications of local infection or bleeding occur in about 2 in every 1,000 cases. Local anesthetic reduces the pain of circumcision and is now recommended. Generally, circumcision is not recommended for sick infants.

If you do have your son circumcised, after the procedure apply petroleum jelly liberally to the head of the penis at each diaper change to prevent the scab from sticking to the diaper. Wash the penis by dripping warm water over it (do not use alcohol or baby wipes). Pat dry with a soft towel. Some redness at the circumcision site is normal. Call your doctor if the redness extends down the shaft of the penis, or if there is more than a small amount of blood on the diaper.

If you choose not to have your son circumcised, wash his penis as you would any other body part. Do not try to pull back (retract) the foreskin before age 3, and never forcibly retract the foreskin. Most boys' foreskins are fully retractable by age 5, but some may not fully retract until puberty. Once the foreskin is fully retractable, teach your son to wash his penis well at every bath and to gently retract and wash beneath the foreskin. After puberty he should wash the area under the foreskin daily.

Toilet Training

Every child has a unique timetable for becoming toilet-trained. Most children are ready to begin toilet training between 24 and 30 months of age. Look for these signs of readiness in your child:

• Passes stools at about the same time each day.

• Is able to have a dry diaper for at least 2 hours at a time during the day.

• Makes certain facial expressions when urinating or passing stools.

• Lets you know when a diaper is dirty and asks to have it changed.

• Seems eager to please and can follow simple instructions.

• Tells you that he or she wants to use the toilet or wear adult underwear.

If you think your child is ready to begin toilet training, the following tips may make it go more smoothly:

• Get your child a potty chair. Let the child get used to using the chair by having him or her sit on it with a diaper on when he or she is passing stools or urinating.

• Let your child watch you or a sibling of the same sex use the toilet. Talk with your child about what you are doing.

• Select clothing for your child that is easy to take off. Clothes with elastic waistbands or easy-to-open fasteners, such as Velcro, work best. Pull-on diapers are also helpful.

• Reward every success with hugs and words of praise. Accidental wetting and soiling are common in the first few weeks, but don't scold or punish your child when they happen. Keep a casual attitude.

Bladder control may take longer than bowel control. If the child is aware of when his or her bladder is full, try putting the child on the potty chair every 30 to 60 minutes. Praise the child for success and give gentle encouragement when the child wets his or her pants.

Sleep Habits

Babies have both deep and light sleep cycles. In each sleep cycle, there are 60 minutes of light sleep, 60 to 90 minutes of deep sleep, and another 30 minutes of light sleep. At the end of this cycle, the baby is semi-alert and can be wakened easily.

Parents can help their baby sleep through the night by helping the baby learn to soothe him- or herself back to sleep during the light sleep cycles.

For babies age 4 to 6 months:

• Put the baby in the crib when he or she is drowsy but awake.

• Make middle-of-the-night feedings short and boring.

• As the baby gets older, delay the middle-of-the-night feeding, and discontinue it sometime after age 6 months.

It is safer for a baby to sleep on his or her back to prevent sudden infant death syndrome (SIDS). Do not force a baby into a sleeping position. Babies are capable of moving themselves.

Bed-Wetting

Bed-wetting (enuresis) in children who have never been dry is common, and most children will outgrow it between the ages of 6 and 10. In almost all cases, bed-wetting is really not a disease, but rather a normal variation in development.

In some cases, a child who has been dry for several months or longer may start to wet the bed again. This can happen without a clear cause, or it may be caused by a urinary tract infection or emotional problems.

Home Treatment

 There are a number of ways to deal with bed-wetting. Ask your doctor for advice in managing bed-wetting until your child outgrows it.

• Do not punish, embarrass, or blame your child.

• Have your child empty his or her bladder before bed.

• Remind the child to get up during the night to urinate. Providing a bedside potty chair and night light may help.

• Do not force your child to wear diapers at night. Try waterproof, extra-absorbent underwear instead. A thick pad or a vinyl mattress cover will protect the mattress.

• Encourage the child to take responsibility for changing his or her clothes after wetting, for putting a dry towel down on the bed, and for helping wash bed linens.

• Wash underwear and bedding with ½ cup vinegar to eliminate odor.

When to Call a Health Professional

Your doctor can rule out or treat any physical causes of bed-wetting and help you and your child manage the problem. Call your doctor:

• If bed-wetting occurs with pain or burning during urination or other signs of a urinary tract infection. See page 103.

• If bed-wetting occurs in a child older than 6 years, and home treatment is not successful after 4 to 5 weeks.

• If bed-wetting becomes more frequent or severe despite home treatment.

• If bed-wetting occurs in a child who had previously been dry for several months.

- If a child age 4 or older is wetting the bed and leaking stool.

- If a child over age 3 has daytime bladder control problems after having been toilet-trained.

Chickenpox

Chickenpox (varicella) is usually a relatively minor illness. For the first couple of days, your child will feel ill, with fever, loss of appetite, headache, and fatigue. Then a rash of red, pimplelike spots will appear. A child may have as few as 30 spots, but usually there are hundreds. The rash may cover the child's entire body, including the throat, mouth, ears, groin, and scalp.

The spots turn into clear blisters that become cloudy, break open, and crust over. The rash itches a lot. Spots continue to appear for 1 to 5 days and subside over 1 to 2 weeks.

Chickenpox is very contagious. After exposure to the chickenpox virus, symptoms usually appear in 14 to 16 days. The contagious period starts 1 to 2 days before the rash appears and lasts until all the spots have crusted over. Children can usually return to school or day care after the sixth day of the rash as long as any blisters that have not crusted over are covered with clothing. Encephalitis (see page 162) is a rare complication of chickenpox.

Prevention

The chickenpox vaccine can be given to children age 12 months and older and to teens and adults who have not had the illness. See page 18. It is especially important to immunize teens and adults who have not had chickenpox, because the disease is more severe in adulthood.

Adults who have not been vaccinated and who have not had chickenpox should avoid exposure to children who have it and avoid exposure to people who have shingles (see page 205). Pregnant women who have never had chickenpox and have not been vaccinated should also avoid exposure, since the illness can harm the developing fetus. The vaccine cannot be given during pregnancy.

Home Treatment

- Use acetaminophen to relieve fever. Do not give aspirin to anyone younger than 20 who may have chickenpox because aspirin use is related to Reye syndrome (see page 221).

- Control itching (see page 204). Oral Benadryl and warm baths with baking soda or Aveeno colloidal oatmeal added to the water will help. Avoid Benadryl creams because it is difficult to control the dosage when the medicine is applied to the skin.

- Cut your child's fingernails to prevent scratching. If scabs are scratched off too early, the sores may become infected.

When to Call a Health Professional

- If the child is at risk for complications from chickenpox (is taking steroid medications or receiving cancer chemotherapy, or has a weakened immune system).

- If a child age 3 months to 3 years has a fever of 103° or higher for 24 hours. See Fever on page 228.

- If severe itching cannot be controlled by oral Benadryl and warm baths.

- If bruising appears without injury.

- If sores appear in a child's eyes.

- If you notice signs of encephalitis (see page 162):

  - Fever, severe headache, and stiff neck

  - Unusual sleepiness or lethargy

  - Persistent vomiting

- If a teenager or adult gets chickenpox.

Colic

Colic is not a disease; it is a condition that causes otherwise healthy babies to cry inconsolably, usually in the evening and at night. Doctors aren't sure what causes colic. It is often thought to be caused by abdominal pain due to intestinal gas, but this has not been proven.

Reye Syndrome

Reye syndrome is a rare, serious disease that occurs most often in children 6 to 12 years old. It is rare in people over 18. The cause of Reye syndrome is unknown. It usually occurs after aspirin is given to a child who has a viral illness such as chickenpox or flu. Reye syndrome is not contagious.

Reye syndrome causes changes in the body that affect all the organs but are most harmful to the brain and liver.

Symptoms of Reye syndrome include:

- Sudden onset of persistent vomiting that is not related to having flu.

- Drowsiness and lack of energy.

- Rapid, deep breathing (hyperventilation).

- Behavior changes such as extreme irritability, aggressiveness, or confusion.

If Reye syndrome is not treated immediately, it can lead to seizures, coma, and, in severe cases, death.

Early treatment of Reye syndrome increases the chance for full recovery. Most people have no long-lasting complications and gradually get better after a few weeks. However, some people may have permanent brain damage.

To prevent Reye syndrome, never give aspirin to anyone younger than 20. Give ibuprofen or acetaminophen instead.

All babies cry, so how do you know if your baby has colic? Colic usually follows the "rule of three": Crying starts in the first 3 weeks to 3 months after birth and continues more than 3 hours a day, more than 3 days a week, for more than 3 weeks.

Fortunately, colic goes away as the baby matures, almost always by the end of the fourth month—sooner for many babies. Although no single method always works to relieve colicky babies, there are a number of things you can try. Unfortunately, what works one time may not work the next. Be creative and persistent.

Home Treatment

- Most important: Stay calm and try to relax. If you start to lose control, take a minute to calm down. Never shake a baby; it can cause permanent brain damage and even death.

- Make sure your baby is getting enough to eat, but not too much. The problem may be hunger, not colic.

- Make sure your baby isn't swallowing too much air while eating. Feed the baby slowly, holding him or her almost upright. Burp your baby periodically. Prop your baby up for 15 minutes after feeding.

- If your baby is bottle-fed, use nipples with holes large enough to drip cold formula at least 1 drop per second. Babies will swallow more air from around the nipple if the hole is too small.

- Heat formula to body temperature. Don't overheat.

- Babies may need to suck on something for up to 2 hours a day to be satisfied. If feedings aren't enough, use a pacifier.

- Keep a regular routine for meals, naps, and playtime. Mealtime should be quiet and undisturbed by bright lights and loud noises.

- Make sure your baby's diaper is clean, that he or she isn't too hot, and that your baby isn't bored.

- Don't overstimulate your baby. Some babies cry because there is too much light, noise, activity, or too many people around them.

- Try rocking or walking your baby. Putting him or her stomach-down over your knee or forearm may be helpful.

- Calm your baby with a car ride or a walk outside. Placing your baby near the hum of a clothes dryer, dishwasher, or bubbling aquarium may have a soothing effect.

- Don't worry about spoiling a baby during the first few months; comforting a baby makes both of you feel better.

- Don't leave your baby alone while he or she is crying for more than 5 to 10 minutes. After 10 minutes, try the above suggestions again.

When to Call a Health Professional

 <u>Colic</u> generally does not require professional treatment unless it is accompanied by vomiting, diarrhea, or other signs of a more serious illness. If the baby looks healthy and acts normally between crying episodes, and if your emotions can stand the noise for the first 3 to 4 months, you have little cause for worry.

However, if colic lasts more than 4 hours a day, or if you feel like you need help, contact your doctor for advice.

In rare cases, colic may be so severe that you and your doctor may consider a medication for the baby. Ask about side effects.

Cradle Cap

Cradle cap is an oily, yellow scaling or crusting on a baby's scalp. It is caused by a buildup of normal oils on the skin.

Home Treatment

- Wash your baby's head with baby shampoo once a day. Gently scrub the scalp with a soft-bristled brush (a soft toothbrush works well) for a few minutes to remove the scales. Rinse well.

- You can also rub mineral oil on your baby's scalp an hour before shampooing to loosen the scales.

- If scrubbing with baby shampoo doesn't work, try using a dandruff shampoo, such as Selsun Blue, Head & Shoulders, or Sebulex. Use these products carefully because they can irritate your baby's eyes.

- If the rash looks irritated and red, applying a mild hydrocortisone cream (such as Cortaid) may help.

Croup

Croup is a respiratory problem that develops most often in children from 6 months to 4 years of age. Croup usually accompanies a viral infection, such as a cold. The main symptom is a harsh cough that sounds like a seal's bark and may cause the child to become very frightened. A fever up to 101° is also common. Croup may last 2 to 5 days. Symptoms usually get worse at night, but they generally improve with each passing night.

Home Treatment

- Do whatever you can to calm your child. Crying can make breathing more difficult.

- Get moisture into the air to make it easier for your child to breathe. Use a cool humidifier (do not use a hot vaporizer). Use only water in the humidifier. Set your child in your lap, and let the cool vapor blow directly into your child's face.

• If your child does not improve after several minutes, take him or her into the bathroom and turn on all of the hot water faucets to create steam. Close the door, and sit with your child while he or she breathes in the moist air for several minutes.

• If your child's breathing still does not improve, bundle him or her up and go outside into the cool night air.

When to Call a Health Professional

Call 911 or other emergency services if the child stops breathing or begins to turn blue. Give rescue breathing (see page 40) until help arrives.

Call a health professional:

• If these signs of respiratory distress appear and persist despite home treatment:

  - Squeaky or raspy sound as the child inhales (stridor).

  - Sucking in or retraction between ribs as the child inhales.

  - Flaring nostrils.

• If the child is so short of breath that he or she can't walk or talk.

• If the child drools or is breathing with the chin jutting out and the mouth open.

• If the child is not calm enough to sleep after being in a room with a humidifier or breathing cold outdoor air for 20 minutes.

• If the child has a fever of 102° or higher or any fever that doesn't go away after 48 hours.

• If you or the child becomes hysterical and cannot calm down.

• If this is the first case of croup in your family and you need reassurance.

• If croup lasts longer than 3 nights without improving.

Diaper Rash

Diaper rash is a skin reaction, usually to the moisture and bacteria in a baby's urine and stools, to the soap used to wash diapers, or to disposable diapers. While it is uncomfortable, diaper rash is usually not dangerous.

Symptoms of the rash are a red bottom and thighs. It will be easier for you to recognize diaper rash after you have seen it the first time.

Prevention

• Change diapers as soon as possible after they have been soiled or wet. Check the diaper at least every 2 hours.

• As often as possible, leave your baby's skin open to the air for 5 to 10 minutes before applying a clean diaper.

• Wash cloth diapers with mild detergent and rinse twice. Do not use bleach or fabric softeners.

• If your baby has frequent diaper rash, avoid using plastic pants for a while. They trap moisture against the baby's skin.

• When your baby has diarrhea, protect the diaper area with zinc oxide or another cream (such as Desitin or A & D Ointment).

Home Treatment

• Change diapers frequently. Using a washcloth and water, rinse the skin in the diaper area at every diaper change. Allow the diaper area to air dry if possible. Wash the area with a mild soap once a day.

• Stop using plastic pants when the rash appears.

• Protect healthy skin near the rash with Desitin, Diaparene, A & D Ointment, or zinc oxide cream. Apply cream only to dry, unbroken skin. Discontinue creams if a rash develops or they appear to slow healing.

• Try another brand of disposable diapers. Some babies tolerate one kind better than another. Unscented, noncolored diapers may be less irritating to the skin.

• Avoid bulky or multilayered diapers.

• Try changing detergents if the rash does not clear.

When to Call a Health Professional

• If the diaper rash becomes very red, raw, or sore-looking, or if it has blisters, pus, peeling areas, or crusty patches.

• If the rash is mainly in the skin creases, because this may indicate a yeast infection.

• If a significant rash lasts longer than 3 days.

Diarrhea and Vomiting

Diarrhea and vomiting may be caused by viral stomach flu or by eating unusual kinds or amounts of food. An infant's developing digestive system sometimes will not tolerate large amounts of juice, fruit, or even milk. Breast-fed babies are less likely to develop diarrhea.

Stomach flu often starts with vomiting that is followed in a few hours (sometimes 8 to 12 hours or longer) by diarrhea. Sometimes there is no diarrhea.

Infants and young children, especially those younger than age 1, need special attention when they have diarrhea or are vomiting, because they can quickly become dehydrated. Careful observation of the child's appearance and fluid intake can help prevent problems. For diarrhea in children age 12 and older, see Diarrhea on page 86. For vomiting in children age 4 and older, see Vomiting on page 95.

Home Treatment

Diarrhea in babies up to 1 year:

- If your baby is breast-fed, continue breast-feeding at more frequent intervals to replace lost fluids.

- If your baby is formula-fed, give small feedings at more frequent intervals to make up for lost fluids.

- Supplement feedings with a children's oral electrolyte solution (such as Pedialyte, Ricelyte, or a store brand) only if signs of dehydration develop (see page 84). The amount of electrolyte solution your baby needs depends on his or her weight and degree of dehydration. Call your doctor if your baby shows signs of dehydration.

- You can give the oral electrolyte solution a little at a time in a dropper, spoon, or bottle. For children over 6 months of age, you can improve the taste by adding a pinch of NutraSweet or sugar-free Kool-Aid or Jell-O powder.

- Don't use sports drinks, fruit juice, or soda to treat dehydration. These drinks contain too much sugar and not enough of the minerals (electrolytes) that are being lost. Do not give your baby plain water.

- Don't use oral electrolyte solutions as the sole source of fluid for more than 12 to 24 hours.

- Offer your baby easily digestible solid foods (cereal, strained bananas, mashed potatoes) if he or she was eating them before.

- Protect the diaper area with Desitin, Diaparene, A & D Ointment, or zinc oxide cream. Diaper rash is common after diarrhea.

Diarrhea in children 1 year through 11 years:

- Give ½ cup to 1 cup of a children's oral electrolyte solution, half-strength orange juice, or plain water (if the child is eating food) each hour. Add Nutra-Sweet flavorings if needed. Allow your child to drink as much as he or she wants.

- Don't give your child apple juice, chicken broth, sports drinks, soft drinks, or ginger ale. These drinks do not contain the right mixture of minerals and sugar to restore lost fluids and may make the diarrhea worse.

- Give your child frequent small meals of easily digestible foods (cooked cereal, crackers, mashed potatoes, applesauce, bananas). Avoid foods that contain a lot of sugar. Don't use an electrolyte solution as the sole source of fluids and nutrients for more than 24 hours.

As the child gets better, the stools will become smaller and less frequent. Some types of diarrhea may cause watery stools for 4 to 6 days. Watch for signs of dehydration (see page 84). You can treat the illness at home as long as the child is taking in enough fluids and nutrients, is urinating normal amounts, and seems to be improving.

For home treatment of diarrhea in children 12 and older, see page 86.

Vomiting in babies up to 6 months:

• Do not feed your baby anything for 30 to 60 minutes after he or she has vomited. Watch your baby closely for signs of dehydration.

• Do not give your baby plain water.

• If your baby is breast-fed, offer short but frequent feedings.

• If your baby is formula-fed, switch to an oral electrolyte solution (such as Pedialyte or Ricelyte). Offer 1 tablespoon every 10 minutes for the first hour, and double the amount every 20 minutes each hour that your child does not vomit. You can return to regular feedings once 6 hours have passed without your child vomiting.

Vomiting in children 7 months through 3 years:

• After 1 hour has passed since your child last vomited, give 1 ounce of a clear liquid (not plain water) every 20 minutes for 1 hour. Double the amount every 20 minutes each hour that your child does not vomit. Clear liquids that are safe include children's oral rehydration solution, fruit juice mixed to half strength with water, clear broth, and gelatin dessert.

• Do not use sports drinks (such as Gatorade or Allsport), undiluted fruit juice, or soda. These drinks contain too much sugar. Do not offer plain water or diet soda

because they lack the calories and essential minerals your child needs.

• Offer your child regular foods after 6 hours with no vomiting. Avoid high-fiber foods (such as beans) and foods with a lot of sugar, such as candy or ice cream.

For home treatment of vomiting in children 4 and older, see page 95.

When to Call a Health Professional

• If vomiting occurs with severe headache, sleepiness, lethargy, or a stiff neck. See "Encephalitis and Meningitis" on page 162.

• If the diarrhea is bloody, tarry, or dark red.

• If the urine becomes bloody or cola-colored.

• If there is blood in the vomit.

• If signs of severe dehydration appear (also see page 84):

  - Sunken eyes, no tears, dry mouth and tongue.

  - Sunken soft spot (fontanelle) on an infant's head.

  - Little or no urine for 8 hours.

  - Skin that is doughy or doesn't bounce back when pinched.

  - Rapid breathing and heartbeat.

  - Sleepiness, lethargy, listlessness, and extreme irritability.

- If a child with diarrhea or vomiting refuses to drink or cannot take in enough liquid to replace lost fluids.

- If severe vomiting (vomiting most or all clear liquids and feedings) occurs in an infant younger than 3 months of age. In older children, call if severe vomiting continues:

  - Longer than 4 hours in an infant age 3 to 12 months.

  - 8 hours in a child age 1 to 3 years.

- If occasional vomiting occurs without other symptoms and the child is able to keep fluids down between vomiting episodes. Call if this continues longer than:

  - 1 to 2 days in an infant under 3 months of age.

  - 2 to 4 days in an infant age 3 to 6 months.

  - 1 to 2 weeks in a child age 7 months to 3 years.

- If severe diarrhea (large loose stools every 1 to 2 hours) continues for longer than:

  - 4 hours in an infant under 3 months of age.

  - 8 hours in an infant age 3 to 6 months.

  - 24 hours in a child age 7 months to 4 years.

- If mild to moderate diarrhea continues without obvious cause or other symptoms for longer than:

  - 24 hours in an infant under 3 months of age.

  - 1 to 2 days in an infant age 3 to 6 months.

  - 4 days in a child age 7 months to 4 years.

- If the child has a fever of 103° or higher or a lower fever with diarrhea for more than 12 hours.

- If the child has stomach pain that:

  - Is severe.

  - Is persistent, with frequent vomiting for more than 12 hours but little or no diarrhea.

  - Starts several hours before the vomiting begins and seems like more than just stomach cramps.

  - Is localized to one part of the abdomen, especially the lower right section. See illustration on page 79. This may be difficult to determine in a small child.

Fever

Fever is usually defined as a rectal temperature above 100.4°.

For information about taking accurate temperatures in infants and children, see page 340. All temperatures listed in this section are rectal temperatures. Rectal temperatures are the most accurate for checking for fever in a child.

In most but not all cases, fever indicates that an illness is present. By itself, a fever is not harmful; in fact, it may help the body fight infections more effectively.

In children, viral infections, such as colds, flu, and chickenpox, can cause high fevers. Flu (see page 161) can cause a high fever for 5 days or longer. Bacterial infections, such as strep throat and ear infections, also cause fevers. Teething does not cause a fever. If a baby is teething and has a fever, other symptoms may be present that need to be evaluated. Body temperature can also rise above normal when an infant is overdressed or in a room that is too warm.

Children tend to run higher fevers than adults do. Although high fevers are uncomfortable, they do not often cause medical problems. Seizures from fever occur only occasionally. See page 230.

There is no medical evidence that fevers from infection can cause brain damage. The body limits a fever caused by infection from going above 106°. However, heat from an external source (like sunshine on a parked car) can cause the body temperature to go above 107°, and brain damage can occur rapidly.

Home Treatment

It can be hard to know when to call your doctor when your child has a fever, especially during the cold and flu season.

The height of a fever may not be related to the seriousness of the illness. The way your child looks and acts is a better guide than the thermometer is.

Most children will be less active when they have a fever. If your child is comfortable and alert, eating well, drinking enough fluids, urinating normal amounts, and seems to be improving, home treatment is all that is needed.

- Encourage the child to drink extra fluids or suck on frozen fruit pops.

- Dress the child lightly, and do not wrap him or her in blankets.

If the fever is higher than 102° and your child is uncomfortable:

- Give acetaminophen or ibuprofen. Do not give aspirin to anyone younger than 20 because of the risk of Reye syndrome (see page 221).

- Keep encouraging the child to drink extra fluids, and watch for signs of dehydration (see page 84).

When to Call a Health Professional

- If fever occurs with vomiting, severe headache, sleepiness, lethargy, stiff neck, or a bulging soft spot on an infant's head. See "Encephalitis and Meningitis" on page 162.

- If fever is accompanied by these symptoms:

  - Rapid, difficult breathing.

  - Drooling or inability to swallow.

- Purple rash that does not lighten when you press on it.

- Vomiting, diarrhea, and stomach pain (see page 225).

- Signs of dehydration (see page 84).

- Unexplained skin rash (see page 216 for common childhood illnesses that cause rashes).

- Ear pain (babies often pull at painful ears). See Ear Infections on page 179.

- Pain when urinating (crying when urinating), not caused by painful diaper rash.

- New swelling, pain, redness, or warmth in one or more joints.

- Any unusual or severe pain.

• If an infant younger than 3 months of age has a fever of 100.4° or higher.

• If a child age 3 months to 3 years has a fever that:

- Is 105° or higher.

- Is 104° or higher and does not come down after 4 to 6 hours of home treatment.

- Is 102° to 104° and does not come down after 12 hours.

- Is 100.4° to 102° and does not come down after 24 to 48 hours.

• If the child has a fever and seems sicker than you would expect from a viral illness, such as a cold or the flu.

• If the child becomes delirious or has hallucinations.

• If the child's fever began after he or she took a new medication.

For fever in children age 4 and older, see page 159.

Fever Seizures

Fever seizures are uncontrolled muscle spasms that can happen while a child's temperature is rapidly rising (sometimes the seizure occurs before you are even aware that the child has a fever). Once a child's fever has reached a high temperature, the risk of a seizure is probably over.

A child who is having a fever seizure will lose consciousness. The child's muscles will stiffen, and his or her teeth will clench. Then the child's arms and legs will start to jerk. The child's eyes may roll back, and he or she may stop breathing for a few seconds. The child might also vomit, urinate, or pass stools. Seizures usually last 1 to 5 minutes.

Although frightening, fever seizures in children age 6 months to 5 years are seldom serious and do not cause harm. Two to 4 percent of children in this age group are prone to fever seizures. About 30 percent of children who have a fever seizure will have another one in the future.

Child Car Seats

Infant and child car seats save lives. Many states require them for all children under age 4 and those weighing less than 40 pounds. Children who are not in car seats can be seriously injured or killed during crashes or even abrupt stops at low speeds. For maximum safety, follow the manufacturer's recommendations for car seat use.

All children under age 12 should be in the backseat, especially if the car has air bags.

Infants under 20 pounds, regardless of age: Use an infant car seat that reclines and faces the rear.

Infants younger than 1 year, regardless of weight: Use an infant car seat that reclines and faces the rear.

Children over 20 pounds and older than 1 year: Use a toddler seat that faces the front of the car and has a shield or harness. Some infant seats can be converted to toddler seats.

Children over 40 pounds and over age 4: Use a booster seat that raises the child so that the regular lap and shoulder belts fit properly. Adjust the shoulder belt to fit across the shoulder, not the neck. Use the booster seat until your child is big enough to use the seat belt properly.

Set a good example for your children by always wearing your own seat belt, and always insist that they buckle up.

Home Treatment

During a seizure:

- Try to stay calm, because that will help calm the child.

- Protect the child from injury. Ease the child to the floor, or hold a very small child facedown on your lap. Do not restrain the child.

- Turn the child onto his or her side. This will help clear the mouth of any vomit or saliva and will keep the airway open so the child can breathe.

- Do not put anything in the child's mouth to prevent tongue biting, because it may injure the child.

- Time the length of the seizure, if possible.

After a seizure:

- If the child is having difficulty breathing, turn his or her head to the side and, using your finger, gently clear the mouth of any vomit or saliva so the child can breathe.

- Check for injuries.

- Give acetaminophen or ibuprofen and lukewarm sponge baths if the fever is higher than 102° and your child is uncomfortable. Do not give aspirin to anyone younger than 20.

- Put the child in a cool room to sleep. Drowsiness is common following a seizure. Check the child often. The child should return to his or her normal behavior and activity level within 60 minutes after the seizure.

When to Call a Health Professional

Call 911 or other emergency services:

- If the child stops breathing for longer than 30 seconds or has difficulty breathing. Begin rescue breathing (see page 40).

- If a seizure lasts longer than 10 minutes, or if a second seizure occurs.

Call your health professional:

- If the child is younger than 6 months of age, is 5 years old or older, or if the seizure only affects one side of the body.

- If fever occurs with vomiting, severe headache, sleepiness, lethargy, stiff neck, or a bulging soft spot on an infant's head. See "Encephalitis and Meningitis" on page 162.

- If a seizure occurs without fever.

- If it is the child's first seizure, or if you haven't discussed with your doctor what to do if there is another one.

See page 229 for information on when to call a doctor because of fever.

Impetigo

Impetigo is a bacterial infection that is much more common in children than in adults. It often starts when a small cut or scratch becomes infected. Symptoms are oozing, honey-colored, crusty sores that often appear on the face between the upper lip and nose, especially after a cold. Scratching the sores may spread impetigo to other parts of the body.

Prevention

- Wash all scratches and sores with soap and water.

- If your child has a runny nose, keep the area between the child's upper lip and nose clean to prevent infection.

- Keep your child's fingernails short and clean.

Home Treatment

Small areas of impetigo may respond well to prompt home treatment.

- Remove crusts by soaking the area in warm water (use a warm washcloth for the face) for 15 to 20 minutes; then scrub gently with a washcloth and antibacterial soap. Pat dry gently; do not rub. Repeat several times a day.

- Apply an antibiotic ointment. Cover the area with gauze taped well away from the sores. This will help keep the infection from spreading and prevent scratching.

- Adult men with impetigo should shave around the sores, not over them, and use a clean blade daily. Do not use a shaving brush.

• To prevent spreading the infection, do not share towels, washcloths, or bath water.

When to Call a Health Professional

• If impetigo covers a total area larger than 2 inches in diameter.

• If impetigo does not improve after 3 to 4 days of home treatment, or if any new infected areas appear. Your doctor may prescribe an antibiotic.

• If there is facial swelling or tenderness, especially near the nose and lips.

• If other signs of infection develop. See page 67.

Pinworms

Pinworms are tiny, threadlike worms that infect the digestive tract. Pinworms are most common in school-age children, although anyone can become infected. The worms live in the upper end of the large intestine, near the appendix, and travel to the outside of the anus to lay their eggs.

The egg-laying almost always occurs at night and usually causes the child to scratch the anal area. When the child later sucks a thumb or licks a finger, the eggs are ingested and the cycle begins again. The eggs are very sticky and can survive on clothing and bedding for days, where they can be picked up by other family members.

Hand-Foot-Mouth Disease

Hand-foot-mouth disease is a viral illness that affects many children under 10 as well as young adults. It usually develops during the summer and fall months. Fever, sore throat or mouth, and loss of appetite are early symptoms. Within 2 days, blisters form in the mouth and on the tongue. In children, a painless, blistering rash often develops on the fingers, palms of the hands, and soles of the feet. Infants may also develop a red rash on the buttocks.

There is no treatment for hand-foot-mouth disease other than to give acetaminophen to reduce fever and mouth pain and to make sure the person drinks plenty of fluids. Do not give aspirin to anyone younger than 20. Offer soft, bland foods and cool or warm (not hot) beverages. Frozen fruit pops may help relieve mouth soreness. Calamine lotion may help soothe the rash on the hands and feet.

The virus that causes hand-foot-mouth disease is easily spread, so a person should not go to day care, school, or work while symptoms are present. All symptoms should go away after about a week. The virus is spread through contact with mouth and nasal fluids and stools, so careful hand washing after blowing a runny nose or changing a diaper is important.

Anal itching, especially at night, is the most common symptom of pinworm infection. If the infection is severe, there may also be loss of appetite, itching in the genital area, and pain when urinating. In many cases, pinworm infection does not cause any symptoms.

Prevention

Pinworms affect many families and are hard to avoid if you have young children. Teach children to wash their hands after using the toilet and before meals.

Follow the home treatment guidelines to prevent reinfection and the spread of pinworms to others.

Home Treatment

- Ask your pharmacist for a nonprescription medication for pinworms. The medication may not be given to children younger than 2 years or used by women who are pregnant.

- Treat every child in the house between the ages of 2 and 10. If infection recurs, consider treating everyone in the family who is older than 2.

- On the first day of treatment, wash all underwear, nightclothes, bedding, and towels in hot water and detergent to get rid of any eggs and prevent reinfection. Sanitize toilet and sleeping areas with a strong disinfectant.

- Trim and keep children's fingernails short.

- Require frequent hand washing, morning showers, and daily changes of pajamas and underwear.

When to Call a Health Professional

- If a person has symptoms of pinworm infection, but you have not seen any worms. If this is the first infection, it is recommended that a health professional confirm the diagnosis.

- If the pinworm medication causes side effects, such as vomiting or pain.

- If you continue to have symptoms of pinworm infection despite using a nonprescription medication. Stronger prescription medications are available.

- If a person who has a pinworm infection develops any of the following:
  - Fever or abdominal pain.
  - Redness, tenderness, swelling, or itching in the genital area.
  - Pain when urinating.

Prickly Heat (Sweat Rash)

Prickly heat, also called heat rash, sweat rash, or miliaria, is a rash of red or pink dots that appears on an infant's head, neck, and shoulders. The dots look like tiny pimples.

Prickly heat often develops when parents dress their baby too warmly, but it can develop in any baby when the weather is hot. An infant should be dressed just as lightly as an adult and will be comfortable at the same temperature. It is normal for a baby's hands and feet to feel cold to the touch.

Prevention

Do not overdress your baby. Place your hand between the baby's shoulder blades. If the skin is hot or moist, the baby is too warm.

Home Treatment

- Dress the baby in as few clothes as possible during hot weather.
- Keep the baby's skin cool and dry.
- Keep the baby's sleeping area cool.

When to Call a Health Professional

- If the rash looks infected or lasts longer than 3 days. See "Signs of Infection" on page 67.
- If the infant looks sick.
- If prickly heat is accompanied by a fever of 100.4° in an infant younger than 3 months of age, and the fever doesn't come down within 20 minutes after you remove extra clothing from the infant.

Fifth Disease

Another common childhood illness that causes a rash is erythema infectiosum, or "fifth disease." The main symptom is a red rash on the face that looks like slapped cheeks and a lacy, pink rash on the backs of the arms and legs, torso, and buttocks. There may be a low fever. The rash may come and go for several weeks in response to changes in temperature and sunlight.

A child with fifth disease is most contagious the week before the rash appears. Once the rash has developed, the child is no longer contagious.

Home treatment for fifth disease consists of keeping the child comfortable and watching for signs that a more serious illness is present (fever over 102°; child seems very sick).

Fifth disease is harmless in children, but it poses a slight risk to developing fetuses. Pregnant women should avoid exposure if possible. If you are pregnant and are exposed to a child with fifth disease, or if you develop a rash similar to the one described above, contact your obstetrician.

Roseola

Roseola (roseola infantum) is a mild viral illness that often starts with a sudden high fever (103° to 105°) and irritability. The fever lasts 2 to 3 days. As the fever drops, a rosy pink rash appears on the torso, neck, and arms. The rash may last 1 to 2 days.

Since the fever is quite high and may come on quickly, fever seizures may occur (see page 230).

Roseola is most common in children from 6 months to 2 years of age. It is rare after age 4.

Home Treatment

• If the child has a fever over 102° and is uncomfortable, give acetaminophen or ibuprofen. Do not give aspirin to anyone younger than 20 because of the risk of Reye syndrome (see page 221).

• Give the child lots of liquids.

• If a fever seizure occurs, see page 231.

When to Call a Health Professional

See When to Call a Health Professional under Fever on page 229.

I live with the expectation that life is not fragile;
that if I push, it will not break.
Andrew Sullivan

12

Chronic Conditions

Most of the conditions described in this book are acute illnesses, which means that they get better after a short while. Chronic conditions, on the other hand, last long periods of time or come and go, often for the rest of your life. Having a chronic disease does not mean you can no longer enjoy the good things in life. Chronic diseases may not be curable, but they can often be controlled.

Some conditions that can be chronic are covered in other places in this book:

- Allergies, see page 141.

- Arthritis, see page 121.

- Asthma, see page 146.

- Back pain, see page 107.

- Bronchitis (chronic obstructive pulmonary disease, or COPD), see page 149.

- Depression, see page 309.

- Fibromyalgia, see page 134.

- Headaches, see page 187.

- Irritable bowel syndrome, see page 91.

- Neck pain, see page 117.

- Osteoporosis, see page 135.

- Skin conditions such as acne and psoriasis, see pages 195 and 199.

Diabetes

During digestion the starches and sugars in the food you eat are converted to glucose, a sugar that your body uses for energy. Insulin is a hormone produced by the pancreas that helps control the amount of glucose in your blood. Without insulin, your body cannot use or store glucose, so too much sugar stays in your blood. Over a long period of time, high blood sugar levels may damage blood vessels and nerves, increasing your risk for problems that can affect the eyes, heart, kidneys, legs, and feet.

Type 1 diabetes occurs when the pancreas makes little or no insulin. Type 1 diabetes usually develops in childhood or adolescence but can develop at any age. People with type 1 diabetes must give themselves insulin shots every day.

Type 2 diabetes occurs when the pancreas cannot make enough insulin to meet the body's needs or when the body does not use insulin properly. Many people with type 2 diabetes are able to control their blood sugar by getting regular exercise; eating a healthy diet; maintaining a healthy weight; and frequently testing their blood sugar. Some may need insulin shots or oral medications to lower their blood sugar.

Risk factors for type 2 diabetes include:

• Having a family history of type 2 diabetes.

• Being age 45 or over.

• Being overweight (20 percent more than your healthy weight) or having a large percentage of body fat in the abdominal area.

• Having a physically inactive lifestyle.

• Having high blood pressure (above 140/90). See page 243.

• Having an HDL cholesterol level below 40 or triglycerides above 250. See page 240.

• Being of African-American, Hispanic, Pacific Island, Asian-American, or Native American descent.

• Having a history of diabetes during pregnancy (gestational diabetes) or having given birth to a baby over 9 pounds.

• Taking large amounts of steroids.

The symptoms of diabetes vary from person to person and are common to many conditions. A person may believe that his or her symptoms are related to an illness or to aging, not diabetes. Symptoms include:

• Dry mouth and increased thirst.

• Frequent urination (especially at night).

• Increased appetite.

• Unexplained weight loss.

• Weakness, tiredness, and dizziness.

• Frequent skin infections and slow-healing wounds.

• Recurrent vaginal infections.

• Blurry vision.

• Tingling or numbness in the hands or feet.

Your doctor needs to do a blood test to accurately diagnose diabetes.

Prevention

At this time, there is no known way to prevent type 1 diabetes.

The risk for developing type 2 diabetes runs in families and increases with age. However, even if you have a history of type 2 diabetes in your family, you may be able to prevent or delay its onset by maintaining a healthy body weight and exercising regularly.

Home Treatment

- If insulin or other medications are prescribed to keep your blood sugar within a safe range, take them as directed. If you improve your diet and exercise regularly, you may need less medicine. Check with your doctor before making any changes in your medication.

- Eat a healthy diet to help keep your blood sugar within a safe range and maintain a healthy weight. Pay special attention to eating low-fat foods and to the other diet recommendations in the Nutrition chapter starting on page 293.

- Get regular aerobic exercise to help regulate your blood sugar level, reduce your risk for heart disease, and control your weight. Work closely with your doctor to determine how your activity level affects your blood glucose levels and medication needs.

- It may help you to keep your blood sugar level within the safe range if you track the following daily:

  - The time and content of each meal you eat.

  - The kind and amount of exercise you get.

  - How tired or energetic you feel.

- Check and record your blood sugar level as often as directed by your doctor. This record will help you understand how your body reacts to different foods and exercise, so you can keep your blood sugar level in the safe range.

- Take good care of your feet, and check them daily for blisters, cracks, and sores. Diabetes may damage nerves and reduce blood flow to your feet, increasing your risk for infection while making you less likely to notice a problem.

- Have an eye exam every year. Eye changes caused by diabetes often have no symptoms until they are quite advanced. Diabetic retinopathy is one form of diabetic eye disease that can cause blindness. Early detection and treatment of diabetic retinopathy may slow its progress and save your sight.

- Have regular medical checkups. Talk to your doctor about how often you need them.

- Wear a medical alert bracelet in case of an emergency.

- Attend a diabetes education program to learn more about how to take good care of yourself.

 Believe that you can live a healthy life with diabetes. Controlling diabetes requires making significant, long-term lifestyle changes that may seem overwhelming at first. However, if you adopt a "take charge" attitude about your health and focus on making one change at a time, you are more likely to be successful. Work with your doctor to develop a treatment plan that fits your needs.

The National Diabetes Information Clearinghouse (1 Information Way, Bethesda, MD 20892-3560) is a good resource for more information about diabetes.

When to Call a Health Professional

Call 911 or seek emergency services if a person with diabetes is losing consciousness or becomes unconscious.

Call your health professional:

- If these signs of unusually high blood sugar develop in a person who has diabetes:
  - Frequent urination
  - Intense thirst
  - Blurry vision
  - Weakness, drowsiness
  - Fast breathing
  - Fruity-smelling breath

- If these signs of low blood sugar occur often or last longer than 15 minutes after a person who has diabetes has eaten something that contains sugar:
  - Sweating
  - Fatigue, weakness, shakiness, nausea
  - Extreme hunger
  - Blurry vision, dizziness, headache
  - Rapid heartbeat, anxiousness
  - Confusion, irritability, slurred speech

- If your blood sugar level continues to fall outside the range your doctor has recommended.

- If you have been diagnosed with diabetes and are sick, particularly if you are unable to eat or are vomiting.

- If you have diabetes and you suspect or know that you are pregnant.

- To get a blood sugar test if you suspect that you have diabetes but have not yet been diagnosed.

High Cholesterol

Cholesterol is a type of fat that is produced by your body and is also found in foods that come from animal sources (meat and dairy products, poultry, and fish). Your body's cells need cholesterol to function properly. However, excess cholesterol in the blood can build up inside your arteries (atherosclerosis), causing them to narrow. Atherosclerosis is the starting point for most heart and circulation problems.

Good and Bad Cholesterol

Cholesterol travels through your bloodstream attached to protein, in a combination called a lipoprotein. Two lipoproteins are the main carriers of cholesterol: low-density lipoprotein (LDL) and high-density lipoprotein (HDL). High-density lipoproteins contain more protein than fat.

- LDL ("bad cholesterol") carries cholesterol from the liver to other parts of the body. Under certain conditions, LDL cholesterol can build up on the walls of the arteries. Having a high LDL cholesterol level increases your risk for coronary artery disease (CAD), heart attack, and stroke.

- HDL ("good cholesterol") helps clear LDL cholesterol from the body by picking up cholesterol from the bloodstream and taking it back to the liver for disposal. Increasing your HDL cholesterol level may reduce your risk for heart disease, stroke, and peripheral vascular disease.

Triglycerides are another type of fat that can be found in the bloodstream. A high triglyceride level may increase your risk of coronary artery disease and stroke.

What Do the Numbers Mean?

There are guidelines doctors rely on to evaluate your cholesterol numbers and assess your risk for heart disease. The importance of the numbers varies from person to person, depending on whether a person has additional risk factors for heart disease or actually has heart disease. The following ranges apply to people who are at average risk for heart disease.*

Total cholesterol

Desirable: Less than 200

Borderline high: 200 to 239

High: 240 and above

HDL cholesterol

High (desirable): Above 60

Acceptable: 40 to 60

Low (not desirable): Less than 40

LDL cholesterol

Optimal: Less than 100

Near optimal: 100 to 129

Borderline high: 130 to 159

High: 160 to 189

Very high: 190 and above

Triglycerides

Normal: Less than 150

Borderline high: 150 to 199

High: 200 to 500

Very high: Above 500

Figures provided by the National Cholesterol Education Program (NCEP) of the National Institutes of Health (NIH).

Cholesterol Screening

Basic cholesterol screening tests are easy, quick, and inexpensive. Call your local health department to find out when free or low-cost cholesterol tests may be available.

You and your doctor can determine the schedule that is best for you based on your risk factors for coronary artery disease. Most healthy adults who are not at high risk should have their cholesterol tested every 3 to 5 years. Another recommendation is to start cholesterol screening at age 35 for men and age 45 for women.

If your total cholesterol is over 200 mg/dl (milligrams per deciliter), or if you have any of the following risk factors for coronary artery disease, you may want to have your cholesterol checked more often:

- Having a family history of early heart attack (before age 55 in father or brother; before age 65 in mother or sister)
- Being a cigarette smoker
- Having high blood pressure (over 140/90) or taking high blood pressure medication
- Having diabetes
- Having an HDL level below 40
- Having a triglyceride level over 150

If your total cholesterol is over 200 mg/dl, and you don't know what your HDL and LDL levels are, more extensive testing can help you better estimate your actual risk.

How to Reduce Your Cholesterol

 For most people, a diet low in saturated fat and regular exercise are all that are needed to lower cholesterol. People who have very high cholesterol, diabetes, or coronary artery disease (or who are at very high risk for CAD) may need medication as well as exercise and a low-fat diet to lower their cholesterol.

To reduce your cholesterol:

- Eat less total fat, especially saturated fat. Follow the guidelines for eating less fat on page 297.
- Attend a nutrition workshop or consult a registered dietitian to learn ways to lower your saturated fat intake to 7 percent or less of total calories and your dietary cholesterol to less than 200 mg per day. Your total fat intake can be up to 35 percent of total calories, as long as most of it is unsaturated fat.
- Eat 2 to 3 servings (4 to 6 ounces) of baked or broiled fish per week. The safety and value of fish oil supplements is not yet known.
- Eat more soluble fiber (fruit, dry beans and peas, cereal grains). See page 296.

MORE INFO **For more information, see the back cover.**

- Exercise more. Exercise increases your HDL cholesterol level and may lower your LDL level.

- Quit smoking. Smoking increases the risk of heart attack and stroke, even in people with low cholesterol.

- Lose weight. Losing even 5 to 10 pounds can lower triglyceride levels and raise HDL levels. In some people, LDL levels may fall as well.

High Blood Pressure

Blood pressure is a measurement of the force of blood against the walls of the arteries. Blood pressure readings include two numbers, for example, 130/80. The first number in the reading is called the systolic pressure. It is the force that blood exerts on the artery walls as the heart contracts. The second number in the reading is the diastolic pressure. It is the force that blood exerts on the artery walls between heartbeats, when the heart is at rest.

If an adult's blood pressure readings are consistently above 140 systolic and 90 diastolic, he or she is said to have high blood pressure (hypertension).

Despite what a lot of people think, high blood pressure usually does not cause headaches, dizziness, or lightheadedness. Often called the "silent killer," high blood pressure usually has no symptoms. High blood pressure increases your risk for heart attack, stroke, and kidney or eye damage. Your risk of developing these problems increases as your blood pressure rises.

Risk factors for high blood pressure and its complications include:

- Smoking.

- Being overweight.

- Having a family history of high blood pressure.

- Being of African-American descent.

- Having an inactive lifestyle.

- Drinking too much alcohol.

- Having too much salt or not enough potassium, calcium, or magnesium in the diet.

- Using certain medications, including birth control pills, steroids, decongestants, and anti-inflammatory drugs.

Prevention

 Changes in your lifestyle may help you prevent high blood pressure or help you lower your blood pressure if it's too high.

- Maintain a healthy weight. This is especially important if you tend to put on weight around the waist rather than in the hips and thighs. Losing even 10 pounds can help you lower your blood pressure.

- Be physically active for at least 30 minutes on most days of the week. This will help you lower your blood pressure (and may also help you lose weight).

- Drink alcohol only in moderation.

- Use salt moderately. Too much salt in the diet can be a problem for some people who have high blood pressure and are also salt-sensitive.

- Make sure you get enough potassium, calcium, and magnesium in your diet. Eating plenty of fruits (such as bananas and oranges), vegetables, legumes, whole grains, and low-fat dairy products will ensure that you get enough of these minerals.

- Reduce the saturated fat in your diet. Saturated fat is found in animal products (milk, cheese, and meat). Limiting these foods will help you lose weight and also lower your risk for coronary artery disease. See page 297.

- Stop using tobacco products. Tobacco use increases your risk for heart attack and stroke. See page 26 for tips to help you quit.

- Learn how to check your blood pressure at home. See page 353.

Home Treatment

- Follow the prevention tips above even more closely if you already have high blood pressure.

- Take any prescribed blood pressure medications exactly as directed, and see your doctor at least once a year. Realize that these medications help control high blood pressure but do not cure it. If you stop taking them, your blood pressure may go back up.

- If you are taking blood pressure medication, talk to your doctor before taking decongestants or anti-inflammatory drugs, because they can raise your blood pressure.

When to Call a Health Professional

- Call immediately if you have high blood pressure and:

  - Your blood pressure rises suddenly.

  - Your blood pressure is 180/110 or higher.

  - You have a sudden, severe headache.

  - You develop chest pain or discomfort.

- Call if your blood pressure is higher than 140/90 on two or more occasions (taken at home or in a community screening program). If one blood pressure reading is high, have another taken by a health professional to verify the first reading.

- Call if you develop uncomfortable or disturbing side effects from any medication taken for high blood pressure.

Behind every successful woman is herself.
New American Proverb

13

Women's Health

This chapter focuses on health problems that are unique to women. If you are looking for general guidelines for making healthy lifestyle choices to prevent illness and injury, see Living Healthwise starting on page 15. Specific tips for developing a fitness plan, eating a healthy diet, maintaining a healthy body weight, managing stress, and preventing sexually transmitted diseases are included in other chapters. Use the index to find the information you need.

Breast Health

Breast cancer is the second leading cause of cancer deaths in women. The good news is that breast cancer can often be cured if it is detected early. There are three methods of early detection: mammography, clinical breast exam, and breast self-exam.

One of the most important risk factors for breast cancer is age. The risk goes up significantly after age 50. Women younger than 50 are at lower risk for breast cancer. However, if your mother or a sister had breast cancer before menopause, talk with your doctor about starting mammography and other screenings before age 40.

Mammography

A mammogram is a breast X-ray that can reveal breast tumors that are too small to be detected by breast self-exam or a clinical breast exam.

Studies have shown that mammograms save lives. In women over 50, mammograms reduce breast cancer death rates by up to one-third. Mammograms reduce breast cancer deaths in women under 50 as well, but the total number of deaths prevented is small because breast cancer is rare before age 50.

Breast Pain

Breast pain is common and, fortunately, is rarely a serious problem. Many women's breasts become achy, heavy, or sore a week or so before their menstrual periods start. This is called cyclic pain. It is caused by hormonal changes that occur during the menstrual cycle. The symptoms usually go away at the end of a woman's period. Cyclic breast pain usually ends after a woman completes menopause.

Noncyclic breast pain, which is not associated with a woman's periods, is usually described as sharp or burning. This pain usually occurs on one side only; it may go up towards the armpit; and it may come and go. Pain in one spot that does not go away should be checked by a health professional.

Stress, estrogen therapy, and the use of certain medications can make breast pain worse. Sore breasts can also be a sign of pregnancy.

If breast pain occurs with other premenstrual symptoms (such as bloating and weight gain), avoid salty foods before your period starts, and try taking 400 to 500 mg of magnesium daily. There is some evidence that taking evening primrose oil reduces breast pain. Wearing a support bra, especially when exercising, may also help.

If pain or any other changes in your breasts concern you, talk to your health professional. If you are over 40 or have a family history of breast cancer, discuss breast cancer screening with your doctor.

Your doctor may tell you how often he or she would like you to get a mammogram. The following is a schedule that a doctor may recommend for a woman who is not at high risk for breast cancer:

- Younger than 40: mammograms not usually done for routine screening.

- Age 40 to 49: mammograms according to a schedule agreed upon by the woman and her doctor.

- Age 50 and older: mammograms every 1 to 2 years.

Yearly mammograms are recommended for any woman who has had cancer in one breast. If you have a female relative (especially your mother or a sister) who had breast cancer before menopause, talk to your doctor about when to start and how often to have mammograms.

 MORE INFO Getting all the facts and thinking about your own needs and values will help you make a wise decision about <u>mammography</u>. Always see your health professional if you find a lump or change in your breast.

Preparing for a Mammogram

- Arrange to have your mammogram 1 to 2 weeks after your period ends.

- Do not wear deodorant, perfume, powder, or lotion, because they can affect the quality of the X-ray.

- Wear clothing that allows you to easily undress from the waist up.

MORE INFO **For more information, see the back cover.**

- If you had a previous mammogram at a different facility, have it sent or bring it with you on the day of your mammogram.

Clinical Breast Exam

During a clinical breast exam, a doctor or nurse looks at your breasts and gently feels them for lumps or other unusual changes. During the exam, the doctor or nurse can also teach you how to examine your breasts yourself.

A clinical breast exam is recommended every year after age 40. A clinical breast exam is also done whenever a woman has symptoms indicating that there may be a problem with her breasts.

Breast Self-Exam

The breast self-exam is a simple way for you to learn what is normal for your breasts and how to notice changes in them. It is useful for finding lumps (most of which are not cancerous), cysts, and other noncancerous problems. Once you know what your breasts normally look and feel like, you will be better able to recognize any changes in your breasts and know when to get help early instead of waiting until your next checkup.

Few women have breasts that match exactly. It is normal for one breast to be slightly larger than the other. Most women's breasts have some lumpiness or places where the tissue feels thicker. If the lumpiness is the same in both breasts, it is probably normal. If you find a lump that feels different or much harder than the rest of your breast tissue, or if you find anything else that worries you, have it checked by your health professional.

Establish a regular time each month to examine your breasts. A good time is a few days after your period ends, when your breasts are less likely to be swollen or sore. Women who do not menstruate can examine their breasts at any time of the month.

The breast self-exam takes place in two stages. Ask your health professional for help in learning the technique.

Stage 1: In front of the mirror

Stand in front of a well-lighted mirror and examine your breasts carefully: first with your arms at your sides; then with your hands pushing firmly on your hips to tighten your chest muscles; then with your arms raised overhead; and finally while bending forward (arms at sides).

Look for changes in the shape of your breasts (indentations, flattening, or puckering of the skin) as you move your arms. Both breasts should change in the same way. Also check to see if either nipple appears to be turning inward when it never did before, and look for changes in the skin of the nipple. Squeeze each nipple carefully between your thumb and index finger to feel for lumps. A milky discharge that happens only when you squeeze your breast or nipple is usually normal.

Look at your breasts in a mirror.

Put your hands on your hips.

Raise your arms.

Bend forward, still looking
in the mirror.

Stage 2: Lying down

To examine your right breast, place a pillow or folded towel under your right shoulder. Put your right arm under your head and use your left hand to examine your breast. Using the pads of your fingers (not just the fingertips), move your fingers in dime-sized circles over your skin, and push down gently to feel for lumps, thickening, or changes of any kind. Be sure to feel all of your breast, including the nipple, as well as your breastbone, the area under the breast, and the armpit.

Move the pillow or towel to the left shoulder. Use your right hand to examine your left breast.

Instead of lying down, some women like to do the second stage of the exam while standing in the shower. If your skin is wet and soapy, it may be easier to feel your breast tissue.

Stand with one arm raised (hand behind your head) and feel the breast with your other hand.

Prevention and Early Detection of Breast Cancer

- Limit alcohol to 1 drink per day. Moderate to heavy drinking increases your risk for breast cancer.

- Eat a low-fat diet. Fat in the diet is linked to an increased risk for breast cancer. Cut down on fried foods and high-fat meats and dairy products. Choose lean meats and low-fat dairy products instead.

- Eat foods that contain vitamins A and C, such as dark green and orange vegetables and fruits. Eat more cruciferous vegetables (broccoli, cabbage, kale). There is some evidence that a diet that includes these foods may reduce your risk for breast cancer.

- Have a clinical breast exam every year after age 40.

- Have a mammogram every 1 to 2 years starting at age 50. If you are age 40 to 49, discuss an appropriate mammogram schedule with your doctor.

- If you have a strong family history of breast cancer, talk with your doctor about tamoxifen, a medication that may lower your risk of developing breast cancer.

When to Call a Health Professional

- If you find a lump that concerns you, particularly if it is hard and unlike other tissue in your breasts.

- Any time you find a breast lump if you are past menopause.

- If you have a bloody or greenish discharge from a nipple, or a watery or milky discharge that occurs without pressing on the nipple or breast.

- If one of your breasts changes shape, or if it seems to pucker or "pull" when you raise your arms.

- If the skin of one breast becomes dimpled (like an orange peel).

- If you notice a change in the color or feel of the skin of a breast or the darker area (areola) around a nipple.

- If you have a new pain in one breast, not caused by an injury, that lasts longer than 1 or 2 weeks.

- If you have any signs of infection in a breast. See page 67.

- If you are a man and you find a lump.

Gynecological Health

Regular pelvic exams and Pap tests are vital components of women's health. These exams can give you early indications of any abnormalities in your reproductive organs. It is better to catch any disease in its early stages, when it may be easier to treat.

Self-Exam

Self-exams will help you better understand your own body and what is normal for you. Periodically examine your entire genital area for any sores, warts, red swollen areas, or unusual discharge. A normal vaginal discharge may be white to yellowish white and smell slightly like vinegar. It can be either thick or thin and may vary in amount throughout your menstrual cycle; every woman is different. During ovulation (the midpoint between periods), there is often a large amount of clear, slippery mucus. If your discharge seems unusual in amount, smell, or texture, see Vaginitis on page 262.

There should be no pain or straining when you urinate, and the urine should come out in a fairly steady stream. The urine should be pale yellow, and it should not have a strong ammonia smell. If you experience pain or burning when you urinate, see Urinary Tract Infections on page 103 or Vaginitis on page 262. If you have problems with bladder control, see Urinary Incontinence on page 101.

Pelvic Exam and Pap Test

A pelvic exam given by a health professional will generally include an external genital exam, a Pap test, and a manual exam.

The Pap test is the screening exam for cancer of the cervix (the opening of the uterus). The Pap test detects 90 to 95 percent of cervical cancers, making it a reliable and important test. To do the test, your health professional will insert an instrument (speculum) into your vagina to spread apart the vaginal walls. Then,

using a cotton swab, small brush, or wooden spatula, your health professional will gather several samples of cells from your cervix. The cells are put on a slide and sent to a lab for classification. Your health professional should let you know the results of your Pap test when they return from the lab. Ask for an explanation of your results if you don't understand them.

Female pelvic organs

 If your Pap test results are abnormal, you will be asked to return for more testing. You may have another Pap test, or your doctor may try to find the area in your cervix that contains abnormal cells using a special magnifying device (colposcope).

To do a manual exam, your health professional will insert two gloved and lubricated fingers into your vagina and press on your lower abdomen with his or her other hand to feel for any abnormalities in the shape or size of your ovaries and uterus.

Scheduling a Pelvic Exam

It is recommended that you have your first Pap test when you become sexually active. After that, Pap tests are recommended every 1 to 3 years, depending on whether you have risk factors for cervical cancer. You may not need annual Pap tests if:

• You have had several normal Pap tests in a row (done annually).

• You have only one sex partner.

• You do not smoke.

• You do not have a history of abnormal Pap tests, cervical cancer, or a sexually transmitted disease such as genital warts.

• You have had a hysterectomy for a reason other than cancer.

If you do have risk factors for cervical cancer or a history of abnormal Pap tests, it is recommended that you have a Pap test each year. Discuss the best schedule for Pap tests for you with your doctor.

Arrange to have the test 1 to 2 weeks after your period ends. Do not douche, have sexual intercourse, or use feminine hygiene products for at least 24 hours before a Pap test, because doing any of these things can alter the test results.

Pregnancy: How to Make a Healthy Baby

You can increase the chances that your baby will be healthy. The following guidelines will help.

Before Conception

Your health, both before conception and during the first weeks after, is particularly important for your baby's health. Start helping your baby even before you become pregnant.

• Get a thorough physical checkup. If any problems or needs are found, deal with them early. Have a blood test to check your rubella immunity. If you test negative, you will need an immunization. Wait at least 3 months after being vaccinated before you get pregnant. Exposure to rubella during early pregnancy can harm your baby.

• During this checkup, you may want to ask for a "pre-pregnancy exam," which can help determine any risks to you or your children from pregnancy. Knowing the possible risks may help you decide whether you wish to see a family practitioner, a midwife, or an obstetrician for care during your pregnancy. It may also help you decide what tests you want to have done during pregnancy.

• You and your partner may want to be screened for potential genetic problems, such as sickle cell anemia if you are of African-American descent, or Tay-Sachs disease if you are of Jewish-European or French-Canadian descent.

- If you have diabetes, high blood pressure, seizure disorders, or any inherited diseases, talk with your doctor before getting pregnant. Your doctor may want to modify your treatment and may be able to prescribe medicine that is safer for the developing baby.

- See your dentist and have any necessary fillings or other work done before you get pregnant.

- If you have symptoms of a sexually transmitted disease or are unsure of your partner's sexual history, arrange for an examination and testing. See Sexually Transmitted Diseases on page 278.

- Eat well. Make sure your diet includes plenty of green, leafy vegetables and legumes.

- Take a multivitamin supplement that contains 0.4 mg of folate (folic acid). Folic acid helps prevent certain birth defects such as spina bifida. Other good sources of folic acid include fortified cereal and whole-wheat bread.

- Exercise and control your weight as advised by your doctor.

- Stop smoking and cut down on caffeinated drinks, such as coffee, tea, and cola.

- Stop drinking alcoholic beverages, such as beer, wine, and hard liquor.

- Stop all illegal drug use and eliminate any medications that are not absolutely essential.

- If you are anxious or depressed, get help. See pages 308 and 309.

- Buy a good book on pregnancy and start reading.

Morning Sickness

Many women experience nausea and vomiting during the first few months of pregnancy. Morning sickness, which can occur at any time of day, is a normal result of the body's adjustment to pregnancy. The following home treatment can help.

- Eat five or six small meals a day to avoid having an empty stomach. Include some protein in each of the meals.

- Eat crackers or dry toast as soon as you get up in the morning.

- Increase your intake of vitamin B_6 by eating more whole grains and cereals, wheat germ, nuts, seeds, and legumes. Talk with your health professional before taking vitamin supplements during early pregnancy.

- Avoid foods or smells that make you nauseous.

- Get plenty of rest.

Call your health professional if your symptoms are so severe that you cannot hold down food or liquids, if you are vomiting more than 3 times a day, or if you are losing weight.

Early Pregnancy (Weeks 1 to 14)

- Continue to avoid smoking, alcohol, and drugs.

- Make the first visit to your caregiver in the first 10 to 12 weeks of your pregnancy.

- Get tested for HIV infection.

- Continue to improve your nutrition. Call your local WIC (Women, Infants, and Children) agency to learn whether you are eligible for this program. WIC provides vouchers for nutritious food, nutrition education, and breast-feeding support to pregnant women, women with new babies, and children younger than 5.

- Continue taking a multivitamin supplement containing 0.4 mg of folate.

- Avoid touching cat feces and litter boxes. Also, wash your hands after handling raw meat and cook all meat well before you eat it. Cat feces and raw or undercooked meat can carry toxoplasmosis, an infection that can cause a miscarriage or brain damage in the fetus.

- Avoid all chemical vapors, paint fumes, and poisons.

- If you drink coffee or soda with caffeine, cut back to 2 cups or less per day.

Middle Pregnancy (Weeks 15 to 28)

- Continue with the guidelines described above.

- Reduce your risk for injury and falls:

  - Wear sensible shoes.

  - Continue moderate levels of your regular exercises, but do not become exhausted or significantly short of breath.

  - Avoid sports with a high risk for falls or impact, such as skiing or horseback riding.

- Increase your calcium intake by drinking more milk (1 quart of skim or low-fat milk per day) or through other sources of calcium. See page 299.

Late Pregnancy (Weeks 29 to 40)

- Follow all of the guidelines listed above.

- Get plenty of rest.

- Take childbirth classes with your partner or designated coach.

- Educate yourself about early signs of labor.

- Have your other children take a class to help them adjust to the new baby.

- Practice relaxation exercises (see page 323). They will be helpful during labor.

• Develop a written birth plan with your health professional that outlines your wishes and expectations throughout the labor and delivery.

• Maintain a good sense of humor.

Cesarean Deliveries

Most babies are delivered vaginally, just as nature intended. However, when the health of the baby or mother is at risk, doctors can deliver the baby through an incision in the mother's abdomen. This is called a cesarean delivery or a C-section.

There are three main concerns with cesarean deliveries:

• More risk. Many mothers who have C-sections develop infection or bleeding that requires additional medications or treatment. A C-section is a major surgery, which always carries risks.

• Longer recovery. You can usually go home within 1 day after a vaginal delivery. The hospital stay after a cesarean delivery may be 2 to 4 days. After a C-section, you must limit your activity over the next 4 to 6 weeks to allow the incision to heal.

• Less involvement. The mother and other family members can be more involved with a vaginal delivery. Cesarean delivery is a surgery, which limits family involvement.

 C-sections are a good idea when either the baby or the mother is in danger. A cesarean delivery should not be done just because it is easier to schedule. If you previously had a C-section delivery, you may be able to have a vaginal delivery with your next pregnancy. Ask your caregiver to discuss this option with you.

Breast-Feeding

Breast milk is the ideal food for your new baby. Consider taking a breast-feeding class before your baby is born. See page 217.

A nursing mother needs to consume 500 more calories per day than she did before becoming pregnant. Although you don't need to drink milk to make milk, extra calcium and protein are important, and your doctor may prescribe a vitamin supplement. Avoid smoking and drinking alcohol, and limit caffeine to one or two beverages per day. Do not take any medication while breast-feeding unless it is prescribed by a health professional.

Bleeding Between Periods

Many women experience bleeding or spotting between periods. It does not necessarily mean a serious condition is present. Use of an intrauterine device (IUD) may increase your chances of spotting.

Some minor bleeding is common during ovulation and during the first few months of using birth control pills. Other hormonal birth control methods, such as Norplant implants and Depo-Provera injections, can cause bleeding between periods. Women who are breast-feeding often have irregular vaginal bleeding or spotting. Stress and hormonal imbalances are other common causes of irregular bleeding. In all of these situations, if the bleeding is not heavy and occurs only occasionally, there is probably no cause for concern. Avoid aspirin, which may prolong the bleeding.

There are other, less common causes of bleeding between periods that may be more serious:

- In a woman who is pregnant, bleeding may indicate a problem with the pregnancy.

- A woman who is having a miscarriage usually will have cramping, lower abdominal pain, and vaginal bleeding.

- Ectopic pregnancy (when a fertilized egg attaches somewhere other than the uterus, also called tubal pregnancy) usually causes lower abdominal pain, and there may be vaginal bleeding.

- Noncancerous uterine growths (uterine fibroids) can cause spotting or bleeding between periods in some women.

- A pelvic infection may cause bleeding between periods. Fever, cramping pain, painful sexual intercourse, and a bad-smelling vaginal discharge are other symptoms.

- If the opening of the uterus (cervix) is inflamed or has an abnormal growth on it, there may be bleeding, especially after sexual intercourse or douching.

- A woman who has gone through menopause and is not on hormone replacement therapy should not have any vaginal bleeding. If she does, she may have an abnormal growth in her uterus and should see a health professional. Women taking hormones may have some postmenopausal bleeding, which they should discuss with their health professional.

When to Call a Health Professional

Call 911 or other emergency services if you have severe vaginal bleeding (soaking more than 8 pads or super tampons in 8 hours) and signs of shock (see page 69).

Call a health professional:

- If you are pregnant and have any vaginal bleeding.

- If you have new lower abdominal pain with unexpected vaginal bleeding.

- If the bleeding is severe.

- If you have irregular vaginal bleeding and a fever of 100° or higher.

- If bleeding between periods lasts longer than 1 week or occurs 3 months in a row.

- If bleeding occurs after sexual intercourse or douching.

- If you are over 35 and have any bleeding between periods or prolonged bleeding with periods.

- If you are using a hormonal method of birth control and your periods are different from what your doctor told you to expect.

- If bleeding occurs after you have gone through menopause.

Hormone Therapy

During and after menopause, a woman's body produces much less of the hormone estrogen. Hormone therapy is often prescribed to treat symptoms of menopause and to reduce a woman's risk for osteoporosis. There are two types of hormone therapy:

- Estrogen replacement therapy (ERT). ERT is estrogen alone. Because ERT may increase the risk of cancer in the lining of the uterus (endometrial cancer), it is usually prescribed only for women who have had a hysterectomy.

- Hormone replacement therapy (HRT). HRT combines estrogen with progestin, another female hormone. Progestin reduces the effect of estrogen on the uterine lining and protects against cancer of the uterus.

Hormone therapy reduces the discomfort of menopausal symptoms such as hot flashes and vaginal dryness. However, hormone therapy can have unpleasant side effects, including bloating, cramping, nausea, breast tenderness, and irregular vaginal bleeding.

Hormone pills are taken every day. Some forms of hormone therapy are available as skin patches or creams. There is very little risk in taking hormone therapy for 1 year or less to manage symptoms of menopause. However, hormone therapy is not recommended for women who have had breast cancer, trouble with blood clots, liver disease, or undiagnosed uterine bleeding.

 The sooner hormone therapy is started and the longer it is used, the more protection it gives against osteoporosis (and possibly heart disease). Evaluate your risk for osteoporosis (see page 135) and talk to your doctor before deciding whether hormone therapy is a good idea for you.

Menopause

For most women, menopause occurs between the ages of 45 and 55, when the production of female hormones (estrogen and progesterone) begins to decline. These hormonal changes may cause irregular menstrual periods before periods stop altogether. You may also experience hot flashes, vaginal dryness, or mood changes. Every woman is unique and will experience menopause differently. Menopause can also occur as the result of having a hysterectomy.

Osteoporosis is also directly linked to the decrease in estrogen that comes with menopause. See page 135.

Most women can expect to live one-third of their lives after menopause, so it is important to manage any problems related to menopause.

Irregular periods. The hormonal changes that occur during menopause may cause you to have irregular periods before your periods stop altogether. This may mean that your menstrual flows will be lighter or heavier than usual; that the intervals between your periods will be shorter or longer; or that you will have spotting between periods. Some women have regular periods until their periods stop suddenly, and others have irregular periods for a long time until menopause.

Birth control. Although you may be less fertile during the years just before the onset of menopause, you continue to release eggs (ovulate) and could become pregnant. If you do not wish to become pregnant, continue to use birth control until your doctor confirms that you have reached menopause or until you have not had a menstrual period for 12 months.

Hot flashes. Hot flashes are sudden periods of intense heat, sweating, and flushing. A hot flash usually begins in the chest and spreads out to the neck, face, and arms. Seventy-five to 80 percent of women going through menopause will have hot flashes. Hot flashes may occur as frequently as once an hour and can last from a few minutes to an hour. If they occur at night, they may disrupt your sleep patterns. Disrupted sleep can lead to insomnia, fatigue, irritability, or inability to concentrate.

Hot flashes usually stop within 1 or 2 years but may persist for several years. They are rarely noticed by others.

Vaginal changes. Vaginal changes that occur during menopause include vaginal dryness caused by the loss of lubrication and moisture in the vagina; thinning of the vaginal walls and loss of elasticity in them; and shrinkage of the outer lips (labia) of the vagina. These vaginal changes can lead to soreness during and after sexual intercourse and may also increase your risk for vaginal infections and urinary incontinence. See Vaginitis on page 262 and Urinary Incontinence on page 101.

Mood changes. The hormonal and physical changes of menopause can cause mood changes. Symptoms such as nervousness, lack of energy, insomnia, moodiness, or depression are common.

Many women think that menopause means emotional upset and the loss of sexuality. Other women feel positive about the changes that occur with menopause, such as freedom from menstruation and the need for birth control. Understanding what is happening to you and having a plan for dealing with symptoms will help you through menopause.

Home Treatment

Irregular periods

Keep a written record of your periods in case you need to discuss them with a health professional.

Hot flashes

Hot flashes usually improve after 1 to 2 years. In the meantime:

- Keep your home and workplace cool, or use a fan.

- Wear layers of loose clothing that can be easily removed. Wear natural fibers such as cotton and silk.

- Drink cold beverages rather than hot ones, and limit your intake of caffeine and alcohol.

- Eat smaller, more frequent meals to avoid the heat generated by digesting large amounts of food.

- Try the relaxation tips on page 323.

Vaginal dryness

Use a water-soluble vaginal lubricant, such as Astroglide or Replens, to ease discomfort during sexual intercourse. Vegetable oil will also work. Do not use Vaseline or other petroleum-based products.

Mood changes

The best thing you can do for yourself is realize that you are not alone. Discuss your symptoms with other women. Give yourself, and ask others for, abundant amounts of love, caring, and understanding. Try to develop a relaxed attitude about menopause. Tension and anxiety may make your symptoms worse.

Hormone therapy may improve hot flashes, vaginal dryness, and mood changes, in addition to protecting you from osteoporosis. See page 256. Certain antidepressants can also help with hot flashes and mood swings.

When to Call a Health Professional

- If your menstrual periods are unusually heavy, irregular, or prolonged (1½ to 2 times longer than usual).

- If bleeding occurs between periods when your periods have been regular.

- If bleeding recurs after periods have stopped for 6 months.

- If your symptoms are interfering with your life and home treatment does not help.

- If you are considering hormone therapy or other medical treatment.

- If you have unexplained bleeding (different from what your health professional told you to expect) while you are taking hormones.

Menstrual Cramps

Many women suffer from painful menstrual cramps (dysmenorrhea). Symptoms include mild to severe cramping in the lower abdomen, back, or thighs; headaches; diarrhea or constipation; nausea; dizziness; and fainting. During the menstrual cycle, the lining of the uterus produces a hormone called prostaglandin. This hormone causes the uterus to contract, often painfully. Women who get severe cramps may produce higher-than-normal amounts of prostaglandin or may be more sensitive to its effects.

An intrauterine device (IUD) can cause increased cramping during your period for the first few months of use. If menstrual cramping persists or gets worse, you may need to consider having the IUD removed and choosing another birth control method. Pain caused by endometriosis (a condition in which cells from the lining of the uterus become implanted on other pelvic organs) usually occurs 1 to 2 days before menstrual bleeding begins and continues through the period. Pelvic infections may cause pain at any time, but the pain often occurs after menstrual bleeding has begun. Some women who have noncancerous uterine growths (uterine fibroids) have severe menstrual cramps.

Home Treatment

- Ibuprofen and naproxen sodium generally help ease cramps better than aspirin and acetaminophen do. Take either ibuprofen or naproxen sodium the day before your period starts, or at the first sign of pain. Take these products with milk or food. Otherwise, they may upset your stomach.

- Exercise. Regular workouts decrease the severity of cramps. See Fitness starting on page 285.

- Use heat (hot water bottles, heating pads, or hot baths) to relax tense muscles and relieve cramping.

- Herbal teas (such as chamomile, mint, raspberry, and blackberry) may help soothe tense muscles and anxious moods.

- If symptoms other than cramping (such as weight gain, headache, and tension) occur before your period begins, see Premenstrual Syndrome on page 261.

When to Call a Health Professional

- If sudden, severe pelvic pain occurs, with or without menstrual bleeding.

- If your menstrual cramps have become worse.

- If pelvic pain seems unrelated to your menstrual cycle.

- If you have cramps and a fever of 100° or higher.

- If cramps begin 5 to 7 days before your period starts or continue after your period stops.

- If cramps do not respond to home treatment for 3 cycles, or if they interfere with your normal activities.

- If you suspect that your intra-uterine device (IUD) is causing cramps, and the pain is more than you can stand or is worse than what your doctor told you to expect.

Missed or Irregular Periods

Missed or irregular periods have many possible causes. Pregnancy is usually the first cause to be considered, but other common causes include:

- Stress; weight loss or weight gain; increased exercise (missed periods are common in endurance athletes); and travel.

- Use of hormonal birth control methods, such as birth control pills, Depo-Provera injections, and Norplant implants, all of which may cause lighter, less frequent, or skipped periods.

- Menopause.

- Menarche (the start of menstrual periods). For the first few years of menstruation, periods may be irregular.

- Medications, including steroids, tranquilizers, and diet pills, or recreational drugs.

- Hormonal imbalance or problems in the pelvic organs.

- Breast-feeding.

- Untreated thyroid disease.

If you've skipped a period, try to relax. Restoring your life to emotional and physical balance may help. Many women miss periods now and then. Unless you are pregnant, chances are your cycle will return to normal next month. If you could be pregnant, treat yourself as if you are until you know for sure.

Home Treatment

- If you had sex during the previous month, do a home pregnancy test. See page 353.

- Avoid fad diets that greatly restrict calories and food variety, and avoid rapid weight loss. To maintain a healthy weight, focus on eating a variety of low-fat foods. See Nutrition starting on page 293.

- Increase exercise gradually. If you are an endurance athlete, cut back on training and talk with a doctor about hormone and calcium supplements to protect against bone loss.

- Learn and practice relaxation techniques to reduce and cope with stress. See page 323.

- If you are age 45 or older, you may be starting menopause. See page 257.

When to Call a Health Professional

- Call your doctor immediately if it is possible that you may be pregnant and you are having lower abdominal pain.

- If it is possible that you may be pregnant, see a doctor to confirm your home pregnancy test and begin pregnancy counseling and prenatal care.

- If you have missed 2 regular periods, and there is no obvious cause such as those listed previously.

- If you are an endurance athlete who is unable to cut back on training. You may need to take hormones or calcium supplements.

- If you miss 2 or 3 periods while taking birth control pills, and you have not skipped any pills.

- If you have not started having menstrual periods by age 16.

Premenstrual Syndrome

Many women have mild symptoms related to menstruation, such as cramps and breast tenderness. These symptoms are considered a normal part of the menstrual cycle. A diagnosis of premenstrual syndrome (PMS) is reserved for symptoms that occur during the 2 weeks before a woman's period begins and that are severe enough to disrupt her life.

About 40 percent of women are affected by PMS at some time in their lives. PMS occurs most often in women in their 20s and 30s and is rare in teenagers.

Many physical and psychological symptoms have been attributed to PMS. Symptoms vary greatly from woman to woman. They can include physical changes such as breast swelling, water retention, bloating, weight gain, and acne; mood and behavior changes such as irritability, depression, difficulty concentrating, decreased sex drive, and aggression; painful symptoms such as headaches, breast tenderness, and muscle aches; and other symptoms such as food cravings, lack of energy, and sleep disturbances.

If you suspect that you have PMS, keep a menstrual diary in which you record:

- Your symptoms and how severe they are.

- Dates when symptoms occur.

- Days when you have your period.

If symptoms consistently appear shortly before your period and end shortly after your period, you may want to follow the home treatment recommendations. Many women find that making small changes in their lives significantly improves their PMS symptoms.

Home Treatment

- Eat small meals every 3 to 4 hours that include plenty of whole grains, fruit, and vegetables. Limit fats and sweets, and reduce salt to help limit bloating.

- Eliminate tobacco, alcohol, and caffeine. This may help relieve some symptoms.

- Exercise regularly to help minimize PMS symptoms.

- Try a nonprescription PMS medication such as Midol or Pamprin. Many products contain a combination of drugs to help relieve symptoms of cramps, bloating, and headache.

- Be good to yourself. Reduce your stress level as much as possible. Try yoga (see page 335) or other relaxation techniques (see page 323).

- Create a support system. Talk with your family, friends, and any others who may be affected by your symptoms. Join a support group for women who have PMS.

- Try taking calcium (1200 mg daily), magnesium (400 mg daily), or vitamin B_6 (no more than 100 mg daily). These may improve your mood, reduce fluid retention and pain, and help with other PMS symptoms.

When to Call a Health Professional

- If PMS symptoms regularly disrupt your life and keep you from doing your regular activities.

- If you feel out of control because of PMS symptoms.

- If PMS symptoms do not end within a few days after your menstrual bleeding starts.

 If PMS symptoms are severely disrupting your life, make an appointment with your doctor. He or she may prescribe medication to reduce these symptoms.

Vaginitis

Vaginitis is any vaginal infection, inflammation, or irritation that causes a change in normal vaginal discharge. General symptoms include a change in the amount, color, odor, or texture of vaginal discharge; itching; painful urination; and pain during sexual intercourse. Common causes of vaginitis include yeast infection (see page 265), bacterial vaginosis, and trichomoniasis, which is caused by a parasite spread through sexual contact (see page 282). Some other sexually spread diseases can cause unusual vaginal discharge or vaginal irritation. See page 278. In addition, irritation caused by douching frequently, wearing tight clothing, or using strong soaps, perfumed feminine hygiene products, or spermicides may contribute to vaginal irritation or infection.

If you have burning and pain when you urinate and feel the need to urinate often, see Urinary Tract Infections on page 103.

Symptoms of bacterial vaginosis often include a thin, grayish white, fishy-smelling vaginal discharge. The odor is often worse after sex. Bacterial vaginosis is commonly associated with having multiple sex partners, using an intrauterine device (IUD) or diaphragm, exposure to a sexually transmitted disease (STD), or frequent douching, but it may occur in women who don't have these risk factors.

Symptoms of trichomoniasis may include a large amount of frothy, foamy, white, yellow, green, or gray vaginal discharge; vaginal redness, irritation, and swelling; and vaginal odor.

Prevention

- Limit the number of your sex partners and use condoms during sexual intercourse. Having multiple sex partners may increase your risk for vaginitis by changing the normal environment of your vagina.

- If you think frequent vaginal infections may be related to use of a diaphragm or IUD, spermicidal foams or jellies, or condoms, discuss other birth control options with your health professional.

- Wipe from front to back after using the toilet. This will help you avoid spreading bacteria from your anus to your vagina.

- Wash your vaginal area once a day with plain water or a mild, nonperfumed soap. Rinse well and dry thoroughly. Do not douche unless your health professional advises you to do so.

- Avoid the use of feminine deodorant sprays and other perfumed products. They irritate and dry tender skin.

- During your period, change tampons at least 3 times a day, or alternate tampons with pads. Remember to remove the last tampon used during your period.

- Antibiotic medications can kill the healthy bacteria that grow in your vagina. If you are taking an antibiotic, drink acidophilus milk or eat yogurt that contains live *Lactobacillus* cultures to help prevent vaginitis.

- Avoid panty hose and tight nylon underwear, which limit air circulation to your vaginal area.

Hysterectomy Guidelines

Hysterectomy is the surgical removal of the uterus. It is generally done to treat disease. However, there are times when other treatments may work as well with fewer risks.

Hysterectomy is often the best treatment for:

• Uterine, ovarian, or cervical cancer.

• Severe uterine bleeding that cannot be controlled by other treatments.

• Severe endometriosis.

• Large, noncancerous tumors (fibroids) that cause severe bleeding and pain or press on the bladder.

• Severe uterine prolapse (uterus falls into the opening of the vagina).

Conditions that may respond to nonsurgical treatments include:

• Abnormal uterine bleeding.

• Fibroids that cause mild symptoms.

• Mild to moderate uterine prolapse.

• Pelvic pain or mild endometriosis.

• Pelvic inflammatory disease.

 MORE INFO Getting all the facts and thinking about your own needs and values will help you make the best decision about <u>hysterectomy</u>.

Home Treatment

A vaginal infection may clear up without treatment in 3 or 4 days. If your symptoms do not improve, call your doctor.

• Follow the Prevention guidelines.

• Avoid sexual intercourse to give irritated vaginal tissues time to heal.

• Do not scratch. Relieve itching with a cold water compress or cool baths.

• Make sure the cause of vaginitis is not a forgotten tampon or another foreign object.

• If you think you may be pregnant, do a home pregnancy test. See page 353. Bacterial vaginosis can be more serious if it occurs during pregnancy.

• If itching is the most bothersome symptom, try a nonprescription vaginal cream or suppositories for yeast infections. See Yeast Infections on page 265. If you are pregnant, talk with your doctor before using a nonprescription treatment.

When to Call a Health Professional

• If you have pelvic or lower abdominal pain, fever, and unusual vaginal discharge.

• If you have pain or bleeding after sexual intercourse (and the pain is not eased by using a vaginal lubricant such as Astroglide).

MORE INFO **For more information, see the back cover.**

- If you have an unusual or foul-smelling vaginal discharge.

- If you have vaginal itching that does not go away after you use a nonprescription medication for yeast infections.

- If you think you've been exposed to a sexually transmitted disease (see page 278). Your sex partner may need to be treated too.

If you plan to see a health professional, do not douche, use vaginal creams, or have sexual intercourse for 48 hours before your appointment. Doing these things may make your problem more difficult to diagnose.

Yeast Infections

A vaginal yeast infection (candidiasis) is caused by an excess growth of yeast organisms in the vagina. Yeast infections are common in women of childbearing age. They can cause severe discomfort but rarely cause serious problems.

Common symptoms of yeast infection include vaginal itching (often severe); white, curdy, usually odorless vaginal discharge; and pain when urinating and during sexual intercourse. The skin around the vagina (labia) may be red and irritated. If you have burning and pain when urinating and feel the need to urinate often, see Urinary Tract Infections on page 103.

Yeast infections are not spread by sexual contact. However, some doctors feel that treating your sex partner with antifungal medications may help prevent recurrent yeast infections.

Yeast infections are commonly associated with antibiotic or steroid use, pregnancy, diabetes, and illnesses that weaken the immune system. In addition, douching frequently, wearing tight clothing, or using strong soaps or perfumed feminine hygiene products may contribute to vaginal irritation or infection.

Prevention

- Drink acidophilus milk or eat yogurt that contains live *Lactobacillus* organisms. Some studies suggest that yogurt may help prevent vaginal yeast infections.

- Wear cotton or cotton-lined underwear. Avoid tight-fitting pants and undergarments. They increase heat and moisture in the vaginal area, which may allow yeast to grow more easily in your vagina.

- Avoid feminine sprays, talcs, or perfumes in your vaginal area, because they may affect the balance among the microorganisms in your vagina. Do not douche unless your health professional advises you to do so.

- Wipe your vaginal area from front to back after using the toilet and when bathing.

• Eat a well-balanced diet. This helps maintain a normal balance in your vagina.

• If you have diabetes, keep your blood sugar level within the range recommended by your doctor.

Home Treatment

Left untreated, vaginal yeast infections often clear up on their own, usually when your period begins. Be sure you have a yeast infection before you try self-treatment. If you are pregnant, talk to your doctor first.

• Follow the Prevention guidelines.

• Use a nonprescription antifungal medication for yeast infections (such as Monistat 7, Gyne-Lotrimin, or a store brand) as directed.

• Douche with yogurt that contains live *Lactobacillus* cultures. Talk with your doctor before using a yogurt douche.

• Avoid excessive cleaning of your vaginal area. Wash once a day with plain water or a mild, nonperfumed soap.

• Don't use tampons while using topical cream or vaginal suppositories for a vaginal yeast infection. The tampons can absorb the medication. Use sanitary pads instead.

• If sexual intercourse causes discomfort, avoid it until your symptoms go away.

When to Call a Health Professional

• If you develop lower abdominal pain or a fever greater than 100° along with symptoms of a vaginal yeast infection.

• If you think this is the first time you've had a yeast infection, or if you aren't sure whether your symptoms are being caused by a yeast infection.

• If home treatment with a nonprescription antifungal product fails to clear up a yeast infection within 3 or 4 days, or if you are using antifungal creams repeatedly.

• If you have symptoms of a urinary tract infection. See page 103.

• If you are or may be pregnant and you have symptoms of a vaginal infection.

• If symptoms of a yeast infection return within 2 months and you have not been taking antibiotics.

If you plan to see a health professional, do not douche, use vaginal creams, or have sexual intercourse for 48 hours before your appointment. Doing these things may make your problem more difficult to diagnose.

The man who says it cannot be done should not
interrupt the man doing it.
Old Chinese Proverb

14

Men's Health

This chapter focuses on health problems that are unique to men. If you are looking for general guidelines for making healthy lifestyle choices to prevent illness and injury, see Living Healthwise starting on page 15. Specific tips for developing a fitness plan, eating a healthy diet, maintaining a healthy body weight, managing stress, and preventing sexually transmitted diseases are included in other chapters. Use the index to find the information you need.

Genital Health

Daily cleansing of the penis, particularly under the foreskin of an uncircumcised penis, can prevent bacterial infection and reduces the already low risk of penile cancer. Boys should be taught by age 3 or 4 to start to gently pull back (retract) the foreskin and wash beneath it. The foreskin may not be fully retractable until puberty. Do not forcibly retract a child's foreskin if it is painful or difficult to do so.

Erection Problems

Erection problems are common and can often be solved with self-care. By definition, an erection problem is difficulty in getting or maintaining an erection capable of intercourse.

Erection problems are often caused by stress, tension in relationships, depression, fatigue, lack of privacy, physical injury, or side effects of medications. These causes are generally temporary and will usually

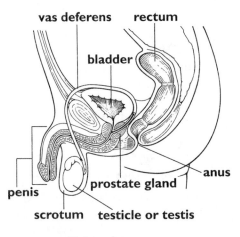

vas deferens   rectum

bladder

anus

penis

prostate gland

scrotum   testicle or testis

Male pelvic organs

267

resolve with home treatment. Other, less reversible causes include diabetes, a long history of smoking, nerve damage, and vascular disease.

The ease of gaining and sustaining erections generally decreases with age. However, with the right foreplay and environment, there is no age limit to the ability of healthy men to have erections.

Prevention

Most erection problems can be prevented or resolved by taking a more relaxed approach to lovemaking and watching for possible side effects from medications or illnesses.

Home Treatment

- Rule out medications first. Many drugs, especially blood pressure medicines, water pills (diuretics), and mood-altering drugs, can cause erection problems. Ask your doctor or pharmacist to check your medications for possible effects on sexual function, or look it up yourself.

- Avoid alcohol and smoking, which can make erection problems worse.

- Cope with stress (see page 321). Tension in your life can distract you and make getting erections difficult. Regular exercise and other stress-relieving activities may help ease tension.

- Talk to your partner about your concerns, and take time for more foreplay. Let your partner know

that you would enjoy some stroking. Slow down; then slow down some more.

- Make sure you're ready. If you have recently experienced a loss or change in a relationship, you may not yet be emotionally ready for erections. Generally, your stress will subside and your erection problem will disappear over time. Do what you can to relax.

- Find out if you can have erections at other times. If you can have an erection during masturbation or on awakening, the problem is probably stress-related or may be caused by an emotional problem.

When to Call a Health Professional

- If you think that a medication may be causing the problem. Your doctor may be able to prescribe a different medication for you.

- If you are unable to have an erection at all, or think that your problem may be a physical one.

- If you have other symptoms such as urinary problems, pain in the lower abdomen or lower back, or fever.

- If your symptoms develop after a recent injury.

 If you have tried home treatment for a few months but your symptoms have not improved, you may wish to talk with your doctor about erection-producing medications or injections, a vacuum device, or a penile implant. Getting all the facts and thinking about your own and your partner's needs and values will help you make a wise decision about treatment for erection problems.

Prostate Infection (Prostatitis)

The prostate is a doughnut-shaped gland that lies under the bladder, about halfway between the rectum and the base of the penis. It encircles the urethra, the tube that carries urine from the bladder out through the penis. The prostate produces some of the fluid that transports sperm during ejaculation.

There are several types of prostatitis. They include acute and chronic bacterial prostatitis, inflammatory chronic pelvic pain, and noninflammatory chronic pelvic pain. Symptoms are similar for all forms of prostatitis. With the exception of acute bacterial prostatitis (in which the symptoms are severe, come on suddenly, and may include fever and chills), it is difficult to determine the kind of prostatitis a man has based on symptoms alone.

Symptoms may include:

- Frequent urge to urinate, but passing only small amounts of urine.
- Burning sensation when urinating; inability to empty the bladder completely.
- Difficulty starting urination; interrupted or weaker-than-normal urine flow; and dribbling after urinating.
- Urinating excessively at night.
- Pain or discomfort in the lower back; the scrotum; the area between the scrotum and the anus; the lower abdomen; the upper thighs; or above the pubic area.
- Pain or vague discomfort during or after ejaculation.

Bacterial prostate infections usually respond well to self-care and antibiotics. If the infection recurs, long-term antibiotic treatment may be needed. Prostate infections that are not caused by bacteria usually respond to home treatment.

Prevention

- Practice good hygiene, and wash your penis daily.
- Drink enough water and other fluids so that you urinate regularly.
- If you develop symptoms of a urinary tract infection, seek treatment early.
- Take the full amount of the antibiotic prescribed by your doctor for bacterial prostatitis. This can reduce your risk of having another infection in the future.

Home Treatment

- Avoid alcohol, caffeine, and spicy foods, especially if they make your symptoms worse.

• Take hot baths to help soothe pain and reduce stress.

• Eat plenty of high-fiber foods, and drink enough water to avoid constipation. Straining to pass stools can be very painful when your prostate is inflamed.

• Take aspirin, ibuprofen, or acetaminophen to help relieve pain. Do not give aspirin to anyone younger than 20.

When to Call a Health Professional

• If urinary symptoms occur with fever, chills, vomiting, or pain in the back or abdomen.

• If your urine is bloody, red, or pink and there is no dietary reason for this (see page 105).

• If symptoms continue for 5 days despite home treatment.

• If your symptoms suddenly change or get worse.

• If you have pain during urination, ejaculation, or bowel movements. If there is also an unusual discharge from your penis, see pages 278 to 282.

• If you have urinary symptoms, such as trouble starting to urinate, inability to empty your bladder completely, or frequent urination (especially at night), that are not related to drinking more fluids.

Prostate Enlargement

As a man ages, the prostate may enlarge (benign prostatic hyperplasia or hypertrophy). This seems to be a natural process and is not really a disease. However, as the gland gets bigger, it tends to squeeze the urethra and cause urinary problems, such as:

• Difficulty getting the urine stream started and completely stopped (dribbling).

• Frequent urge to urinate, or being awakened by the urge to urinate.

• Decreased force of the urine stream.

• Having the sense that the bladder is not completely empty after urinating.

An enlarged prostate gland is not a serious problem unless urination becomes difficult or backed-up urine causes bladder infections or kidney damage. Some dribbling after urination is very common and not necessarily a sign of prostate problems.

 Surgery is usually not necessary for an enlarged prostate. Many men find that their symptoms are stable, and sometimes symptoms even clear up on their own. In these cases, the best treatment may be no treatment at all. Drugs are available that may help improve symptoms in many men. Your doctor can advise you about the various treatment options.

Home Treatment

- Avoid antihistamines, decongestants, and nasal sprays, which can make urinary problems worse.

- If you are bothered by a frequent urge to urinate at night, cut down on beverages before bedtime, especially those that contain alcohol or caffeine. Continue to drink at least 8 glasses of water and other fluids during the day.

- Don't postpone urinating, and take plenty of time. Try sitting on the toilet instead of standing.

- Also see Urinary Incontinence on page 101.

When to Call a Health Professional

- If you are unable to urinate, or if you feel as if you cannot empty your bladder completely.

- If you develop fever, back or abdominal pain, or chills.

- If there is blood or pus in your urine.

- Water pills (diuretics), tranquilizers, antihistamines, decongestants, and some antidepressants can aggravate urinary problems. If you take any of these drugs, ask your doctor if there are other medications you could use that do not cause these urinary side effects.

Prostate Cancer

Prostate cancer is the second leading cause of cancer deaths in men. When detected early, before it has spread to other organs, prostate cancer may be curable. Most cases develop in men over 65. Since prostate cancer tends to develop late in life and usually grows slowly, it does not usually shorten a man's life. However, the younger you are and the larger or more advanced the cancer is, the more serious the disease may be.

There are no specific symptoms of prostate cancer. Most men have no symptoms at all. In a few cases, it can cause urinary symptoms very similar to those of prostate enlargement (see page 270). Other symptoms, such as pain, may develop if the cancer spreads to other organs or to the bones.

Prostate cancer sometimes runs in families, is more common in African-American men, and tends to be more common in men who eat a high-fat diet.

Prevention

There is no known way to prevent prostate cancer. However, you may reduce your risk of developing prostate cancer by:

- Eating a low-fat diet that includes plenty of fruits and vegetables.

- Adding foods that contain tomato or tomato sauce in your diet.

- Increasing your intake of soy products.

• Taking a vitamin E supplement. In one recent study, men who took 50 extra units of vitamin E a day were about one-third less likely to develop prostate cancer. Talk to your health professional about whether you should take vitamin E (or any other nutritional supplements).

 MORE INFO Early detection may be the most important part of prevention, but there is controversy about the value of using digital rectal exams and the prostate-specific antigen (PSA) blood test to screen all men for prostate cancer. Detecting early prostate cancer may not improve quality of life or prolong life, especially in men who are older or have other serious health problems. Therefore, many experts are uncertain whether routine screening is appropriate for all men. Talk with your doctor for more information about prostate cancer screening.

Home Treatment

Prostate cancer treatment is tailored to each individual. Work with your doctor to be sure that you will receive the long-term benefits from the treatment you choose.

Learn all you can about the available treatment options, which may include watchful waiting, so that you and your doctor can select the one best suited for you. Your age, overall health, other medical conditions, and the characteristics of the

cancer are all important factors to consider when you make treatment decisions.

When to Call a Health Professional

• If you have blood or pus in your urine.

• If any urinary symptoms (see Prostate Enlargement on page 270) come on quickly, are bothersome enough that you want help, or last longer than 2 months.

Testicular Problems

The testicles produce sperm and male hormones. Males normally have two testicles, located behind the penis inside a sac of skin called the scrotum. It is normal for one testicle to be slightly larger than the other.

Each testicle is suspended at the end of a spermatic cord, which consists of blood vessels, nerves, and a tube called the vas deferens. Sperm cells leave the testicle through the epididymis (a coiled tube located at the top of the testicle). Then they move through the vas deferens and are deposited in the seminal vesicles, which are near the prostate gland. Sperm mix with fluids produced by the seminal vesicles and the prostate to create semen, which exits the body through the penis during sexual activity.

MORE INFO **For more information, see the back cover.**

The location of the testicles makes them prone to injury, especially during contact sports. Pain caused by a testicular injury should go away within an hour or so.

Testicular torsion occurs when one of the testicles rotates, twisting the spermatic cord and cutting off blood flow to the testicle. Testicular torsion can occur at any age, but it is most common in teenage boys. It may occur after strenuous physical activity or after an injury, but it often has no specific cause and may occur while a boy is sleeping.

Symptoms of testicular torsion include sudden, severe pain in one testicle that may spread to the lower abdomen; swelling high in the scrotum; nausea and vomiting; and fever.

Testicular torsion is a medical emergency. Surgery is often needed to restore blood flow to the testicle. If the procedure is not done within a few hours after the onset of symptoms, the testicle can be permanently damaged and may have to be removed.

Epididymitis is inflammation of the epididymis. It can be caused by a bacterial infection (including chlamydia, which is spread through sexual contact, see page 279) or by irritation resulting from a bladder infection or injury. Epididymitis causes pain and swelling in the scrotum that develops gradually, over hours or days, and can become severe. The scrotum may feel hot and be tender to the touch, and the person may have a fever. Bacterial epididymitis is usually treated with antibiotics.

Orchitis is inflammation of the testicle. It may be caused by a bacterial infection or by a virus, most often the mumps. Orchitis can also occur with epididymitis or a prostate infection (prostatitis). Symptoms include scrotal pain; swelling (usually on one side of the scrotum); and a feeling of heaviness in the scrotum. If it is not treated, orchitis can cause infertility.

Testicular cancer is rare and most often affects males between the ages of 15 and 35. Those at highest risk include males whose testicles have not descended or did not descend until after age 6, and males with a family history of testicular cancer. Testicular cancer usually affects only one testicle and responds well to treatment if detected early. Symptoms of testicular cancer may include a painless lump or swelling or a feeling of heaviness in one testicle.

Prevention

- Prevent testicular injury by wearing a protective athletic "cup" when you play sports.

- Prevent bacterial infections that are spread through sexual contact by following the safer sex guidelines on pages 282 and 283.

Gently feel each testicle for hard lumps or a change in size.

- Make sure your child has completed the measles, mumps, and rubella (MMR) vaccination series. See page 17.

- Teenage boys and men should do a testicular self-exam once a month. After taking a warm bath or shower:

  - Stand and place your right leg on an elevated surface such as the side of the bathtub or the toilet seat.

  - Examine the surface of your right testicle by gently rolling it between the thumb and fingers of both hands. Feel for any hard lumps or nodules. The testicle should feel round and smooth.

  - Feel for any enlargement of the testicle or a change in its consistency. It is normal for one testicle to be slightly larger than the other. Report any major size differences or any changes in feeling or appearance to a health professional.

  - Repeat the exam on your left testicle.

Home Treatment

- Elevating the scrotum with a pillow and applying ice may help relieve pain caused by an injury.

- Wearing a jock strap daily may relieve scrotal pain.

- Take aspirin or acetaminophen to relieve pain caused by orchitis. Do not give aspirin to anyone younger than 20. Warm baths may also help relieve pain.

When to Call a Health Professional

- If pain in a testicle or the scrotum comes on suddenly and is severe. This may be a sign of testicular torsion, which requires immediate treatment.

- If you find a lump in a testicle.

- If you notice any enlargement in a testicle or a change in its consistency.

- If pain or swelling in a testicle or the scrotum worsens over a period of several hours or days or does not lessen after a few days.

- If pain or swelling in a testicle or the scrotum is accompanied by fever.

- If pain or swelling in the scrotum develops after exposure to the mumps virus.

- If you have a feeling of heaviness in one testicle.

*I wasn't kissing her, I was
whispering in her mouth.*
Groucho Marx

15

Sexual Health

This chapter covers specific health issues of concern to people who are sexually active, from birth control to sexually transmitted diseases (STDs), including infection with the human immunodeficiency virus (HIV), which causes AIDS.

Birth Control

Birth control can help prevent unplanned pregnancies. However, no birth control method (except abstinence) is 100 percent effective and without risks. The text that follows and the chart on page 276 briefly describe the most common birth control methods.

 Review each of the birth control methods presented in this chapter with your partner before deciding which one meets your needs. Your health professional can help you better understand the effectiveness and risks of each method.

Use all birth control methods exactly as your doctor or the package instructions recommend. Proper use helps ensure effectiveness.

Hormonal methods of birth control for women either prevent the ovaries from releasing an egg each month (ovulation) or thicken the mucus at the opening of the uterus so sperm can't get to the uterus to fertilize an egg. All hormonal birth control methods require a doctor's prescription. Hormonal methods of birth control do not protect against STDs.

Oral contraceptives (the Pill) are taken daily. Norplant is a set of small plastic cylinders that are inserted under the skin in the upper arm. The cylinders release hormones continuously for up to 5 years and can be removed whenever you decide you want to get pregnant. Depo-Provera and Lunelle are hormone injections given by a health professional once every 3 months (for Depo-Provera) or once every month (for Lunelle).

Birth Control		
Method	**Pregnancies***	**Comments**
Sterilization Tubal ligation (women) Vasectomy (men)	Fewer than 1	Consider it permanent.
Hormonal Methods Oral contraceptives (the Pill)	5	Increased risk of circulatory disorders and high blood pressure in women who smoke.
Norplant (implant) Depo-Provera and Lunelle (shots)	Fewer than 1 Fewer than 1	Both Norplant and Depo-Provera may cause irregular menstrual bleeding.
Intrauterine Device (IUD)	Fewer than 1 to 2 depending on type of IUD used	May cause bleeding and cramping. May be expelled without being noticed. Increased risk of pelvic infection.
Barrier Methods Condom (male)	14	For maximum protection against STDs, use latex or polyurethane condoms every time you have sex.
Condom (female)	21	
Diaphragm (with spermicide)	20	
Cervical cap (with spermicide)	20 to 40	
Spermicides Jelly, cream, foam, suppositories	26	Use with a condom for best protection.
Used with condom	6	
Periodic Abstinence (natural family planning: basal body temperature, mucus, or rhythm/calendar method)	25	
Withdrawal	19	
No method (chance)	85	
*Typical number of accidental pregnancies per 100 women in 1 year. When birth control methods are used exactly as directed, pregnancy rates are lower. Adapted from: R. Hatcher et al., *Contraceptive Technology, 1998.*		

The intrauterine device (IUD) is a plastic or metal device that is inserted into the uterus by a doctor. Some IUDs release a hormone to prevent conception. Other IUDs are made of copper, which appears to kill sperm. IUDs do not provide any protection against STDs.

Barrier methods of birth control kill sperm or keep sperm from entering the uterus and reaching the egg. Barrier methods work best when two methods are combined (for example, male condoms used with spermicidal foam).

The male condom is a thin, flexible tube of latex rubber or animal skin that is placed over the man's erect penis before sexual intercourse to catch ejaculated semen. There are also condoms for women that fit inside the vagina. Latex or polyurethane condoms provide the most reliable, but not total, protection against STDs, including HIV. Lambskin condoms are not effective in preventing STDs. Condoms are available without a doctor's prescription. Many condoms are lubricated with a spermicide. Condoms can be used with other birth control methods for added protection against STDs.

Spermicides are foams, jellies, and suppositories that contain chemicals which kill sperm. Spermicides are available without a doctor's prescription. Most spermicides contain nonoxynol-9. Some people are allergic to nonoxynol-9 and may develop sores in the vagina or on the penis after coming in contact with it. Sometimes the allergic reaction is triggered by other chemicals in the spermicide, and switching to a different product solves the problem.

The diaphragm and cervical cap are small rubber caps that are filled with spermicide and inserted into the vagina to cover the opening of the uterus (cervix) before sexual intercourse begins. They are left in place for 6 hours or longer after sexual intercourse. Both the diaphragm and the cervical cap require a doctor's prescription. When used alone, these barrier methods provide minimal protection against STDs.

Surgical methods are the most effective forms of birth control. During a vasectomy, the tubes (vas deferens) that carry a man's sperm from his testes are clamped or cut off, thus preventing sperm from being ejaculated in semen. Tubal ligation procedures close off or cut the tubes (fallopian tubes) that carry a woman's eggs from her ovaries to her uterus. This prevents eggs from being fertilized or implanting in the uterus. Both vasectomy and tubal ligation should be considered permanent, but in some cases they can be successfully reversed with surgery. Surgical methods of birth control do not protect you against STDs.

Emergency Contraception

Emergency contraception either prevents the release of an egg from a woman's ovaries (ovulation) or prevents a fertilized egg from implanting in the uterus. It can be very effective for preventing unwanted pregnancy if you use it soon after you have unprotected sex.

Sometimes called the "morning-after pill," emergency contraceptive pills (usually a high-dose form of regular birth control pills) can be taken anytime within 72 hours after you have unprotected sex. Inserting a copper-bearing intrauterine device (IUD) within 5 to 7 days after intercourse is another method of emergency contraception.

Regardless of method, the sooner you use emergency contraception, the more effective it is in preventing pregnancy.

If you have sexual intercourse and are concerned about a possible pregnancy because you did not use birth control or because your birth control may have failed (for instance, if a condom or diaphragm tore), call your health professional immediately for information about emergency contraception.

Natural family planning (fertility awareness) methods help a couple estimate when the woman is most likely to become pregnant (during ovulation) so they can avoid sexual intercourse during that time or have intercourse to get pregnant. To estimate when ovulation occurs, a woman records her temperature, examines her vaginal mucus discharge, and tracks her menstrual periods. Like any birth control method, natural family planning is most effective when used correctly. Couples who do not receive or follow proper instruction in using the method have a much higher rate of accidental pregnancy. Natural family planning does not provide protection against STDs.

Sexually Transmitted Diseases

Sexually transmitted diseases (STDs) or venereal diseases (VD) are infections passed from person to person through sexual intercourse, genital contact, or contact with fluids such as semen, vaginal fluids, and blood (including menstrual blood). Many of these diseases can also be spread by sharing needles and other items that may be contaminated with infected blood or body fluids. Chlamydia, genital herpes, genital warts, gonorrhea, hepatitis B, HIV (which causes AIDS), syphilis, and trichomoniasis are among the most common STDs.

Chlamydia, gonorrhea, hepatitis B, herpes simplex virus, HIV, and syphilis can be spread from an infected mother to her unborn baby or infant. Treatment during pregnancy can prevent the spread of many of these diseases from mother to child. If you are infected with any of these diseases, talk to your doctor about how you can protect your baby before and after it is born.

Chlamydia

Chlamydia is a bacterial infection that affects millions of men and women. It may be difficult to detect chlamydia; about 80 percent of women and 50 percent of men with the disease have no symptoms, but they can still infect their sex partners. If symptoms do show up, they occur 1 to 3 weeks after exposure to the bacteria. In women, symptoms may include vaginal discharge or irregular menstrual bleeding, pain when urinating, or lower abdominal pain. In men, there may be a discharge from the penis and pain when urinating.

Chlamydia is easily treated with antibiotics. If undetected and untreated, chlamydia can cause pelvic inflammatory disease (infection in the ovaries and fallopian tubes), which may lead to sterility (inability to conceive a child). Both partners need to be treated.

Genital herpes

Genital herpes is caused by the herpes simplex virus, which also causes cold sores (see page 202).

Genital herpes is easily spread through sexual contact and any other direct contact with genital herpes sores.

Symptoms of the first genital herpes outbreak occur 2 to 7 days after contact with an infected person. It is also possible to be infected with genital herpes and have no symptoms.

The first case of genital herpes may be quite severe, with many painful sores or blisters. Fever, swollen glands, and headache or muscle aches may also occur. If the sores develop inside the urethra (the tube that carries urine out of the body) or the vagina, there may be pain when urinating or vaginal discharge. The sores crust over and disappear in 2 to 3 weeks.

 There is no known cure for genital herpes, although medication can reduce pain and speed healing of sores during an outbreak. Most people with genital herpes have recurrent outbreaks. Having 4 outbreaks per year is typical. Outbreaks tend to become less frequent and less severe over time. Itching, burning, or tingling may occur at the place where the sores will later appear. If you have frequent or severe outbreaks, taking medication every day can help reduce how often outbreaks occur and how long they last.

Genital warts

Genital warts are caused by the human papillomavirus (HPV), which is spread through sexual contact. The warts generally look like small, fleshy bumps or flat, white patches on the lips around the vagina (labia), inside the vagina, on the penis or scrotum, or around the anus. A person infected with HPV may never develop genital warts, or the warts may be too small to be seen. Certain types of HPV seem to increase the risk of cervical cancer in women, but these may not cause visible warts. A Pap test can occasionally detect the virus.

 MORE INFO If genital warts are bothersome or develop on the cervix, they can be removed by a health professional. However, wart removal does not cure HPV infection, and the warts may recur. There does not appear to be an effective cure for HPV infection at this time. However, in many people the infection goes away by itself and does not cause further problems.

Gonorrhea

Gonorrhea is a bacterial infection that is spread through sexual contact. Symptoms, which appear 2 days to 2 weeks after infection, may include painful or frequent urination, vaginal discharge, irregular menstrual bleeding, or a thick discharge from the penis. Many people who are infected have no symptoms.

Untreated gonorrhea can lead to pelvic inflammatory disease and sterility in women; it can lead to prostate infection (see page 269) in men. Gonorrhea sometimes spreads to a person's joints, causing arthritis. Antibiotic treatment cures the infection. Both sex partners need to be treated to keep from passing the infection back and forth.

Hepatitis B

Hepatitis B is a viral infection that is spread through contact with infected blood, semen, or vaginal fluid (see page 94). The hepatitis B virus (HBV) is very contagious and may be spread to household contacts (other than sex partners) by sharing such things as razors and toothbrushes. Most people with hepatitis B recover completely after 4 to 8 weeks, but a small percentage of adults remain infected for months or years. Chronic infection can lead to life-threatening liver damage or cancer. Drug treatment for chronic HBV infection is not very effective.

People at risk for HBV infection (those with more than one sex partner; men who have sex with men; people who use intravenous drugs and share needles; and health care workers) should receive the hepatitis B vaccine. The vaccine is also recommended for all infants and for people under 18 who have not already been vaccinated. See page 18.

Human immunodeficiency virus (HIV)

Human immunodeficiency virus (HIV) is spread when blood, semen, or vaginal fluids from an infected person enter someone else's body. Once a person becomes infected, the

MORE INFO **For more information, see the back cover.**

virus attacks and gradually weakens his or her immune system. AIDS (acquired immunodeficiency syndrome) is the last phase in HIV disease, when the body is no longer able to fight infection or disease. Without treatment, AIDS develops in most people 12 to 13 years after they first become infected with HIV. With treatment, AIDS may be delayed for many more years.

A person is said to be HIV-positive if antibodies to the virus are detected in his or her blood. It may take up to 6 months after infection for the antibodies to appear. However, the virus can be spread to others before antibodies or symptoms are apparent.

The specific behaviors that spread HIV include:

• Having more than one sex partner.

• Having unprotected sex, especially unprotected sex between men (other than in a relationship in which both sex partners have sex only with each other and neither is infected).

• Sharing needles, syringes, or other "drug works" with someone who is HIV-positive.

• Having a sex partner with any of the above risk factors.

Babies born to or breast-fed by women who are HIV-positive are also at high risk for becoming infected with the virus.

Because all donated blood has been tested for HIV since 1985, the risk of getting the virus from transfused blood or blood products is extremely low.

HIV is not spread by mosquitoes; toilet seats; being coughed on by an infected person; casual contact with someone who is HIV-positive or who has AIDS; or by donating blood. Being touched, hugged, or lightly kissed by someone who is HIV-positive will not transfer the virus to you.

A simple, confidential blood test can determine if you are HIV-positive. You can have the test done in your doctor's office or at the local health department. A home test kit is available as well. If you engage in activities that put you at risk for HIV infection, have an HIV test every 6 months. Early diagnosis and treatment of HIV are important even before symptoms develop. If you think you have been exposed to HIV, but you test negative, you should be tested again 6 months after your last known exposure to HIV.

If you are pregnant and have any reason to believe that you may ever have been exposed to HIV, getting tested is the most important thing you can do for your baby. If you are HIV-positive, drug treatment during pregnancy can greatly reduce the likelihood that you will pass the infection on to your baby.

MORE INFO People who educate themselves about <u>HIV</u> infection learn how to make wise health decisions about preventing the spread of the virus and seek treatments that may improve their chances for staying healthy longer.

Syphilis

Syphilis is a bacterial infection spread through sexual contact, through sharing needles contaminated with an infected person's blood, or from an infected mother to her unborn baby. When syphilis is spread through sexual contact, symptoms appear about 3 weeks after infection occurs. The first symptom is a red, painless sore that appears on the genitals, rectal area, or mouth. The sore may go unnoticed. Swollen lymph nodes near the sore are another possible symptom.

If syphilis is not treated, it can proceed to a second phase after about 2 months. Symptoms of the second phase include a rash, patchy hair loss, fever, swollen lymph nodes, and flulike symptoms that are easily confused with other illnesses. Syphilis can be treated with antibiotics. If untreated, syphilis may cause serious health problems and death. Both partners need to be treated.

Trichomoniasis

Trichomoniasis is a bacterial infection that is spread through sexual contact. In women, the bacteria usually infect the vagina or urethra. In men, infections can develop in the urethra or under the foreskin of the penis.

Up to 50 percent of women who have trichomoniasis have no symptoms, and symptoms in infected men are rare. If symptoms do appear, they do so 4 to 28 days after infection occurs. Symptoms in women may include vaginal discharge, itching, and irritation and pain during sexual intercourse and when urinating. In men there may be a discharge from the penis and pain when urinating.

Trichomoniasis usually does not lead to serious illness. However, the infected person and his or her sex partner need to be treated with antibiotics to keep from passing the infection back and forth. Condoms should be used until treatment is completed.

Prevention

Preventing a sexually transmitted disease is easier than treating an infection once it occurs. Only monogamy (you and your partner have sex only with each other) between uninfected partners or sexual abstinence completely eliminates the risk of HIV infection and other sexually transmitted diseases. The following safer sex guidelines will help you reduce your risk.

- If you are beginning a new sexual relationship:

  - Take time before having sex to talk about HIV and other STDs. Find out if your partner has ever been exposed to or infected with an STD or if your partner's behavior puts him or her at risk for HIV infection. Tell your partner if you've ever engaged in high-risk behavior. Remember that it is possible to be infected with an STD without knowing it.

  - Use latex condoms and spermicide every time you have sex (vaginal, anal, or oral) until you are certain that neither you nor your partner has any STDs and that neither of you will have unprotected sexual contact with anyone else while your relationship lasts.

  - If you plan to use HIV testing to decide whether it is safe to have unprotected sex, have the test done 6 months after the last time you engaged in high-risk behavior. In the meantime, use condoms every time you have sexual contact.

- Avoid unprotected sexual contact with anyone who has symptoms of or who has been exposed to an STD, or whose behavior puts him or her at risk for HIV infection. Keep in mind that a person may still be able to transmit STDs even if no symptoms are present.

- Avoid unprotected vaginal, anal, or oral sex with anyone whose sexual history may not be risk-free or who has sores on the genitals or mouth. Use latex condoms from the beginning to the end of sexual contact. "Natural" or lambskin condoms do not protect against HIV infection or other STDs.

- Avoid sexual contact while you or your partner is being treated for an STD.

- If you or your partner has genital herpes, avoid sexual contact when a blister or an open sore is present. Use condoms unless you are in a stable, monogamous relationship and you have considered the risks associated with having unprotected sex with a person who has genital herpes.

- Do not rely on spermicides or a diaphragm to protect against STDs. Latex condoms provide the best protection against STDs, including HIV.

In addition to the guidelines above, taking the following precautions will reduce your risk of getting HIV and hepatitis B:

- Avoid activities that may spread HIV (see page 280). Safer activities include closed-mouth kissing, hugging, massage, and other pleasurable touching.

- Never share needles, syringes, razors, or other personal items that could be contaminated with blood.

If your job or behavior puts you at risk for HIV infection, or if you come in contact with HIV-infected blood (for example, an accidental needle stick), contact a health professional immediately. In some cases, medications may prevent HIV infection if they are started within a few hours after you are exposed to the virus. Have a blood test 6 months after any activity or accident that puts you at risk for HIV infection.

For more information, call the National AIDS Hotline at 1-800-342-AIDS.

When to Call a Health Professional

All STDs need to be diagnosed and treated by a health professional. Your doctor or a clinician at your local health department can diagnose and treat STDs. Your sex partner may also need to be treated, even if he or she has no symptoms. Otherwise, your partner may reinfect you or develop serious complications.

Call a health professional:

- If you suspect that you have been exposed to an STD.

- If you notice any unusual discharge from the vagina or penis or any sores, redness, or growths on the genitals.

- If your behavior puts you at risk for exposure to HIV, or if your sex partner has high-risk behavior or is HIV-positive.

- If you are pregnant and have any reason to believe that you may have been exposed to an STD, especially HIV.

- If you have symptoms, including fatigue, weight loss, fever, diarrhea, cough, or swollen glands, that do not go away after a short period of time and do not seem to be related to another illness.

- If you are HIV-positive and you develop any of the following:

  - Fever higher than 103°.

  - Fever higher than 101° that lasts 3 days or longer.

  - Increased outbreaks of cold sores or any unusual skin or mouth sores.

  - Severe numbness or pain in the hands and feet.

  - Unexplained weight loss.

  - Unexplained fever and night sweats.

  - Severe fatigue.

  - Diarrhea or other bowel changes.

  - Shortness of breath and a persistent dry cough.

  - Swollen lymph nodes in the neck, armpits, or groin.

  - Personality changes, difficulty concentrating, confusion, or severe headache.

If exercise could be packed into a pill, it would
be the single most widely prescribed,
and beneficial, medicine in the nation.
Robert Butler, MD

16

Fitness

Do you want to feel less stressed? Less tired? More in control of your weight and appearance? More healthy? Do you want to reduce your risk of heart disease, diabetes, and many other health problems? Believe it or not, there is one thing that can help you do all of this, and it doesn't come in a bottle. It's regular physical activity.

If just thinking about exercise makes you sweat, you may be pleasantly surprised by the information in this chapter. If you have already made physical activity a routine part of your life, you may find new reasons to keep your body moving.

Your Personal Fitness Plan

No one can prescribe the perfect fitness plan for you. You have to figure it out based on what you enjoy doing and what you will continue to do. The next few pages can be a big help.

Consistency is the most important, the most basic, and the most often neglected part of people's efforts to become more fit. No matter which activities you choose to do, in order to get the most benefit you need to do them consistently.

Don't forget the important role that nutrition plays in your healthy lifestyle. A balanced diet and regular physical activity go hand in hand to help you maintain a healthy weight. For information about how active people can get adequate nutrition, see Nutrition starting on page 293.

A good fitness plan has three parts: aerobic fitness, muscle strengthening, and flexibility. Many physical activities stress two or all three of these aspects of fitness. Read the sections that follow to learn about each aspect of fitness; then see Setting Your Fitness Goals on page 291.

Aerobic Fitness

Aerobic conditioning improves the function of your heart and lungs. Its purpose is to increase the amount of oxygen that is delivered to your muscles, which allows them to do more work.

Generally speaking, anything that raises your heart rate can be considered aerobic exercise. Some of the more common aerobic exercises include brisk walking, running, bicycling, swimming, and dancing.

You don't have to go out of your way to improve your aerobic fitness. Many activities that you do each day will help you become more fit if you do them regularly and long enough. The following ordinary activities all count as aerobic activity:

• Sweeping or mopping floors (perhaps to fast-paced music).

• Raking leaves, shoveling snow, or pushing a lawn mower.

• Walking the dog.

• Taking the stairs to your office instead of taking the elevator.

• Walking to a nearby restaurant for lunch instead of driving there.

How Hard Should I Exercise?

In order to benefit from aerobic exercise, you need to work hard enough to increase your heart rate. Work hard enough to feel the effort, but not so hard that you become out of

breath. Above all, listen to your body. If the exercise feels too hard, slow down. You will reduce your risk of injury and enjoy the exercise much more.

Try the "talk-sing test" to determine your ideal exercise pace:

• If you can't talk and exercise at the same time, you are going too fast.

• If you can talk while you exercise, you are doing fine.

• If you can sing while you exercise, it would be safe to increase your pace a little.

Target Heart Rate	
Age	10-second heart rate
20	20–27
25	20–26
30	19–25
35	19–25
40	18–24
45	18–23
50	17–23
55	17–23
60	16–22
65	16–21
70	15–20

Target heart rate is 60 percent to 80 percent of maximum heart rate. (Maximum heart rate = 220 minus your age.)

Target Heart Rate

Another way to see how hard you are exercising is to check your heart rate. You get the most benefit from aerobic exercise when your exercising heart rate is 60 percent to 80 percent of your maximum heart rate. After exercising for about 10 minutes, stop and take your pulse for 10 seconds (see page 58). Compare the number to the chart on page 286. Adjust the intensity of your exercise so that your heart rate stays between the two numbers. Remember, the target heart rate is only a guide. Everyone's body is different, so pay attention to how you feel.

Muscle Strengthening

Strengthening your muscles enables you to do more work and to work longer before you become exhausted. Strong muscles also help protect your joints.

Muscles become stronger through a three-step process:

1. Stress

2. Recovery (rest)

3. Repeated stress

A program for increasing your muscle strength can be as formal or informal as you'd like it to be. You may choose to do resistance training with free weights, weight-training equipment, inexpensive rubber tubing, or even canned goods.

Other simple, safe, and effective strengthening exercises include bent-knee curl-ups, chin-ups, push-ups, side leg-lifts, and other exercises that improve abdominal, neck, arm, shoulder, and leg strength.

Flexibility

Like aerobic fitness and muscle strengthening, flexibility is a result of physical activity. Flexibility comes from stretching. Your muscles are repeatedly shortened when they are used, especially during exercise. They need to be slowly and regularly stretched to counteract the repeated shortening that happens during other activities.

Stretching can increase your range of motion and reduce stiffness and pain. Being flexible also helps you have a better sense of balance. Stretching is particularly important during the cool-down phase of exercise when your muscles are warm. See the stretches on page 288.

• Stretch slowly and gradually. Don't bounce. Maintain a continuous tension on the muscle.

• Relax and hold each stretch for a count of 10.

• Exhale as you stretch to further relax your muscles. If stretching hurts, you have gone too far or you are doing something incorrectly.

groin stretch

calf stretch

quadriceps stretch

triceps stretch

hip stretch

latissimus stretch

hamstring stretch

Stretching exercises. Shaded areas show where stretches are felt.

Try to stretch a little every day. Take a stretch break instead of a coffee break, or take dance, martial arts, or yoga classes, which may appeal to your sense of fun and adventure as well as improve your flexibility.

How Often and How Long Should I Exercise?

The three factors that you need to consider when planning a fitness routine are:

1. Frequency (how often you exercise).

2. Duration (how long you exercise).

3. Intensity (how hard you exercise).

Achieving a balance between these three factors will give you better results than if you take any one of them to an extreme. You may choose to do a vigorously paced physical activity (such as swimming, fast dancing, or cycling) 3 times a week for 30 minutes per session. Or you may choose to exercise at a moderate intensity (such as walking or doing yardwork) 5 to 6 times a week for 30 minutes per session. The first routine stresses intensity while the second stresses frequency. Both routines are probably equally effective for improving your overall fitness.

Warm Up and Cool Down

For the first 5 or 10 minutes of your activity routine, go slowly and easily, gradually increasing your pace, so your muscles have a chance to warm up. After a few minutes of warm-up, do some stretches to prepare your muscles for the workout.

End your activity with a cool-down period of about 8 to 10 minutes. Gradually slow your pace for about 5 minutes; then do a few stretches (see page 288) to improve flexibility.

Drink water before, during, and after the activity.

Making Progress

As you build aerobic endurance, your heart rate will not rise as high as it once did during the same activity. You will need to do the activity longer or harder to get the same benefits from it. You can use your target heart rate to decide how much harder your workout needs to be. You can also add some new element of difficulty or variety to your current workout, such as increasing your pace, alternating between an aerobic activity and a strength-training activity (cross-training), or trying a new aerobic activity that is slightly harder for you.

As your muscles grow stronger, you will notice that you can work longer without tiring. If a muscle-strengthening activity starts to feel too easy, gradually add more resistance. Remember to work slowly, and move your muscles through their full range of motion.

Overcoming Barriers to Exercise

There are many barriers to getting regular physical activity, some of which are easier to overcome than others. Here are a few common barriers and some suggestions for getting past them.

1. No time? Try shorter periods of activity spread throughout the day, such as walking 3 times a day for 10 minutes each time.

2. Too tired? It's often lack of exercise that makes you tired. Exercise gives you energy. Try it.

3. Embarrassed? Many people are, especially at first. Be proud that you're taking care of your body.

4. No partner? Yes, it's more fun to exercise with a friend. If your regular exercise partner quits, find another one.

5. Bad weather? Too hot, too cold, too wet, too windy—it never seems right for exercise. Lots of people exercise come rain or shine. You can too; just dress properly. Try a variety of indoor and outdoor activities.

6. Too costly? You had to let the fitness club membership expire. You can't afford a mountain bike. You panic at the price of running shoes. It all costs money. But can you afford not to exercise? Try a low-cost option, such as walking, riding a bicycle, or dancing.

7. Not the athletic type? Physical activity doesn't require any special athletic skill. Everyone's body is made to move.

Exercise Cautions

Moderate exercise is safe for most people. However, if you can answer "yes" to any of the following questions, talk with your doctor before starting an exercise program.

- Do you have heart trouble?

- Do you often have pains in your heart or chest?

- Do you have high blood pressure?

- Do you often feel faint or have dizzy spells?

- Do you have arthritis or other bone or joint problems that might be made worse by exercise?

- Do you have diabetes? (Increased exercise affects your insulin needs.)

- Are you over age 40 with 2 or more risk factors for heart disease*?

- Are you older than 60 and not used to hard exercise?

*Cholesterol over 200 mg/dl; blood pressure over 140/90; smoking; diabetes; family history of heart disease before age 50.

Setting Your Fitness Goals

Are you as strong, flexible, and physically fit as you would like to be? If you are, good for you. We hope this chapter has helped reaffirm your commitment to physical fitness and given you ideas to keep you motivated. However, if you want to make some improvements, here's one piece of advice: Try to take it one step at a time.

- Pick one aspect of fitness (aerobic, strength, flexibility) that you want to improve first.

- Pick an activity that you enjoy. You're more likely to keep doing something you like.

- Set a 1-week goal that you think you can reach. For example, plan to walk for 10 minutes at lunch 3 days a week or to stretch for 5 minutes each morning.

- Start today. Keep a record of what you do.

- When you reach your first goal, reward yourself! Then set a new goal. Once you get used to meeting weekly goals, try setting a 1-month goal.

Consistency brings success. Small successes can quickly add up to a level of physical fitness that will make a big difference in your life.

Maintaining the Lifestyle

Staying motivated is essential to making physical activity a long-term lifestyle commitment. If you choose activities wisely, your body will let you know how enjoyable becoming more fit can be.

If you're just starting out with a fitness plan, reaching one goal and then striving for another may be enough to keep you going. Before long, you'll start to notice changes in your endurance, strength, flexibility, energy level, and appearance that will probably encourage you to continue your efforts.

People who are moderately active or very active may become bored with their usual activities and need to find new ways to stay motivated. Vary your activity, or vary when or where you exercise. If you don't already do so, try working out with a partner. Continue to set goals for yourself. You might want to train for a competitive event related to your activity. Another great way to stay motivated is to help someone else who is just starting a fitness program. You will be a role model for that person, you'll have another reason for staying consistently active, and you are more likely to learn ways to vary your routine.

Never eat more than you can lift.
Miss Piggy

17

Nutrition

This chapter gives some guidelines for good eating and some hints on how to help your children establish healthy eating habits. Children learn best by example, so practice good eating habits along with them.

Simple Guidelines for Eating Well

The Dietary Guidelines for Americans are aimed at improving health and reducing the risk of disease, especially high blood pressure, heart disease, stroke, type 2 diabetes, osteoporosis, and certain types of cancer.

1. Aim for a healthy weight. Healthy bodies come in many shapes and sizes. Work toward achieving and maintaining the weight that is best for you by choosing a variety of healthy foods and getting regular physical activity.

2. Be physically active every day. Regular physical activity that is vigorous enough to raise your heart rate has many benefits. When combined with a healthy diet, it is the best way to maintain a healthy body weight.

3. Let the Pyramid guide your choices. The Food Guide Pyramid on page 295 is a simple, flexible guide designed to help you follow a balanced diet. It encourages eating a variety of foods in balance with one another so that your body gets the nutrients it needs every day.

4. Choose a variety of grains daily, especially whole grains. Foods made from grains are the foundation of good nutrition. They provide vitamins, minerals, fiber, and carbohydrates and are often low in fat. Whole grains may help protect against heart disease and high blood pressure.

5. Choose a variety of fruits and vegetables daily. These foods are key parts of your daily diet, but most people eat fewer than the recommended 5 servings. Fruits and vegetables taste great, are easy to prepare, and may help prevent some types of cancer.

6. Keep food safe to eat. Prevent food poisoning by keeping hot foods hot and cold foods cold. See Stomach Flu and Food Poisoning on page 98 for more information on how to store, handle, and prepare food safely.

7. Choose a diet low in saturated fat and cholesterol and moderate in total fat to reduce your risk for heart disease, cancer, and high blood pressure. Choosing more grains, fruits, and vegetables can help your reduce the amount of total fat in your diet.

8. Choose beverages and foods that limit your sugar intake. Added sugars have no other nutrients, and when consumed in excess, they crowd healthier foods out of your diet.

9. Choose and prepare foods with less salt to help reduce your risk of high blood pressure. Reducing your salt intake can also help lower your blood pressure if it is already high. See page 243.

10. If you drink alcoholic beverages, do so in moderation. Alcohol supplies calories but few nutrients. Drinking alcohol is the cause of many health problems and accidents and can lead to addiction. Moderate alcohol consumption is defined as no more than 2 drinks a day for men and no more than 1 drink a day for women. Women who are pregnant or trying to become pregnant should avoid alcoholic beverages altogether.

Eating Well: A Basic Plan

Eat a variety of foods from the Food Guide Pyramid on page 295 each day. Most people who follow the diet outlined by the Pyramid will get all the vitamins, minerals, and other nutrients their bodies need and may have less trouble controlling their weight.

Grain Products

Grains are the foundation of the Food Guide Pyramid. Whole grains, such as whole-wheat breads and pastas, oats, and brown rice, contain large amounts of vitamins, minerals, fiber, and carbohydrates. Carbohydrates are the body's fuel and should provide 55 to 60 percent of total calories for most people.

Fruits and Vegetables

Fruits and vegetables make up the second tier of the Food Guide Pyramid. Notice that the "plant-based" foods in this group and the grain group represent about two-thirds of what you should eat each day. Aim to eat at least 5 daily servings of fruits and vegetables.

Guide to Eating Well

Grains (breads, cereals, rice, pasta) form the foundation of a healthy diet. Serving sizes: 1 slice of bread, 1 oz. of cereal, ½ bagel, ½ cup of pasta or rice.

Eat plenty of fruits and vegetables. Serving sizes: ¾ cup fruit or vegetable juice; ½ cup raw, canned, or cooked fruits or vegetables; 1 medium apple or banana; 1 cup raw leafy vegetables.

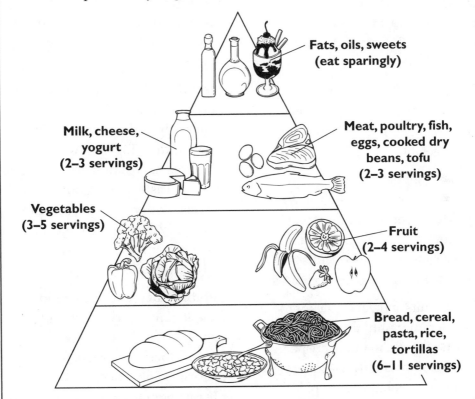

Fats, oils, sweets (eat sparingly)

Milk, cheese, yogurt (2–3 servings)

Meat, poultry, fish, eggs, cooked dry beans, tofu (2–3 servings)

Vegetables (3–5 servings)

Fruit (2–4 servings)

Bread, cereal, pasta, rice, tortillas (6–11 servings)

The Food Guide Pyramid (USDA)

Choose lean meats, fish, or poultry and cooked dry beans to reduce fat. Serving sizes: 2–3 oz. cooked lean meat, poultry, or fish; ½ cup cooked dry beans; 1 egg; 2 tbsp. peanut butter.

Choose nonfat or low-fat dairy products. Serving sizes: 1 cup milk or yogurt, 1½–2 oz. low-fat cheese, ½ cup cottage cheese.

Eat foods from the top of the Pyramid only in moderation. Examples: cooking oil, butter or margarine, high-fat salty snacks, alcohol, candy.

Fruits and vegetables provide vitamins, minerals, fiber, and carbohydrates. They also contain compounds that appear to protect against heart disease, high blood pressure, and some types of cancer. These compounds include antioxidants, such as vitamin C, vitamin A (beta carotene), and other carotenoids, as well as nonnutrient compounds called phytochemicals (see page 302).

To make the most of the nutritents and healthy compounds in fruits and vegetables:

- When shopping for fruits and vegetables, avoid damaged and wilted produce. Choose produce that is in season and locally grown, if possible. Frozen or canned fruits and vegetables are also good choices.

- Store fruits and vegetables at room temperature until they are ripe. Then place them in the crisper drawer of your refrigerator or store them in a cool, dry, dark place.

- Before eating fruits or vegetables, rinse them well but don't soak them. Chop vegetables into large pieces just before cooking. Microwave, steam, stir-fry, or saute vegetables in a small amount of water or oil until they are just tender.

Fiber

Fiber is the indigestible part of plants. It is not absorbed into the bloodstream like other nutrients. However, it plays an important role in keeping your digestive tract healthy by providing "bulk."

There are two types of fiber found in foods: insoluble fiber and soluble fiber.

Insoluble fiber, which can be found in whole-grain products, such as whole-wheat flour, provides bulk for your diet. Together with fluids, insoluble fiber stimulates your colon to keep waste moving out of your bowels. Without fiber, waste moves too slowly, increasing your risk for constipation, diverticulosis, and possibly colon cancer.

Soluble fiber, which is found in fruit, legumes (dry beans and peas), and oats, helps lower blood cholesterol, reducing your risk for heart disease. Soluble fiber, especially the fiber in legumes, can also help regulate your blood glucose level.

Do you need more fiber in your diet? If your stools are soft and easy to pass, you probably get plenty of fiber. If they are hard and difficult to pass, more fiber and water may help. See page 82 for more information about constipation.

To increase fiber in your diet:

- Eat at least 5 servings of fruits or vegetables a day (see the Food Guide Pyramid on page 295). Eat fruits with edible skins and seeds:

kiwi fruit, figs, blueberries, apples, and raspberries. Eat more raw or lightly cooked vegetables.

• Switch to whole-grain and whole-wheat breads, pasta, tortillas, and cereals. The first ingredient listed should be whole-wheat flour.

• Eat more cooked dry beans, dry peas, and lentils. These high-fiber, high-protein foods can replace some of the high-fat, no-fiber meats in your diet.

• Popcorn is a good high-fiber snack. However, avoid added oil, butter, and salt. Use an air or microwave popcorn popper to eliminate oil, and add flavor with salt substitute or herb mixtures.

Sugar

In moderation, sugar does little harm. However, if too many of your calories come from sugar, you will gain weight and may not get enough of the other nutrients you need. Sugar also contributes to dental cavities.

To reduce sugar in your diet:

• Be aware that all sugars are basically alike. Honey and brown or raw sugar have no advantage over other sugars. Corn syrup is another commonly used form of sugar.

• Processed foods and drinks can be full of sugar. Flavored yogurt, breakfast cereals, canned fruits, and desserts often have sugar added. Look for breakfast cereals that have 6 grams or less of added sugar per serving.

• Limit foods and drinks that list sugar among the first few ingredients.

• You can reduce the amount of sugar added to homemade baked goods by up to one-half without affecting the texture. Try using more sweet spices, such as cinnamon and nutmeg, in your recipes.

• Make it a habit to eat a sweet piece of fruit instead of a sugary dessert most of the time.

• Drink water, sparkling water, or milk instead of soft drinks or sweetened fruit drinks.

Fats in Foods

The Dietary Guidelines for Americans recommend that less than 30 percent of your total calorie intake come from fat. Reducing dietary fat to 30 percent will slow the development of heart disease, reduce your cancer risk, and improve your overall diet. No more than 10 percent of total calories should come from saturated fats.

The Food Guide Pyramid is designed to help you eat a low-fat diet. If you need help reducing fat in your diet, a registered dietitian can create a menu plan that will help you meet your goal.

Simple Ways to Reduce Fat
When eating meat:

• Keep serving sizes at 2 to 3 ounces (about the size of a deck of cards), and don't eat second helpings. If you eat red meat, choose the leanest cuts, such as tenderloin, flank steak, chuck, or top and bottom round.

- Eat more poultry (without skin) and fish. They contain less saturated fat than red meat does.

- Remove all visible fat from meat, poultry, and fish before cooking. Remove poultry skin either before or after cooking.

- Bake, broil, or sauté meats, poultry, and fish instead of frying in butter or fat.

- Occasionally serve a combination of legumes (dried beans, peas, lentils) and grains in place of a meat entree.

When using dairy products:

- Use skim, ½, or 1 percent milk.

- Choose cheeses made with skim or part skim milk, or look for cheeses that have no more than 5 grams of fat per ounce (read the label).

- Try low-fat cottage cheese or yogurt in place of cream and sour cream; or use fat-free sour cream and fat-free cream cheese.

When cooking:

- Steam vegetables. If you choose to sauté them, use 1 tablespoon of oil (or less), or try using other liquids such as wine, defatted broth, or cooking sherry.

- Use nonstick pans, or add a small amount of oil to a preheated pan (less oil goes farther this way).

The 80-20 Rule

If you are generally healthy, you don't need to worry about maintaining a perfect diet. If you make healthy eating choices 80 percent of the time, occasionally eating high-fat or high-calorie foods the remaining 20 percent of the time won't be a problem.

- Season vegetables with herbs and spices instead of butter and sauces; or try a butter substitute such as Butter Buds or Molly McButter. Dress salads with lemon juice, fat-free mayonnaise, or fat-free dressing.

- Use a cooking oil that is liquid at room temperature (such as canola, olive, or peanut oil) and use it sparingly (1 teaspoon at a time).

- Experiment with using less oil than is called for in recipes. You may need to increase other liquids. Use applesauce, prune puree, or mashed bananas to replace some of the fat in baked goods.

Cholesterol

For many people, a diet high in saturated fat raises the amount of cholesterol in the blood, which increases your risk of heart attack and stroke. (See page 240.) Review the tips on how to reduce fat in your diet on page 297.

Protein

Protein is important for maintaining healthy muscles, tendons, bones, skin, hair, blood, and internal organs. Most adult Americans get all the protein they need in their diets. If you eat animal products (milk, cheese, eggs, fish, meat), your diet will contain plenty of protein. However, if you eat little meat, poultry, or fish and use no dairy products, your diet will require careful planning in order for you to get all the protein and other nutrients you need.

Vitamins

Vitamins are tiny elements of food that have no calories, yet are essential to good health. Vitamins A, D, E, and K are fat-soluble and can be stored in the liver or in fat tissue for a relatively long time. Other vitamins, including all the B vitamins and vitamin C, are water-soluble, and your body can only retain them for a short time, so it is important that you consume them often.

Most people who eat a variety of foods from the Food Guide Pyramid (page 295) get all the necessary vitamins. However, if you typically eat fewer than 1,500 calories per day, you may want to consider taking a vitamin-mineral supplement. Choose a balanced, multivitamin-mineral supplement rather than a specific vitamin or mineral, unless your doctor prescribes a specific supplement. Avoid taking much more than 100 percent of the recommended dietary allowance of any vitamin or mineral unless it is prescribed by a doctor.

Certain vitamins found in foods have been shown to prevent some diseases. However, researchers are still trying to determine whether those vitamins have the same preventive effects when taken as supplements. If possible, add more variety and balance to your diet rather than trying to make up for a poor diet by taking supplements.

Minerals

Minerals have many important roles in the structure and function of your body. You need minerals to build and maintain healthy teeth and bones; to carry nerve signals to and from your brain; to carry oxygen to your cells; to regulate blood sugar levels; and to maintain a healthy immune system.

A total of 60 minerals have been discovered in the body, and 22 are essential to health. Eating a variety of foods is the best way to get all the minerals you need.

Calcium

Calcium is the primary mineral needed for building and maintaining strong bones. Calcium is especially important for growing children and for women, especially in the peak bone-building years between the teens and early 30s. Calcium also helps women prevent osteoporosis, which can occur after menopause. See page 135.

Children from 1 to 3 years of age need 500 mg of calcium per day; those from 4 to 8 years of age need 800 mg per day; and those from 9 to 18 years of age need 1,300 mg per day. Adults between 19 and 50 years of age need 1,000 mg per day. Adults age 51 and older need 1,200 mg per day.

Fat-free or low-fat milk products are the best source of dietary calcium. Each serving provides about 300 mg of calcium. Milk products provide other nutrients in addition to calcium, such as protein and vitamin D. Other foods, such as tofu, fortified soy milk, broccoli, certain greens, and calcium-fortified orange juice, provide calcium in varying amounts.

While dietary calcium is preferred, low-dose calcium supplements (such as Tums) can also help keep bones strong. If you are not sure you are getting enough calcium in your diet, talk to your health professional about whether a calcium supplement would be helpful.

Salt

Most people get far more salt (sodium) than they need. For some people, excess salt causes high blood pressure. See page 243.

In general, processed foods contain the most salt, while unprocessed foods, such as fresh fruits and vegetables, have the least. If you want to cut back on the salt in your diet:

- Read the Nutrition Facts labels on foods for sodium content. Choose foods that contain less sodium.

Lactose Intolerance

People whose bodies produce too little of the enzyme lactase have trouble digesting the lactose (sugar) in milk. Symptoms of lactose intolerance include gas, bloating, cramps, and diarrhea after drinking milk or eating milk products.

If you have mild to moderate lactose intolerance:

- Eat small amounts of milk products at any one time.

- Try eating cheese. Most of the lactose in cheese is removed during processing.

- Eat yogurts made with active cultures, which provide their own enzymes that digest the lactose in milk.

- Drink pretreated milk (such as Lactaid), or try enzyme tablets (such as Lactaid or Dairy Ease), which will help you digest lactose.

- You may be able to tolerate milk if you drink it with snacks or meals.

If you have severe lactose intolerance:

- Read labels to avoid any form of lactose in foods.

- Be sure to include nondairy sources of calcium in your diet. See page 299. You may need calcium supplements to get enough calcium. Ask your doctor or a dietitian.

- Find ways to get enough of the nutrients supplied by the milk group from the rest of your diet.

• Limit ready-mixed sauces and seasonings, frozen dinners, and canned or dehydrated soups. These foods are usually packed with salt. Products labeled "low sodium" contain less than 140 mg of sodium per serving.

• Eat lots of fresh or frozen fruits and vegetables. These foods contain very little sodium.

• Don't put the salt shaker on the table, or get a salt shaker that allows very little salt to come out. Use salt substitute or "lite salt" sparingly.

• Always measure the salt in recipes, and use half of what is called for.

• Avoid fast foods, which are usually very high in salt. In a restaurant, ask the chef not to salt food during cooking.

Iron

Your body needs small amounts of iron to make hemoglobin, which carries oxygen in your blood. Adult men need 10 mg of iron per day; adult women need 15 mg per day. Infants and young children have higher iron needs relative to their size than other age groups. People who have increased blood loss caused by ulcers or heavy menstrual periods or who take arthritis medications (such as aspirin) are at high risk for iron deficiency anemia. Symptoms of iron deficiency anemia include paleness and fatigue. A blood test is needed to confirm the diagnosis, and further testing may be needed to determine the cause of the blood loss.

To get more iron in your blood:

• Eat foods with vitamin C along with iron-rich foods. Vitamin C helps you absorb more iron from food. To get the most iron from a bowl of iron-enriched cereal, drink a glass of orange or other citrus juice when you eat the cereal. High-iron cereals have at least 25 percent of the Daily Value (DV) of iron.

• Eat meat and vegetables or grains together. The iron in animal tissues (heme iron) improves absorption of the iron in other foods.

• Avoid caffeinated tea with meals. It interferes with iron absorption.

Iron Supplements

Women who menstruate and who eat fewer than 1,500 calories per day may wish to consider taking a multivitamin-mineral supplement that contains iron. (Men are much less likely to need iron supplements.) A low-dose ferrous-form iron supplement containing no more than 20 mg is safe for most women to take daily. However, too much iron can cause a number of serious medical problems or mask the development of others. Do not take more than 20 mg of iron per day without consulting your doctor first. Take iron supplements between meals, at bedtime, or on an empty stomach. Keep iron supplements away from children.

Nonnutrients in Foods

In addition to the essential nutrients, foods also contain nonnutrient compounds that act on your body in some way. These include phytochemicals (found in plants), many of which protect against cancer.

Some foods contain compounds that have medicinal effects, such as the compound found in cranberries that may flush bacteria from the urinary tract and prevent urinary tract infections.

The nonnutrients in foods are of great interest today, and many of them are just being discovered. Foods are made of hundreds of chemicals that cannot be duplicated in a supplement. Taking a supplement cannot provide "insurance" against a poor or inadequate diet. If you think that your diet is poor, then the best advice is to improve it.

Nutrition for Children

Your whole family can follow the diet outlined in the Food Guide Pyramid (page 295). Offer nutritious foods as well-planned, pleasant meals and snacks. Then sit back and let your child decide how much to eat (or even if he or she wants to eat at all). This is a good division of responsibility that allows children to tune in to their own appetites and takes the pressure off the parents.

Child-Sized Environment

Imagine yourself eating at a giant's table. That's how a child can feel eating at an adult-sized table in an adult-sized chair.

• Provide a booster seat and child-sized utensils. However, fingers are fine until a child can hold utensils easily.

• Give children smaller plates and smaller servings (1 tablespoon per year of age is a good serving size guide). If the child is hungry for seconds, he or she will ask for them.

Healthy Snacks

Young children have small stomachs and high energy needs, so they need frequent snacks to supplement meals. Plan between-meal snacks as part of the day's total food intake. Snacks should provide good nutrition, not just empty calories.

• Fruits and fruit juices are good snacks. Other good choices are raw vegetable sticks with fat-free dressing, cereal, yogurt, cheese, or soup.

• Serve meals and snacks on a regular schedule. Do not serve snacks so close to a meal that they interfere with the child's appetite.

• Choose desserts that are low in fat and high in nutrients. Fruit, yogurt, and other foods found in the Food Guide Pyramid are good choices.

He who laughs, lasts.
Mary Pettibone Poole

18

Mental Health Problems and Mind-Body Wellness

This chapter is organized in two sections. The first section covers some common mental and emotional health problems and describes what you can do to treat them at home and when you should seek professional help. The second section describes the relationship between your mental health and your physical health.

This chapter does not address all mental health problems. If you have symptoms of a mental health problem that are not described here, contact a health professional.

Mental Health Problems

Mental health problems are similar to other health problems: some can be prevented; others will go away on their own with home treatment; and some need professional attention. Many mental health problems begin

when physical stress (such as an illness or injury) or emotional stress (such as the loss of a loved one) triggers chemical changes in your brain. The goal of treatment for mental health problems—including self-care and professional treatment—is to reduce stress and restore the normal chemical processes in your brain.

In general, it is a good idea to seek professional help for a mental health problem when:

• A symptom becomes severe or disruptive.

• A symptom becomes a continuous or permanent pattern of behavior and does not respond to self-care.

• Symptoms become numerous, affect all areas of your life, and do not respond to self-care or communication efforts.

• You are thinking about suicide.

Alcohol and Drug Problems

The overuse or abuse of alcohol or other drugs is called substance abuse. It is common, costly, and associated with many medical problems.

Alcohol Problems

A person has an alcohol use problem if he or she continues to drink even though alcohol is interfering with his or her health or daily living. Alcoholism is defined as a physical or psychological dependence on alcohol.

Alcohol abuse patterns vary. Some people get drunk every day. Some drink large amounts of alcohol at specific times, such as weekends. Others may be sober for long periods and then go on drinking binges that last for weeks or months.

 Long-term heavy drinking causes liver, nerve, heart, and brain damage; high blood pressure; depression; stomach problems; sexual problems; and cancer. Alcohol abuse can also lead to violence, accidents, social isolation, and difficulties at work, at home, or with the law.

Signs that a person is dependent on alcohol include not remembering what happened while he or she was drinking (blackouts), drinking more and more for the same "high," and being uncomfortable in situations where alcohol isn't served. A person with alcoholism may gulp or sneak drinks, drink alone or early in the morning, and suffer from the shakes.

Are You a Problem User?

Answer the following questions honestly. They refer to your use of alcohol and drugs, including prescribed and illegal drugs.

- Have you ever felt that you ought to cut down on your drinking or drug use?

- Do you get annoyed at criticism of your drinking or drug use?

- Do you ever feel guilty about your drinking or drug use?

- Do you ever take an early morning drink or use drugs first thing in the morning to get the day started or to eliminate the "shakes?"

A person who answers "yes" to any of these questions may have a problem with alcohol or drugs. Call a health professional to arrange for other tests to diagnose alcohol or drug dependence.

A person whose body is dependent on alcohol may suffer serious withdrawal symptoms (such as trembling, delusions, hallucinations, sweating, and seizures) if he or she stops drinking suddenly or tries to reduce his or her alcohol intake. Once alcohol dependency develops, it is very difficult for a person to stop drinking without outside help. Medical detoxification may be needed.

Drug Problems

Drug abuse includes the use of marijuana, cocaine, heroin, or other "street drugs," and the abuse of legal prescription drugs. Some people turn to drugs as a way to get a "high" or to deal with stress or emotional problems.

Tranquilizers, sedatives, pain-killers, and amphetamines are misused most often, sometimes unintentionally.

Drug dependence (addiction) occurs when a person develops a physical or psychological need for a drug. A person may not be aware that he or she has become dependent on a drug until he or she tries to suddenly stop taking it. Withdrawing from the drug can cause uncomfortable symptoms such as muscle aches, diarrhea, or depression. The usual treatment for drug dependence is to reduce the dose of the drug gradually until it can be stopped completely.

Signs of Drug Use

- Chronic red eyes, sore throat, dry cough, and fatigue (in the absence of allergies)
- Major changes in sleeping or eating habits
- Moodiness, hostility, or abusive behavior
- Work or school problems, absenteeism
- Loss of interest in favorite activities
- Social withdrawal or changes in friends
- Stealing, lying, and poor family relationships

Prevention

- Look for signs of mental stress. Try to understand and resolve sources of depression, anxiety, or loneliness. Don't use alcohol or drugs to deal with these problems.

- Educate your children about the effects of alcohol and drugs. Children are less likely to use alcohol or other drugs if their parents teach them early (during the elementary school years) about their effects.

- If you drink, do so in moderation: not more than 2 drinks a day for men and not more than 1 drink a day for women and older adults. One drink is 12 ounces of beer, 5 ounces of wine, or 1 ounce of hard liquor.

- Don't drink alcohol or use drugs if you are pregnant or trying to become pregnant. Either can seriously harm your baby.

- Ask your pharmacist or doctor if any of your current medications could potentially lead to overuse or dependence. Be especially cautious of painkillers, tranquilizers, sedatives, and sleeping pills. Follow the instructions carefully, and do not exceed the recommended dose.

- Do not suddenly stop taking any medication without your doctor's supervision.

- Avoid alcohol when you are taking medications. Alcohol can react with many drugs and cause serious complications.

Home Treatment

- Recognize early signs that alcohol or drug use is becoming a problem. See "Are You a Problem User?" on page 304.

- Attend an Alcoholics Anonymous meeting (a self-help group devoted to helping members get sober and stay sober).

If you are concerned about another person's alcohol or drug use:

- Never ignore the problem. Discuss it as a medical problem.

- Build up the person's self-esteem and reaffirm his or her value as a person. Help the person see that he or she can be successful without

alcohol or drugs. Let the person know you will support his or her efforts to change.

- Ask if the person will accept help. Don't give up if you get a negative response; keep asking periodically. If the person eventually agrees, act that very day to arrange for help. Call a health professional or Alcoholics Anonymous for an immediate appointment.

- Attend a few meetings of Al-Anon, a support group for family members and friends of alcoholics. Read some 12-step program information.

When to Call a Health Professional

Call 911 or other emergency services:

- If a person loses consciousness after drinking alcohol or taking drugs.

- If a person who has been drinking alcohol or using drugs threatens to commit suicide.

- If a person who suddenly stops using alcohol has withdrawal symptoms (trembling, hallucinations, seizures).

Call a health professional:

- If you answer "yes" to any of the questions under "Are You a Problem User?" on page 304.

- If you recognize an alcohol or drug problem in yourself and are ready to accept help. Both outpatient and inpatient treatment programs are available.

Anger and Hostility

Anger signals your body to prepare for a fight. When you get angry, adrenaline and other hormones are released into your bloodstream. Your blood pressure, pulse, and respiration rate all go up.

Anger is a normal response to daily events. It is the appropriate response to any situation that poses a threat. Anger can be directed to become a positive, driving force behind your actions.

Hostility is being ready for a fight all the time. Continual hostility keeps your blood pressure high and may increase your risk for heart attack and other illnesses. Being hostile also isolates you from other people.

Home Treatment

• Try to understand the real reason why you are angry. Is it the current situation that is making you angry or something that happened earlier in the day?

• Notice when you start to become angry, and take steps to deal with your anger in a positive way. Don't ignore your anger until you "blow up." Express your anger in healthy ways:

- Count to 10 or practice some other form of mental relaxation (see page 323). When you have

calmed down, you will be better able to discuss the conflict rationally.

- Try screaming or yelling in a private place, not at other people.

- Go for a short walk or jog.

- Talk with a friend about your anger.

- Draw or paint to release the anger, or write about it in a journal.

• Use "I" statements, not "you" statements, to discuss your anger. Say "I feel angry when my needs are not being met," instead of "You make me mad when you are so inconsiderate."

• If you are angry with someone, listen to what the other person has to say. Try to understand his or her point of view.

• Forgive and forget. Forgiving helps lower blood pressure and ease muscle tension so you can feel more relaxed.

• Read books about anger and how to handle it. See page 317 for additional information about anger and violent behavior.

When to Call a Health Professional

• If anger has led or could lead to violence or harm to you or someone else.

• If anger or hostility interferes with your work, family life, or friendships.

Anxiety and Panic Disorder

Feeling worried, anxious, and nervous is a normal part of everyday life. Everyone frets or feels anxious from time to time.

Anxiety can cause both physical and emotional symptoms. A specific situation or fear can cause some or all of these symptoms for a short time. When the situation passes, the symptoms go away.

Physical Symptoms

• Trembling, twitching, or shaking

• Lightheadedness or dizziness

• A feeling of fullness in the throat or chest

• Muscle tension, aches, or soreness

• Restlessness

• Fatigue

• Insomnia

• Breathlessness or rapid heartbeat

• Sweating or cold, clammy hands

Emotional Symptoms

• Feeling keyed up and on edge

• Excessive worrying

• Fearing that something bad is going to happen

• Poor concentration

• Irritability or agitation

• Constant sadness

Many people, including children and teens, develop anxiety disorders in which these symptoms occur for no identifiable or rational reason. This type of anxiety can become overwhelming and is not normal. People with an anxiety disorder may develop irrational and involuntary fears (phobias) of common places, objects, or situations.

Panic disorder is a common anxiety-related disorder. People with panic disorder have periods of sudden, intense fear and anxiety when there is no clear cause or danger. These panic attacks can cause frightening (but not life-threatening) symptoms, such as a pounding heart, shortness of breath, a feeling of choking or suffocation, and a sense that you are about to lose control or die. People who have had panic attacks may try to avoid any situations or behaviors that might trigger another attack. This often results in a higher level of anxiety.

Self-care, often combined with counseling and medication, can be effective in managing anxiety and panic disorder.

Home Treatment

The following home treatment tips can relieve simple anxiety and can also help if you are receiving medical treatment for anxiety or panic disorder.

• Recognize and accept your anxiety about specific fears or situations. Then say to yourself, "This is not an emergency. I feel uncomfortable, but I am not in danger. I can keep going even if I feel anxious."

• Be kind to your body:

- Relieve tension by exercising or getting a massage.

- Practice relaxation techniques. See page 323.

- Get enough rest. If you have trouble sleeping, see Sleep Problems on page 314.

- Avoid alcohol, caffeine, and nicotine. They can increase your anxiety level, cause sleep problems, or trigger a panic attack.

• Engage your mind:

- Get out and do something you enjoy, such as going to a funny movie or taking a walk or a hike.

- Plan your day. Having too much or too little to do can make you more anxious.

• Keep a record of your symptoms. Discuss your fears with a good friend or family member, or join a support group for people with similar problems. Confiding with others sometimes relieves stress.

• Get involved in social groups or volunteer to help others. Being alone sometimes makes things seem worse than they are.

When to Call a Health Professional

• If you are seriously considering harming yourself or someone else.

• If anxiety or irrational fear interferes with your daily activities.

• If sudden, severe attacks of fear or anxiety with physical symptoms (shaking, sweating) seem to occur for no reason.

• If symptoms of anxiety are still severe after 1 week of home treatment.

• If you suffer from nightmares or flashbacks to traumatic events.

• If you are unable to feel certain about things (e.g., whether you unplugged the iron) no matter how many times you check, or if repetitive actions that you cannot control interfere with your daily activities.

Depression

Depression is a common problem that affects men and women of all ages, including children and teens. It is more than just the normal, temporary feelings of sadness and moodiness that come with the ups and downs of life. Depression can range from a minor problem to a major life-threatening illness. Fortunately, effective treatments are available for most people who suffer from depression.

Sadness or Depression?

People who are depressed:

- Have persistent feelings of sadness, anxiety, or hopelessness.

- Lose interest in or no longer enjoy their usual activities.

If you have also experienced 5 or more of the following symptoms nearly every day for more than 2 weeks, you may be suffering from depression:

- An unexplained change in your eating patterns that has caused weight gain or loss.

- Restlessness or irritability.

- Insomnia or excessive sleepiness.

- Low energy, fatigue.

- Feelings of worthlessness or guilt.

- Inability to concentrate, remember, or make decisions.

- Frequent thoughts of suicide or death.

Home treatment may be all that is needed for mild depression. However, if you are feeling suicidal or if home treatment doesn't help lift your mood within 2 weeks, contact a health professional. With counseling, medication, and continued home treatment, you can overcome most cases of depression.

Depression is probably caused by a combination of factors, including the genetic traits that a person inherits from his or her parents. Most major depressions involve problems with the chemical messengers (neurotransmitters) in the brain. The amount of stress in a person's life and the way a person copes with stress also contribute to depression. Ongoing depression affects a person's body, mind, and social behavior.

Many things can trigger depression, including:

- Drinking alcohol or using illegal drugs.

- Having a major illness or injury.

- Grieving the death of a loved one.

- Going through major life changes (loss of a job, divorce, children leaving home, retirement).

- Being under long-term stress, such as having a family member with a chronic illness.

- Taking certain medications or having certain health conditions.

- Having recently had a baby (postpartum depression).

Reduced daylight during the winter seems to cause a form of depression called seasonal affective disorder in some people. See page 311.

Everyone gets sad. Gauging how deep and pervasive your sad feelings are can help you decide what to do. See "Sadness or Depression?" on page 310 to help determine if you are depressed.

Because many things can contribute to depression, combining self-care and professional treatment is often most effective. The most common form of treatment combines counseling (psychotherapy) with medication. Inpatient treatment is sometimes needed in severe cases.

Home Treatment

For some people, self-care alone can improve symptoms of mild depression. For more serious depression, self-care can add to the benefits of professional treatment.

- Consider what might be causing or adding to your depression:

  - Are medications causing it? Review your prescription and nonprescription medications with a pharmacist or doctor.

  - If it's wintertime or you haven't been out in the sun for a while, read the information about seasonal affective disorder on page 311.

- Pace yourself according to your energy level. Choose what is most important to get done and do those things first.

- Do not make major life decisions when you are depressed. If you must make a major decision, ask someone you trust to help you.

- Do not drink alcohol or use medications that have not been prescribed by your health professional.

Seasonal Affective Disorder

Seasonal affective disorder (SAD), sometimes called the winter blues, is a mental health problem that usually occurs in the months when there is less sunlight. There is no known cure, but it can be controlled, and it improves in the spring when there are more hours of daylight. The main symptoms include depressed mood, decreased energy, and food cravings. If you notice such a pattern developing during the winter, consider trying the following:

- Go out into the sun as often as possible. Protect your skin—it's your eyes' exposure to the sun that will help.

- Take a vacation to a sunny place.

- Get regular exercise, either outdoors or indoors near a window that lets in sunlight.

 Light therapy (phototherapy) is sometimes successful in treating SAD. It involves sitting, working, or reading in front of special high-intensity lights for up to several hours a day.

Medication can also be helpful, either alone or in combination with light therapy.

- Spend time with other people. Do things you usually enjoy, even if you don't feel like doing them.

- Get enough sleep. If you are having difficulty sleeping, see Sleep Problems on page 314.

- Eat a healthy diet (see Nutrition starting on page 293). If you don't feel like eating, eat small snacks rather than large meals.

- Exercise regularly. Getting 20 to 30 minutes of exercise each day is good for your body and your mind. Go for a walk. Take the stairs instead of the elevator. Dance.

- Believe that this mood will pass. Then look for signs that it is ending.

- Give yourself time to heal. Do not expect too much from yourself too soon.

When to Call a Health Professional

- If you are planning to hurt yourself or someone else.

- If you hear voices.

- If you have a sudden change in your behavior or start to do things that you wouldn't usually do (especially impulsive, irresponsible behavior).

- If symptoms of depression (see "Sadness or Depression?" on page 310) last longer than 2 weeks despite home treatment.

- If grieving continues without improvement for more than 4 weeks. See page 316.

Eating Disorders

In a society where "thin is in," many of us have tried skipping meals or going on diets to lose weight. Unlike typical dieters, people who have eating disorders have medical problems that cause disturbances in their eating behavior.

Anorexia nervosa is a disorder of severe self-imposed dieting. It most often affects teenage girls. Symptoms include refusing to eat; extreme weight loss; loss of menstrual periods; a distorted body image (thinking you're fat when you're actually very thin); a preoccupation with food; low self-esteem; and excessive exercise.

Bulimia nervosa is an eating disorder characterized by eating large amounts of food (binge eating) and then purging the body of that food (by forced vomiting or abuse of laxatives and diuretics). The binges are usually triggered by emotional upset, not hunger. Other symptoms include dry skin and brittle hair; swollen glands under the jaw from vomiting; depression and mood swings; a distorted body image; and secrecy to keep others from discovering your abnormal behavior.

People who have anorexia usually look starved, but most people who have bulimia maintain a normal weight and look healthy. Most people with anorexia deny they have a problem; people with bulimia know they have a problem, but they keep it a secret.

Compulsive overeating is characterized by binging on food. An overeater will consume thousands of calories at a time, quickly and without pleasure. Because there is no purging, a compulsive overeater becomes obese.

 Eating disorders appear to be caused by emotional and psychological factors. They tend to run in families, so there may be a genetic link. Eating disorders require professional treatment. If untreated, they can lead to major health problems or even death. Treatment usually involves nutritional counseling, individual psychotherapy, family therapy, and medication. A hospital stay may be required in extreme cases.

Prevention

- Teach and model healthy eating and exercise habits at home and at school.

- Help young people develop confidence and self-esteem. Accept them for who they are, not how they look.

- Be careful about encouraging a young person to lose weight. Communicate that you love and care for the person, regardless of how much he or she weighs.

- Don't set unrealistic expectations for your child. Striving to live up to them may lead to an eating disorder.

- Be alert to the stress in your child's life. Be available to talk over any problems.

When to Call a Health Professional

Call if you recognize any of these warning signs of an eating disorder:

- Unrealistic body image or an unreasonable fear of gaining weight

- Extreme weight loss in a short period of time

- Forced vomiting or excessive use of laxatives

- Excessive dieting or preoccupation with food

- Excessive, rigid exercise routines

- Loss of menstrual periods in a young woman

- Withdrawal from family and friends

Sleep Problems

The term **insomnia** can mean:

• Trouble getting to sleep (taking more than 45 minutes to fall asleep).

• Frequent awakenings with inability to fall back asleep.

• Early morning awakening.

None of these are problems unless they make you feel chronically tired. If you are less sleepy at night or wake up early in the morning, but still feel rested and alert, there is little need to worry.

Short-term insomnia, lasting from a few nights to a few weeks, is usually caused by worry over a stressful situation. Long-term insomnia, which can last months or even years, is often caused by general anxiety, medications, chronic pain, depression, or other physical disorders.

Sleep apnea is a sleep disorder that is usually caused by a blockage in the upper airways. When airflow through the nose and mouth is blocked, breathing repeatedly stops for 10 to 15 seconds or longer. People who have sleep apnea usually snore loudly and are very tired during the day. They are not aware of waking up at night but do have very restless sleep. Sleep apnea can affect children and adults.

 Mild <u>sleep apnea</u> may be cured by changing some of your pre-bedtime habits. More severe sleep apnea may require medical treatment.

Prevention

• Get regular exercise, but avoid strenuous exercise within 2 hours before bedtime.

• Avoid alcohol and smoking before bedtime. Drink caffeine in moderation and not after noon.

• Avoid foods that upset your stomach.

• Drink a glass of warm milk at bedtime. (But don't drink more than one glass of fluid before going to bed.)

• Make sure your sleeping conditions are comfortable and quiet.

Home Treatment

• Don't take sleeping pills. They can cause daytime confusion, memory loss, and dizziness. Continued use of sleeping pills actually increases sleeplessness in many people.

• Try the following seven-step formula for 2 weeks:

1. Engage in relaxing activities in the evening (e.g., take a warm bath, read, or do some slow, easy stretches).

2. Use your bed for sleeping and sex only. Don't eat, watch TV, read, or work in bed.

MORE INFO **For more information, see the back cover.**

3. Sleep only at bedtime. Don't take naps. (However, naps are fine if you don't have sleep problems.)

4. Go to bed only when you feel sleepy.

5. If you lie awake for more than 15 minutes, get up, leave the bedroom, and do something relaxing .

6. Repeat steps 4 and 5 until it is time to get up.

7. Get up at the same time each day, no matter how sleepy you are.

- Review the sleeping tips for snorers on page 170.

- Review all of your prescription and nonprescription medications with a pharmacist to rule out drug-related sleep problems.

- Read about anxiety on page 308 and depression on page 309. Either condition can cause sleep problems.

When to Call a Health Professional

- If you regularly take sleeping pills and are unable to stop taking them.

- If you suspect medication or a health problem is causing sleep problems.

- If you or your partner snores loudly and feels excessively sleepy during the day.

- If you, your partner, or your child has many episodes of sleep apnea (stops breathing, gasps, and chokes during sleep).

- If your child snores, has difficulty breathing while asleep, sleeps restlessly and awakens frequently, or is very sleepy during the day.

- If you wake up frequently because your legs move or get cramps.

- If a full month of self-care doesn't solve the problem.

Suicide

If you are very depressed or feel overwhelmed, you may sometimes think of taking your own life. Occasional thoughts of suicide are not a problem. However, if thoughts of suicide continue, or if you have made suicide plans, it becomes a very serious matter.

People who are considering suicide are often undecided about choosing life or death. With compassionate help, they may choose to live.

Prevention

When there are significant life crises, when you are depressed, or when someone you know is depressed, be alert to the warning signs for suicide:

- Verbal warning. Most people who commit suicide mention their intentions to someone.

- Preoccupation with death. A suicidal person may talk, read, draw, or write about death.

- Previous suicide attempt. Failed attempts are often followed by a completed attempt.

Grief

Grieving is a natural healing process that helps you adjust to a major change or loss. Grief may be expressed physically or emotionally and may have some of the same symptoms as depression (see page 309). The following tips may help you move through the grieving process.

- Take as much time as you need to grieve. Don't fight the emotions you feel.

- Take care of yourself. Get enough rest, and eat nourishing foods. Exercise to help release pent-up emotions.

- Discuss your feelings with friends who will support you while encouraging you to reconnect with the world. Join a support group, or talk to your clergyperson or a counselor.

- Write your thoughts down in a journal or paint or draw your grief. Or write letters to the person you lost.

- Try to cut back on some of your usual responsibilities until your grieving period is past. Postpone any major decisions.

- As you begin to move beyond your grief, renew old interests and pursue new ones. Do things that give you a sense of control and hope.

There is no easy formula for getting over grief. It can take weeks, months or years. Ask your friends, family, and doctor for help if you are having trouble moving through your grief.

- Giving away prized possessions.

- Depression and social isolation.

If you are troubled by suicidal thoughts, avoid alcohol and illegal drugs. Alcohol and drugs can impair your judgment, which may make you more likely to do things you would not do when sober.

Home Treatment

- Use your common sense and a direct approach to determine if the suicide risk is high. Ask yourself or the person who you feel is at risk:

  - Do you feel there is no other way?

  - Do you have a suicide plan?

  - How and when do you plan to do it?

- Ask someone you trust to stay with you or the suicidal person until the crisis has passed.

- Encourage the person to seek professional help.

- Don't argue with or challenge the person who is thinking of suicide.

- Don't ignore warning signs, thinking that you or another person will "snap out of it."

- Talk about the situation as openly as possible. Show understanding and compassion.

When to Call a Health Professional

Call 911 or other emergency services if you or someone you know is about to attempt or is attempting suicide.

Call your health professional, your local suicide hot line, or the national suicide hot line at 1-800-784-2433 (1-800-SUICIDE):

• If you are considering suicide.

• If you suspect that someone has made suicide plans.

Violent Behavior

Anger and arguments are normal parts of healthy relationships. However, anger that leads to threats or violence, such as hitting or hurting, is not normal or healthy. Physical, verbal, or sexual abuse is not an acceptable part of any relationship.

Violent behavior often begins with verbal threats or relatively minor incidents, but over time it can become more serious, involving physical harm. Violent behavior is learned behavior, so it is especially important to teach your children that violence is not a healthy solution to conflict.

Prevention

• Seek nonviolent ways to resolve conflicts. Arguing is fine, even healthy, so long as it does not turn violent. See page 307 for more information about controlling anger.

• Teach your children that violence is not a solution to conflicts. Do not use physical discipline such as spanking. If you need help with discipline, consider taking a course on parenting skills.

• Do not keep firearms or other weapons in a home where there is someone who has a drug or alcohol problem, is prone to violent behavior, or has threatened suicide.

• Be alert to warning signs, such as threats or drunkenness, so you can avoid dangerous situations. If you cannot predict when violence may occur, have an "exit plan" for use in an emergency.

When to Call a Health Professional

Call 911 or other emergency services:

• If you feel you or someone you know is in immediate danger.

• If you or someone in your family has just been physically or sexually abused or has been the victim of violence. Physical or sexual abuse is a crime, no matter who does it.

Call a health professional:

• If you are concerned about violent behavior (such as physical, verbal, or sexual abuse) in yourself, a family member, a friend, or a co-worker.

• If you suspect abuse, neglect, or maltreatment of a child or if a child reports this kind of treatment to you. You may also call local child protective services or the police.

Check the Yellow Pages for hot lines and other resources for victims of abuse.

The Mind-Body Connection

Medical science is making remarkable discoveries about the relationship between your state of mind and your mental and physical health. Researchers have found that one function of the brain is to produce substances that can improve your health. Your brain can create endorphins, which are natural painkillers; gamma globulin for fortifying your immune system; and interferon for combating infections, viruses, and even cancer. Your brain can combine these and other substances into a vast number of tailor-made prescriptions for whatever ails you.

The substances that your brain produces depend in part on your thoughts, feelings, and expectations. If your attitude about an illness (or life in general) is negative and you don't have expectations that your condition will get better, your brain may not produce enough of the substances your body needs to heal. On the other hand, if your attitude and expectations are more positive, your brain is likely to produce sufficient amounts of the substances that will boost your body's healing power.

Your physical health also has an impact on your brain's ability to produce substances that affect your mental well-being. An illness or injury that causes long-term physical stress can lead to chemical imbalances in the brain. These imbalances may lead to depression and other mental health problems.

Positive Thinking

People with positive attitudes generally enjoy life more, but are they any healthier? The answer is often "yes." Optimism is a resource for healing. Optimists are more likely to overcome pain and adversity in their efforts to improve their medical treatment outcomes. For example, optimistic coronary bypass patients generally recover more quickly and have fewer complications after surgery than do patients who are less hopeful.

Your body responds to your thoughts, emotions, and actions. In addition to staying fit, eating right, and managing stress, you can use the following three strategies to help maintain your health:

1. Create positive expectations for health and healing.

Mental and emotional expectations can influence medical outcomes. The effectiveness of any medical treatment depends in part on how useful you expect it to be. The "placebo effect" proves this. A placebo is a drug or treatment that provides no medical benefit except for the patient's belief that it will help. On the average, 35 percent of patients who receive placebos report satisfactory relief from their medical problem, even though they received no actual medication.

Changing your expectations from negative to positive may enhance your physical health. Here's how to make the change:

- Stop all negative self-talk. Make positive statements that promote your recovery.

- Send yourself a steady stream of affirmations. An affirmation is a phrase or sentence that sends strong, positive statements to you about yourself, such as "I am a capable person" or "My joints are strong and flexible."

- Visualize health and healing. Add mental pictures that support your positive affirmations.

- Don't feel guilty. There is no value in feeling guilty about health problems. While there is a lot you can do to reduce your risk for health problems and improve your chances of recovery, some illnesses may develop and persist no matter what you do. Some things just are. Do the best you can.

2. Open yourself to humor, friendship, and love.

Positive emotions boost your health. Fortunately, almost anything that makes you feel good about yourself helps you stay healthy.

- Laugh. A little humor makes life richer and healthier. Laughter increases creativity, reduces pain, and speeds healing. Keep an emergency laughter kit that contains funny videotapes, jokes, cartoons, and photographs. Put it with your first aid supplies and keep it well stocked.

- Seek out friends. Friendships are vital to good health. Close social ties help you recover more quickly from illness and reduce your risk of developing diseases ranging from arthritis to depression.

- Volunteer. People who volunteer live longer and enjoy life more than those who do not volunteer. By helping others, we help ourselves.

- Plant a plant and pet a pet. Plants and pets can be highly therapeutic. When you stroke an animal, your blood pressure goes down and your heart rate slows. Animals and plants help us feel needed.

3. Appeal to a higher power.

If you believe in a higher power, ask for support in your pursuit of healing and health. Faith, prayer, and spiritual beliefs can play an important role in recovering from an illness. See Healing Touch on page 331.

Your sense of spiritual wellness can help you overcome personal trials and things you cannot change. If it suits you, use spiritual images in visualizations, affirmations, and expectations about your health and your life.

Dealing With Chronic Pain

Long-term, persistent pain (chronic pain) is a problem for many people, especially middle-aged and older adults. Chronic pain is associated with fatigue, sleep problems, irritability, stress, depression, anxiety, and withdrawal from daily activities. Arthritis, back problems, recurring sports injuries, nerve damage, cancer, and many other conditions can result in chronic pain. In many cases the cause of pain is not known. A variety of factors can contribute to it.

Your mind and body are important allies in your efforts to manage chronic pain. Pain often has a mental as well as a physical component. In other words, your thoughts and feelings about pain can affect how much pain you feel. Feeling anxious, angry, frustrated, or out of control about your pain may make pain worse. If you can put your mind to work against the pain, you may find that you can manage pain better and that it interferes less with your life.

There is no magic solution for dealing with chronic pain, no matter what the cause. However, the following tips for dealing with both the mental and physical aspects of chronic pain may help:

• Take control of the pain. This may mean accepting that the pain is not going away, but deciding to take active steps toward managing it and keeping it from affecting your life too much.

• Practice positive thinking (see page 318). Recognize negative or self-defeating thoughts, such as "This pain will never get better" or "I'll never be able to play with the grandkids with this pain." Your thoughts can affect your perception of pain.

• Track how your moods, thoughts, and activities affect your pain. Record your pain level in relation to these factors several times a day for several days. You may find that your pain is worse during or after certain activities or when you are feeling a certain emotion.

• Try to relax. Chronic pain causes stress and tension, which may make the pain worse. Try the relaxation techniques on pages 323 to 325. Learning relaxation skills takes practice, so give each method a 2-week trial. If one doesn't work for you, try another.

• Take any pain medication your health professional has recommended or prescribed on schedule and in the correct dose.

• Exercise regularly. Try gentle, low-impact exercises that don't aggravate your pain, such as swimming, water aerobics, walking, or stationary cycling. Do the stretching exercises on page 288 every day. Ask your health professional about physical therapy, too.

• Experiment with heat, cold, and massage. Find out what works best for you.

- Make sure you are getting enough sleep. See Sleep Problems on page 314. If pain frequently disrupts your sleep, talk to your health professional.

- Change the way you do daily activities so you can do them with less pain. Some people find assistive devices (such as canes, foot supports, or specially designed household tools) helpful.

- Consider complementary therapies such as biofeedback, acupuncture, or yoga in addition to your regular medical care (not as a substitute for it). See Complementary Medicine beginning on page 327.

- Join a support group. By being around others who share your problem, you and your family can learn skills for accepting and coping with pain. You may also feel less isolated. To find a group near you, contact the American Chronic Pain Association at (916) 632-0922.

 No one should have to suffer in uncontrolled pain. Call your health professional if chronic pain is affecting your quality of life. Although treatment will probably not be able to eliminate pain completely, it can help reduce the pain and its impact on your life.

Stress and Distress

Stress is the way you react physically, mentally, and emotionally to various conditions, changes, and demands in your life.

Stress is part and parcel of common life events, both large and small. It comes with all of life's daily hassles as well as with crises and life-changing events. Unless you can regularly release the tension that comes with stress, your risk for physical and mental illness may increase.

What Stress Does to the Body

At the first sign of alarm, chemicals released by the pituitary and adrenal glands and the nerve endings automatically trigger these physical reactions to stress:

- Your heart rate increases to move blood to your muscles and brain.

- Your blood pressure goes up.

- You start to breathe more rapidly.

- Your digestion slows down.

- You start to perspire more heavily.

- Your pupils dilate.

- You feel a rush of strength.

Your body is tense, alert, and ready for action. After the natural "alarm" reaction to a real or perceived threat, your body stays on alert until you feel that the danger has passed. Then your brain signals an "all clear" to your body, and your body stops producing the chemicals that caused the physical reaction and gradually returns to normal.

Problems with stress occur when your brain fails to give the "all clear" signal. If the alarm state lasts too long, you begin to suffer from the consequences of constant stress. You may find it difficult to see the relationship between stress and physical health problems, because the long-term effects of stress are subtle and slow. However, experts in every area of medicine are discovering links between stress, disease, and poor health.

Becoming More Stress-Hardy

Some people seem to be more resistant to stress, and studies indicate that these people are less likely to get sick. Researchers have identified four personality factors that stand out in stress-hardy people:

1. They have a strong commitment to self, work, family, and other values.

2. They have a sense of control over their lives.

3. They generally see change in their lives as a challenge rather than a threat.

4. They have a strong network of support and close relationships.

It's never too late to develop a more stress-hardy personality. The first step is to believe that you can do it (remember, think positive!). Approach one challenging area of your life at a time. Be committed to making things better for yourself and those around you. Identify the things you can control and those you cannot. Accept that changes will occur, and know that you will be able to deal with them. Call upon your support network to get the help you need, whether it's someone to watch your children for a few hours so you can run errands or someone who will just listen to your plans. As you begin to gain control over one challenging area of your life, you will find more time and energy for tackling additional areas.

Recognizing Stress

The signs of stress are classic. You may get a headache, stiff neck, or a nagging backache. You may start to breathe rapidly or get sweaty palms or an upset stomach. You may become irritable and intolerant of even minor disturbances. You may lose your temper more often and yell at your family for no good reason. Your pulse rate may increase and you may feel jumpy or exhausted all the time. You may find it hard to concentrate.

When these symptoms appear, recognize them as signs of stress and find a way to deal with them. Just knowing why you're feeling the way you do may be the first step in coping with the problem. It is your attitude toward stress, not the stress itself, that affects your health the most.

Managing Symptoms of Stress

 Some people try to relieve the symptoms of stress by smoking, drinking, overeating, using drugs, or just "shutting down." Some people become violent or abusive in response to stress. These methods of coping have harmful side effects. By learning other ways to deal with symptoms of stress, you can avoid problems that may affect yourself or others and improve your overall quality of life.

- **Express yourself.** Stress and tension affect your emotions. By expressing those feelings to others, you may be able to understand and cope with them better. Talking about a problem with a spouse or a good friend is a valuable way to reduce tension and stress. Expressing yourself through writing, crafts, or art may also be a good tension reliever.

- **Cry.** Crying can relieve tension. It's part of your emotional healing process.

- **Get moving.** Regular, moderate physical activity may be the single best approach to managing stress. Walking briskly will take advantage of the rapid pulse and tensed muscles caused by stress and release your pent-up energy. After a long walk, your stress level is usually lower and more manageable.

- **Be kind to your body and mind.** Getting enough sleep, eating a nutritious diet, and taking time to do things you enjoy can all contribute to an overall feeling of balance in your life and help reduce stress.

Relaxation Skills

Whatever you do to manage stress, you can benefit from the regular use of relaxation skills.

The following three methods of relaxation and meditation are among the simplest and most effective. They should be done once or twice a day for about 20 minutes each time. Pick a time and place where you won't be disturbed or distracted. Once you've trained your body and mind to relax, you'll be able to produce the same relaxed state whenever you want.

Roll Breathing

The way you breathe affects your whole body. Full, deep breathing is a good way to reduce tension and feel relaxed. The object of roll breathing is to develop full use of your lungs and get in touch with the rhythm of your breathing. It can be practiced in any position, but it is best to learn it while lying on your back, with your knees bent.

1. Place your left hand on your abdomen and your right hand on your chest. Notice how your hands move as you breathe in and out.

2. Practice filling your lower lungs by breathing so that your left hand goes up when you inhale and your right hand remains still. Always inhale through your nose and exhale through your mouth.

3. When you have filled and emptied your lower lungs 8 to 10 times, add the second step to your breathing: inhale first into your lower lungs as before; then continue inhaling into your upper chest. As you do so, your right hand will rise and your left hand will fall a little as your abdomen falls.

4. As you exhale slowly through your mouth, make a quiet, whooshing sound as first your left hand, and then your right hand falls. As you exhale, feel the tension leaving your body as you become more and more relaxed.

5. Practice breathing in and out in this manner for 3 to 5 minutes. Notice that the movement of your abdomen and chest is like rolling waves rising and falling in a rhythmic motion.

Practice roll breathing daily for several weeks until you can do it almost anywhere. Then you'll have an instant relaxation tool any time you need one.

CAUTION: Some people get dizzy the first few times they try roll breathing. If you begin to hyperventilate or become lightheaded, slow your breathing. Get up slowly.

Progressive Muscle Relaxation

The body responds to stressful thoughts or situations with muscle tension, which can cause pain or discomfort. Deep muscle relaxation reduces muscle tension and general mental anxiety too. Progressive muscle relaxation is effective in combating stress-related health problems and often helps people get to sleep.

Muscle Groups and Procedure

You can use a prerecorded audiotape to help you go through all the muscle groups, or you can do it by just tensing and relaxing each muscle group. Choose a place where you can lie down on your back and stretch out comfortably, such as a carpeted floor. Tense each muscle group (hard, but not to the point of cramping) for 4 to 10 seconds; then give yourself 10 to 20 seconds to release it and relax. At various points, check the muscle groups you've already done and relax each one a little more each time.

Hands: Clench them.

Wrists and forearms: Extend them and bend the hands back at the wrist.

Biceps and upper arms: Clench your hands into fists, bend your arms at the elbows, and flex your biceps.

Shoulders: Shrug them. (Check your arms and shoulders for tension.)

Forehead: Wrinkle it into a deep frown.

Around the eyes and bridge of the nose: Close your eyes as tightly as possible. (Remove contact lenses before beginning the exercise.)

Cheeks and jaws: Grin from ear to ear.

Around the mouth: Press your lips together tightly. (Check your facial area for tension.)

Back of the neck: Press the back of your head against the floor.

Front of the neck: Touch your chin to your chest. (Check your neck and head for tension.)

Chest: Take a deep breath and hold it; then exhale.

Back: Arch your back up and away from the floor.

Stomach: Suck it into a tight knot. (Check your chest and stomach area for tension.)

Hips and buttocks: Squeeze your buttocks together tightly.

Thighs: Clench them.

Lower legs: Point your toes toward your face, as if trying to bring your toes up to touch your head. Then point your toes away and curl them downward at the same time. (Check the area from your waist down for tension.)

When you are finished, return to alertness by counting backwards from 5 to 1.

Relaxation Response

The relaxation response is the exact opposite of the stress response. It slows your heart rate and breathing, lowers your blood pressure, and helps relieve muscle tension.

Technique (adapted from Herbert Benson, MD)

1. Lie down in a place where you can stretch out comfortably. Close your eyes.

2. Begin progressive muscle relaxation. See page 324.

3. Become aware of your breathing. Each time you exhale, say the word "one" (or any other word or phrase) silently or aloud. Concentrate on breathing from your abdomen, not from your chest.

Instead of focusing on a repeated word, you can fix your gaze on a stationary object. Any mental stimulus will help you clear your mind.

Continue this for 10 to 20 minutes. As distracting thoughts enter your mind, don't dwell on them. Allow them to drift away.

4. Sit quietly for several minutes, until you are ready to open your eyes.

5. Notice the difference in your breathing and your pulse rate.

Don't worry about becoming deeply relaxed. The key to this exercise is to remain passive, to let distracting thoughts slip away like waves on the beach.

For the times they are a-changin'.
Bob Dylan

19

Complementary Medicine

The term "complementary medicine" broadly describes any health approach that is not part of the conventional medical approach of a particular society or culture. What is considered "complementary" or "alternative" varies from culture to culture. In the United States, many people use complementary therapies like acupuncture or herbal medicine along with mainstream medical treatments (medications or surgery, for instance) to control pain, manage stress, and speed healing.

While complementary treatments are becoming more widely accepted, they are not right for everyone and every situation. As with any other treatment option, the decision to try complementary medicine should be made only after you gather as much reliable information as possible,

understand the benefits and risks, and consider your personal needs and preferences. For more information, see Making Wise Health Decisions starting on page 3.

Here are some important things to consider when deciding whether to try a complementary therapy:

- Think about what you want from complementary medicine. Are you looking for greater comfort and an improved quality of life? Or are you looking for a cure for illness? Seeking a cure through complementary medicine may be disappointing and, in some cases, harmful to your health. Discuss your expectations with the practitioner and make sure they are realistic.

- Do you think that complementary medicine has something special to offer you, or are you seeking complementary treatment because you are fed up with conventional medicine? It is important to recognize the strengths and limitations of both conventional and complementary medicine.

- What is the practitioner's level of expertise? Check with state and local medical licensing agencies and departments of consumer affairs to see if the practitioner is licensed and in good standing. Talk to people who have had experience with the practitioner. Visit the practitioner and ask questions about his or her education, training, licenses, certification, and insurance.

Your primary care doctor may be able to help you make informed decisions about complementary medicine. Some people think their doctors don't want them to try complementary treatment. But more and more doctors are realizing that complementary therapies can work with conventional medicine to improve health and help people feel better. Your doctor may be able to refer you to some qualified complementary medicine practitioners.

If you do decide to try some form of complementary medicine, let your doctor know. Even if your doctor is not comfortable with your decision, it is important for your safety that he or she know what you are doing. Your complementary treatment should at least be safe and at best work in conjunction with your conventional medical treatment.

General Risks and Benefits of Complementary Medicine

All treatments, whether conventional or complementary, have risks and benefits. In general, the risks and benefits of complementary therapies are as follows.

Risks

Overlooking effective conventional medicine: Perhaps greater than the concern for risks of a specific complementary therapy is the concern that a person will forgo effective medical treatment or neglect to get an accurate diagnosis. Some practitioners of complementary therapies do not refer people to conventional doctors even when it is possible that conventional medicine could help. And some people who choose complementary medicine refuse to consider conventional medicine for any problem. This can be dangerous. It is best to get as much information as possible and then make informed decisions, selecting from both conventional and complementary approaches for treatment of a specific health problem.

Health Fraud and Quackery

Millions of people are taken in each year by medical fraud and worthless health products.

Bogus cures are advertised for many chronic health problems, especially arthritis, cancer, baldness, obesity, and impotence. The ads target people who are ready to try anything. Unfortunately, many of these products cause harmful side effects. It is wise to be suspicious of products that:

- Are advertised by testimonials.

- Claim to have a secret ingredient.

- Have not been evaluated in prominent medical journals.

- Claim benefits that seem too good to be true.

- Are available only by mail.

Be suspicious of any practitioner who:

- Prescribes medicines or gives injections at every visit.

- Promises a no-risk cure.

- Suggests something that seems unethical or illegal.

The best way to protect yourself from medical fraud is to be observant and ask questions. If you don't like what you see or hear, find another practitioner or get a second opinion.

Potential dangers: Since many complementary therapies are not well studied, and the manufacture of complementary medicine products and procedures is not well regulated, you may be exposing yourself to unknown effects or possible dangerous interactions. The lack of regulation on products and practitioners may also expose you to additional health risks, especially if you have other medical conditions.

Many options and inadequate evidence: There are many different complementary treatments, and there is lots of evidence about them. Some of it is reliable, some not. Very few complementary treatments have been studied for safety and effectiveness using traditional scientific methods. Unlike conventional medications, herbal medicines and nutritional supplements are not regulated by the Food and Drug Administration (FDA). Little reliable information is available, which makes it difficult to make an informed decision.

Cost: Many health insurance companies do not yet cover the costs of complementary therapies. As with conventional medical treatments, you must decide whether a complementary therapy is working for you and whether its benefits are worth the time and money the therapy requires.

Benefits

Holistic approach: Conventional doctor visits usually last about 10 to 15 minutes. Complementary medicine practitioners often take an hour or more to learn about your lifestyle and background, including information about your family, friends, diet, activities, and work. Many health problems, especially chronic ones, may respond best to treatment that considers the whole person and his or her environment and lifestyle.

Touch: People who provide complementary treatments are often taught to listen to and touch their patients. For many people, being listened to and touched in a caring way is helpful.

Mind-body connection: Science has shown that people's emotional states can affect their health. See page 303. People who describe themselves as happy tend to be healthier than those who see themselves as unhappy. People who have a lot of stress in their lives are more likely to get sick. Conventional medicine offers little help for these kinds of problems. Complementary practices like meditation and tai chi can help ease stress and improve a person's sense of well-being, which may improve the person's health.

Empowerment: Many people find that having the access and freedom to try complementary therapies is empowering. It gives them a stronger sense of control over their bodies and their health.

Choosing the Right Therapy for You

 There are many types of complementary medicine. Choosing between different treatments can be confusing. This section describes several of the most widely available choices. Use this section to learn about different treatments and how they might work for you.

Acupuncture

Acupuncture is an ancient Chinese therapy based on the theory that there is energy called *chi* or *qi* (pronounced "chee") flowing through your body. Your *chi* flows along energy pathways called meridians. If the flow of *chi* is blocked or unbalanced at any point on a meridian, theoretically it may result in illness. Traditional practitioners believe acupuncture unblocks and balances the flow of *chi* to restore health. Western medicine practitioners who have studied acupuncture theorize that it reduces pain by acting on the biological mechanisms that control pain.

Traditional Chinese acupuncture is done by inserting very thin needles into the skin at certain points on the body to stimulate energy flow along the body's energy pathways. Other types of acupuncture may use heat, pressure, or mild electric current in place of the needles.

Acupuncture may be used to relieve pain and treat certain health conditions, including addiction, asthma, headache, menstrual cramps, and joint and muscle problems. Promising results have been found for the use of acupuncture in relieving pain after surgery and in treating nausea and vomiting related to chemotherapy.

Bodywork and Manual Therapy

Bodywork and manual therapy refer to a variety of body manipulation techniques used for relaxation and pain relief. Massage and chiropractic are well-known forms of bodywork. Other common forms are the Alexander technique, the Feldenkrais method, the Trager approach, Rolfing, and deep tissue massage.

The idea behind bodywork is that people learn (or are forced into by injury or stress) unnatural ways of moving or holding their bodies. Theoretically, this unnatural movement or posture changes the natural alignment of bones, which in turn causes discomfort and may contribute to health problems.

The goal of bodywork is to realign and reposition the body to allow natural, graceful movement. Along with identifying possible contributing causes of unnatural movement and posture, bodywork is thought to reduce stress and ease pain.

There has not been much scientific testing of bodywork. A few studies suggest good results for people with arthritis, stress, or low back pain, and for children with cerebral palsy.

Chiropractic Treatment

Chiropractic is a hands-on therapy based on the theory that many medical disorders may be caused by dislocations in the spine. The main goal of chiropractic therapy is to help the body heal itself by correcting misalignments or dislocations of the joints, particularly the bones of the spine (vertebrae).

Chiropractic treatments usually involve adjusting the joints and bones in a person's spine using twisting, pulling, or pushing movements. Some chiropractors use heat, electrical stimulation, or ultrasound to relax the person's muscles before before doing an adjustment.

Chiropractic treatment has been shown to be helpful in treating low back pain, neck pain, and headaches.

Healing Touch

Healing touch, spiritual or energy healing, therapeutic touch, prayer, and distant healing are terms used to describe the conscious focus on another person to promote healing and well-being without physical intervention. Spiritual healing is widespread and may or may not have anything to do with an established religion. Therapeutic touch is taught in many nursing schools, and nurses may use it in conventional medical settings to help comfort their patients.

Like other complementary approaches, healing touch starts with the idea that people are naturally healthy. The way people live and think may disturb their natural health energy, and they become ill. The aim of healing touch is to focus or channel healing energy to restore natural health and balance. Some forms of healing touch use actual physical touch as part of the healing, but many do not.

There has been almost no research on the effects of healing touch. It is a difficult form of therapy to study using traditional scientific methods. However, supporters of healing touch believe it is helpful in healing wounds, curing infection, and relieving pain. At the least, healing touch may help reduce anxiety and stress and provide comfort to a sick person.

The only known risk in using healing touch arises when people forgo effective medical treatment and rely only on healing. Healing touch is not appropriate for acute, life-threatening situations or as a replacement for other treatments that are known to improve a disease. Prayer, healing, and therapeutic touch can always be used along with more conventional treatments.

Herbal Medicine

Plants and other natural products have been used for thousands of years to maintain health and treat illness. They are the basis for many conventional medications. For example, willow bark tea was used for centuries to control fever. Drug companies learned to copy the chemical makeup of willow bark to produce aspirin.

Herbal medicines may do many of the same things that conventional drugs do. They may prevent illness. They may cure infection. They may soothe a fever or help wounds heal. They may keep you regular or ease your pain. They may calm you down or perk you up.

Some herbal medicines may have no effect at all. Others may even be harmful. Like conventional medicines, herbal medicines and natural supplements may cause side effects, trigger allergic reactions, or interact with other medications a person is taking.

There have been thousands of studies on the effects of herbs. Most of the research has been done in Europe and China, where herbal medicine is widely practiced. In the United States, the analysis of this research began fairly recently, and many new studies are underway.

When shopping for herbal supplements, look for the USP (United States Pharmacopeia) or NF (National Formulary) symbols. These symbols indicate that the product has complied with the manufacturing and safety standards set by the USP. The USP symbol further indicates that the product has an FDA or USP endorsement for its intended use.

Be sure to tell your doctor about any herbs or natural supplements you are taking. Pregnant and breast-feeding women and people with serious health problems should not use any herbal medicines or natural supplements without first consulting their doctor.

Homeopathy

Homeopathy, like other complementary treatments, is based on the idea that the body has the ability to heal itself. Sometimes the body needs to be stimulated to start the healing process. In homeopathy, a treatment is chosen because it can cause health problems just like the one that is troubling you. The treatment is given in such a small amount that, in theory, it does not cause the problem but stimulates your body to heal the problem.

Homeopathy has been used to treat allergies, atopic dermatitis, rheumatoid arthritis, irritable bowel syndrome, and other chronic conditions. It is not considered appropriate for treatment of serious illnesses or emergencies.

Homeopathy is widely used in England and other European countries. No one really understands how it works.

Massage Therapy

Massage therapy is based on the idea that touch is healing. There are many different types of massage therapy. Some are very gentle, while some are very active and intense. Some methods use the same ideas as acupuncture: the massage therapist will press on or stroke points on the body where energy is blocked.

Massage therapy has been and continues to be widely studied. Many studies have shown that massage therapy decreases stress and helps control pain. Health problems that are caused by or made worse by stress (such as depression and inflammatory bowel disease) may also improve with massage treatment.

Current research is focusing on the effects of massage in treating conditions such as asthma, diabetes, skin disorders, high blood pressure, behavioral problems, eating disorders, and fibromyalgia.

Naturopathy

Naturopathy blends conventional medicine with complementary medicine. Schools of naturopathy teach anatomy, cell biology, pharmacology, and other sciences studied in conventional medical schools. They also teach herbal medicine, acupuncture, and bodywork. The goal of naturopathy is to help you become and stay well, which is believed to be the natural state of your body.

Naturopathic medicine is used to promote health, prevent disease, and treat all kinds of health problems. Most naturopaths can treat earaches, allergies, and other common medical problems. A properly trained naturopath refers people to other practitioners for diagnosis or treatment when appropriate.

Two of the biggest concerns about naturopathic medicine are the use of fasting and its approach to immunization.

Fasting puts your body under stress and can be dangerous, especially if you have a disease like diabetes. Talk with your conventional doctor before you try fasting. If you start to feel sick while fasting, break your fast with small amounts of fruit or juice and then return to your normal diet.

Some naturopaths do not believe that immunization is necessary. This philosophy is very controversial. Before vaccinations were available, childhood illnesses caused large numbers of deaths and long-term health problems. Talk with your conventional doctor before deciding about immunization.

Tai Chi and *Qi Gong*

Tai chi and *qi gong* (pronounced "chee goong") are traditional Chinese exercises. They are based on the idea that through gentle, graceful, repeated movements, deep concentration, and focused breathing, people can increase and improve the flow of energy (*chi* or *qi*) through their bodies and improve their health.

Tai chi and *qi gong* are also founded on the Chinese belief that nature consists of opposing forces called yin and yang. It suggests that good health results when yin and yang are balanced. Tai chi and *qi gong* movements are done in an attempt to help restore the body's balance of yin and yang.

Tai chi is a series of movements done in a rhythmic pattern, either very slowly or very quickly. *Qi gong* is a lot of different movements that can be done in any order. *Qi gong* is useful to know because you can do it anywhere, anytime, even if you are unable to sit up or stand. Some common *qi gong* movements include raising and lowering your arms, moving your head from side to side, and rubbing your ears, feet, and hands.

Both tai chi and *qi gong* can be done by people of all ages. Their primary benefits are improved muscle strength, balance, coordination, posture, and flexibility. They may help increase stamina, lower blood pressure, and relieve stress. Possible muscle strains and sprains are their only harmful side effect. Gentle stretching before a tai chi or *qi gong* session can prevent most injuries.

Tai chi and *qi gong* usually can be used safely alongside conventional medical treatments for health problems, but they should not replace effective conventional treatment. Talk with your health professional so you can choose the tai chi or *qi gong* program that best suits your needs.

Yoga

Yoga is a meditation program that includes exercises to help improve flexibility and breathing, decrease stress, and maintain health. It has been practiced in India for centuries and is based on the principle of mind-body unity.

Two basic components of yoga are proper posture and breathing. There are many different yoga exercises, called postures. These may be done while standing, lying down, or sitting in a chair; some are done in a headstand position. While practicing a posture, which stretches the body, a person does breathing exercises to help relax muscles, maintain the posture, and focus the mind.

Most people who try yoga find that it improves flexibility and reduces stress. Several studies have shown that yoga helps lower blood pressure and improves a person's sense of well-being. Research has also shown that yoga can help people who have asthma learn to breathe more easily. People with chronic medical conditions like migraine headaches, heart disease, arthritis, or cancer may benefit from combining yoga and their conventional medical treatment.

For more information about these and other complementary treatments, do some research at your local library, or contact the National Center for Complementary and Alternative Medicine (NCCAM) at the National Institutes of Health (NCCAM Clearinghouse, P.O. Box 8218, Silver Spring, MD 20907-8218, 1-888-644-6226).

20

Your Home Health Center

More of your health care takes place in your home than anywhere else. Having the right tools, medicines, supplies, and information on hand will improve the quality of your self-care.

Store all your self-care tools and supplies in one central location, such as a large drawer in the bedroom or family room. Use the charts about tools and supplies in this chapter as checklists for keeping your home health center well stocked.

Note: If small children are around, keep your supplies out of reach or stored in containers or cabinets with childproof safety latches.

Be familiar with the disaster preparation and response plan for your area. Keep the appropriate supplies on hand.

Self-Care Tools

Self-care tools are the basic equipment of your home health center.

Cold Pack

A cold pack is a plastic envelope filled with gel that remains flexible at very cold temperatures. Buy two cold packs and keep them in the freezer. Use them for bumps, bruises, back sprains, turned ankles, sore joints, or any other health problem that calls for ice. A cold pack is more convenient than ice and may become the self-care tool you use the most.

You can make your own cold pack:

• Put 1 pint of rubbing alcohol and 3 pints of water in a 1-gallon, heavy-duty, plastic freezer bag.

• Seal the bag, and then seal it in a second bag. Mark it "Cold pack: Do not eat," and place it in the freezer.

A bag of frozen vegetables will also work as a cold pack.

Humidifier and Vaporizer

Humidifiers and vaporizers add moisture to the air, making it less drying to your mouth, throat, and nose. A humidifier produces a cool mist, and a vaporizer puts out hot steam.

Cool mist from a humidifier may be more comfortable to breathe than hot steam. However, humidifiers are noisy, produce particles that may be irritating to some people, and need to be cleaned and disinfected regularly. This is especially important for people who have mold allergies.

A vaporizer's hot steam does not contain any irritating particles, and you can add medications such as Vicks VapoRub to ease breathing. Steam may feel good when you have a cold, but the hot water can burn anyone who overturns or gets too close to the vaporizer.

Medicine Spoon

Medicine spoons are transparent tubes with marks that indicate typical dosage amounts. A medicine spoon makes it easy to give the right dose of liquid medicine. While the spoons are convenient for anyone, they are particularly helpful for

---

Self-Care Tools

For every household:

• Blood pressure cuff*

• Cold pack*

• Dental mirror

• Eyedropper

• Heating pad

• Humidifier or vaporizer*

• Medicine spoon*

• Nail clippers

• Penlight*

• Scissors

• Stethoscope*

• Thermometer*

• Tweezers

For children younger than 6, add:

• Bulb aspirator/syringe

• Rectal thermometer*

• Otoscope*

*Described in text

---

young children. The tube shape and large lip get most of the medication into a child's mouth without spilling. Buy one at your local pharmacy.

Medicine spoon

Otoscope

An otoscope is a flashlight with a special attachment for looking into the ear. With training, you can use an otoscope to help you decide if an ear infection is present. Inexpensive consumer-model otoscopes are available, but they do not illuminate the ear canal and eardrum as well as the one your doctor uses does. They can also be used as high-intensity penlights.

Penlight

A penlight has a small, intense light that can be easily directed. It is useful for looking into the mouth or throat or examining the skin, and it is easier to handle than a flashlight.

Stethoscope and Blood Pressure Cuff

If you have heart disease or high blood pressure, it's a good idea to have both a stethoscope and a blood pressure cuff (sphygmomanometer) to monitor your blood pressure regularly.

Purchase a flat diaphragm-model stethoscope rather than a bell-shaped one. The flat surface makes it easier for you to hear.

Blood pressure cuffs come in many models. If you have difficulty reading the gauge on a regular cuff, look for a model that uses an upright mercury column, or an electronic digital model. Ask your pharmacist to recommend a blood pressure kit and show you how to use it.

Self-Care Supplies

The supplies listed below are useful to keep on hand in your home health center. The products are inexpensive, easy to use, and generally available in any drugstore or pharmacy.

- Adhesive strips (Band-Aids) in assorted sizes
- Adhesive tape, 1 inch wide
- Butterfly bandages
- Sterile gauze pads, 2 inches square
- Elastic ("Ace") bandage, 3 inches wide
- Roll of gauze bandage, 2 inches wide
- Cotton balls
- Safety pins

Thermometer

Mercury-containing glass thermometers are no longer recommended because of safety concerns. If you have one in your home, consider replacing it with a digital electronic thermometer.

Digital thermometers are accurate, easy to read, and durable. Temperature strips are very convenient and safe but are not as accurate as digital thermometers and should only be used to measure axillary (armpit) temperature. They are inaccurate when used on the forehead. Thermometers that measure the temperature in the ear are fast, easy to use, and quite accurate, but they are expensive.

Rectal thermometers with enlarged bulbs are helpful for children younger than 6 or anyone who cannot hold an oral thermometer in his or her mouth.

How to Take a Temperature

A normal oral temperature ranges from 97.6° to 99.6° and for most people is 98.6°. Temperature varies with time of day and other factors, so don't worry about minor changes.

Whenever a person feels hot or cold to your touch, it is a good idea to take and record his or her temperature. If you have to call your doctor during an illness, knowing your exact temperature will be very helpful.

There are four places where a thermometer can be placed to take a temperature:

1. In the mouth (oral)

2. In the anus (rectal)

3. Under the armpit (axillary)

4. In the ear (tympanic)

Unless otherwise specified, all temperatures in this book are oral Fahrenheit readings. If you take a rectal or axillary temperature, adjust it accordingly (see below).

Oral thermometers are recommended for people age 6 and older.

• Do not drink hot or cold liquids before taking your temperature.

• Clean the thermometer with soapy water or rubbing alcohol.

• If you are using an alcohol or mercury thermometer, hold it firmly at the end opposite the bulb and shake it down to 95° or lower.

• Place the bulb under your tongue and close your lips around it. Do not bite down. Breathe through your nose and don't talk.

• Wait 3 to 5 minutes (or until a digital thermometer beeps).

Rectal thermometers are recommended for children younger than 6 or anyone who cannot hold an oral thermometer in the mouth. Use only a rectal thermometer to take a rectal temperature. Rectal temperature is 0.5° to 1° higher than oral temperature. Rectal temperatures are the most accurate.

• Clean the thermometer. If you are using a mercury or alcohol thermometer, shake it down to 95° or lower.

• Put Vaseline or another lubricant on the bulb.

• Hold the child bottom-up across your lap.

• Hold the thermometer 1 inch from the bulb and gently insert it into the rectum no more than 1 inch. Do not let go. Hold the thermometer right at the anus so it cannot slip in farther.

• Wait for 3 minutes (or until a digital thermometer beeps).

Axillary temperatures are less accurate and are about 1° lower than oral temperatures. Axillary readings are safer for small children who will not hold still while you take a rectal temperature.

• Use either an oral or rectal thermometer. Shake it down below 95°.

• Place the thermometer in the armpit and have the child cross the arm across the chest and hold the opposite upper arm.

• Wait 5 minutes.

How to Read a Thermometer

To read a thermometer that does not have a digital readout:

• Roll the thermometer between your fingers until you can see the thin ribbon of mercury (silver) or alcohol (red). Note that the thermometer is marked from 92° to 108°.

• Each large mark indicates 1° of temperature. Each small mark indicates 0.2°.

Nonprescription Medications and Products

A nonprescription medication (sometimes called an over-the-counter or OTC medication) is any drug that you can buy without a doctor's prescription. However, don't assume that all nonprescription drugs are safe for you. These drugs can interact with other medications and can sometimes cause serious health problems.

Some medications should only be used by adults or older children. Be sure to read the package instructions carefully, or ask a pharmacist before giving any product to an infant or young child.

Carefully read the label of any nonprescription drug you use, especially if you also take prescription medications for other health problems. Ask your pharmacist for help in finding a nonprescription drug best suited to your needs.

Some common nonprescription medications include:

• Antacids and acid reducers.

• Bulking agents and laxatives.

• Antidiarrheals.

• Cold and allergy remedies.

• Pain relievers.

These drugs can be very helpful when used properly but can also cause serious problems if used incorrectly. The following tips will help you use common nonprescription drugs wisely and safely. In some cases, you may find that you don't need to take them at all.

Antacids and Acid Reducers

Antacids are taken to relieve heartburn or indigestion caused by excess stomach acid. While they are safe if used occasionally, antacids may cause problems if taken regularly. There are several kinds of antacids. Learn what ingredients are in each type so you can avoid any adverse effects.

- Sodium bicarbonate antacids (such as Alka-Seltzer and Bromo Seltzer) contain baking soda. Avoid these antacids if you have high blood pressure or are on a salt-restricted diet.

- Calcium carbonate antacids (such as Tums and Alka-2) are sometimes used as calcium supplements (see page 299). However, these products may cause constipation.

- Aluminum-based antacids (such as Amphojel) are less potent and work more slowly than other products do. They may also cause constipation. Some may cause calcium loss and should not be taken by postmenopausal women. If you have kidney problems, check with your doctor before using aluminum-based antacids.

- Magnesium compounds (such as Phillips' Milk of Magnesia) may cause diarrhea.

- Aluminum-magnesium antacids (such as Maalox, Di-Gel, Mylanta, and Riopan) are less likely to cause constipation or diarrhea than are aluminum-only or magnesium-only antacids.

Acid reducers decrease the amount of acid produced by the stomach. There are several types of nonprescription acid reducers on the market. Each has slightly different cautions for use. Read and carefully follow the instructions included with the package.

Antacid and Acid Reducer Precautions

- Try to eliminate the cause of frequent heartburn instead of taking antacids regularly. See Heartburn on page 87.

- Consult your doctor or pharmacist before taking an antacid if you take other medications. Antacids may interfere with the absorption and action of some prescription medications. Also consult your doctor if you have ulcers or kidney problems.

- If you have a problem with the function of your kidneys or liver, you should be careful in using acid reducers. All drugs are broken down and removed from the body by the combined action of the liver and kidneys. If your liver or kidneys are not working correctly, it is possible that too high a dose of the acid-reducing drug will build up in your body.

Bulking Agents and Laxatives

There are two types of products to prevent or treat constipation: bulking agents and laxatives.

Bulking agents, such as bran or psyllium (found in Metamucil, for example), are not laxatives, but they ease constipation by increasing the volume of stool and making it easier to pass. Regular use of bulking agents is safe and helps make them more effective.

Laxatives (such as Correctol, Ex-Lax, Senokot, and Dulcolax) speed up the passage of stool by irritating the lining of the intestines. Regular laxative use is not recommended.

There are many other ways to treat constipation, such as drinking more water. See page 82.

Laxative Precautions

• Take any laxative or bulking agent with plenty of water or other liquids.

• Do not take laxatives regularly. Overuse of laxatives decreases tone and sensation in the large intestine, causing laxative dependence. If you need help keeping regular, use a bulking agent.

• Regular use of some laxatives (such as Correctol, Ex-Lax, and Feen-a-Mint) may interfere with your body's ability to absorb vitamin D and calcium; this can lead to weakened bones.

Antidiarrheals

There are two types of antidiarrheal drugs: those that thicken the stool and those that slow intestinal spasms.

The **thickening** mixtures (such as Kaopectate) contain clay or fruit pectin and absorb bacteria and toxins in the intestine. They are safe because they do not go into the blood, but these products also absorb the bacteria needed for digestion. Long-term use is not advised.

Antispasmodic antidiarrheal products slow the spasms of the intestine. Loperamide (the active ingredient in products such as Imodium A-D and Pepto Diarrhea Control) is an example of this type of preparation. Some products (such as Donnagel and Parepectolin) contain both thickening and antispasmodic ingredients.

Antidiarrheal Precautions

• Diarrhea helps rid your body of an infection, so try to avoid using antidiarrheal medications for the first 24 hours. After that, use them only if cramping and pain continue but there are no other signs of illness, such as fever.

• Be sure to take a large enough dose. Take antidiarrheal preparations until your stools thicken; then stop immediately to avoid constipation.

• Replace lost body fluids. Dehydration can develop when someone, especially an infant, child, or older adult, has diarrhea. See page 85 for a recipe for a rehydration drink you can make at home.

Cold and Allergy Remedies

In general, whether you take drugs or not for your cold, you'll get better in about a week. Rest and liquids are probably the best treatment for a cold (see page 155). Antibiotics will not help. However, medications help relieve some cold symptoms, such as nasal congestion and cough.

Allergy symptoms, especially runny nose, often respond to antihistamines. Antihistamines are also found in many cold medications, often together with a decongestant. However, the value of antihistamines in treating cold symptoms is under debate.

Decongestants

Decongestants make breathing easier by shrinking swollen mucous membranes in the nose, allowing air to pass through. They also help relieve runny nose and postnasal drip, which can cause a sore throat.

Decongestants can be taken orally or used as nose drops or sprays. Oral decongestants (pills) are probably more effective and provide longer relief, but they cause more side effects. Pseudoephedrine (the active ingredient in products such as Sudafed) is an oral decongestant.

Sprays and drops provide rapid but temporary relief. Nasal sprays containing phenylephrine (such as Neo-Synephrine) are effective. Sprays and drops are less likely to interact with other drugs than oral decongestants are.

Decongestant Precautions

• Do not give cold medicines or oral decongestants to infants under 6 months of age. Nonprescription cold medicines have not been proven effective for preschool children.

Saline Nose Drops

Nonprescription saline nasal sprays (such as NaSal and Ocean) are convenient, inexpensive, and sterile. They will keep nasal tissues moist so the tissues can filter the air. Saline nasal sprays will not cause mucous membranes in the nose to swell.

Saline nose drops can also be easily made at home. Mix ¼ teaspoon salt in 1 cup of body temperature water (too much salt will dry nasal membranes). Place the solution in a clean bottle with a dropper (available at drugstores). Use as necessary. Make a fresh solution every 3 days.

Insert the drops while lying on your back on a bed, with your head hanging over the side. This will help the drops get farther back. Try to keep the dropper from touching your nose.

• Do not use medicated nasal sprays or drops more than 3 times a day or for more than 3 days in a row. Continued use will cause a "rebound effect": your mucous membranes swell up more than before you used the spray.

• Drink extra fluids when taking cold medications.

- Decongestants can cause problems for people who have certain health problems, such as heart disease, high blood pressure, glaucoma, diabetes, or an overactive thyroid. Decongestants may also interact with some drugs, such as certain antidepressants and high blood pressure medications. Read the package carefully or ask your pharmacist or doctor to help you choose one.

Cough Preparations

Coughing is your body's way of getting foreign substances and mucus out of your respiratory tract. Coughs are often useful, and you shouldn't try to eliminate them. Sometimes, though, coughs are severe enough to impair breathing or prevent rest.

Water and other liquids, such as fruit juices, are probably the best cough syrups. They help soothe the throat and also moisten and thin mucus so it can be coughed up more easily.

You can make a simple and soothing cough syrup at home by mixing 1 part lemon juice with 2 parts honey. Use as often as needed. This can be given to children older than 1 year of age.

There are two kinds of cough medicines: expectorants and suppressants. **Expectorants** help thin the mucus and make it easier to cough mucus up when you have a productive cough. Look for expectorants containing guaifenesin, such as Robitussin and Vicks 44E.

Suppressants control or suppress the cough reflex and work best for a dry, hacking cough that keeps you awake. Look for suppressant medications containing dextro-methorphan, such as Robitussin-DM or Vicks Dry Hacking Cough.

Don't suppress a productive cough too much (unless it is keeping you from getting enough rest).

Cough Preparation Precautions

- Cough preparations can cause problems for people with certain health problems, such as asthma, heart disease, high blood pressure, or an enlarged prostate. Cough preparations may also interact with some drugs, such as sedatives and certain antidepressants. Read the package carefully or ask your pharmacist or doctor to help you choose one.

- Cough suppressants can stifle breathing. Use them with caution if you give them to someone who is very old or frail or if you have chronic respiratory problems.

- Read the label so you know what the ingredients are. Some cough preparations contain a large percentage of alcohol; others contain codeine. There are many choices. Ask your pharmacist to advise you.

Antihistamines

Antihistamines dry up nasal secretions and are commonly used to treat allergy symptoms and itching.

If your runny nose is caused by allergies, an antihistamine will help. For cold symptoms, home treatment and perhaps a decongestant (see page 344) will probably be more helpful. It is usually best to take only single-ingredient allergy or cold preparations, instead of those containing many active ingredients.

Products such as Chlor-Trimeton (chlorpheniramine) and Benadryl (diphenhydramine) are single-ingredient antihistamine products.

Products such as Dristan, Coricidin, and Triaminic contain both a decongestant and an antihistamine.

Antihistamine Precautions

- Do not give antihistamines to infants younger than 4 months of age. For children between 4 months and 1 year, ask your doctor first.

- Use of antihistamines to treat the stuffiness of a cold will often thicken the mucus, making it harder to get rid of.

- Drink extra fluids when taking antihistamines.

- Antihistamines can cause problems for some people with health problems such as asthma, glaucoma, epilepsy, or an enlarged prostate. Antihistamines may also interact with some drugs, such as certain antidepressants, sedatives, and tranquilizers. Read the package carefully or ask your pharmacist or doctor to help you choose one that will not cause problems.

- The drowsiness that antihistamines often cause usually lessens with continued use. If it continues, or if the medication isn't helping your allergies after 1 week, call your doctor for advice.

- Antihistamines that don't cause drowsiness are available by prescription. Ask your health professional if these are appropriate for you.

Pain Relievers

There are dozens of pain reliever products. Most contain either aspirin, ibuprofen, or acetaminophen. These three drugs, as well as ketoprofen and naproxen sodium, relieve pain and reduce fever. Aspirin, ibuprofen, ketoprofen, and naproxen sodium also relieve inflammation. They belong to a class of drugs called nonsteroidal anti-inflammatory drugs (NSAIDs).

When purchasing pain relievers, keep in mind that generic products are chemically equivalent to more expensive brand-name products, and they usually work equally well.

Aspirin

Aspirin is widely used for relieving pain and reducing fever in adults. It also relieves minor itching and reduces swelling and inflammation. Most tablets contain 325 mg of aspirin. Although it seems familiar and safe, aspirin is a very powerful drug.

Aspirin Precautions

- Keep all aspirin, especially baby aspirin, out of children's reach.

- Aspirin can irritate the stomach lining, causing bleeding or ulcers. If aspirin upsets your stomach, try a coated brand, such as Ecotrin. Talk with your doctor or pharmacist to determine what will work best for you.

- Aspirin increases the risk of Reye syndrome in children. See page 221. Do not give aspirin to anyone younger than 20 unless your doctor tells you to do so.

- Some people are allergic to aspirin. (They may also be allergic to ibuprofen.)

- Throw aspirin away if it starts to smell like vinegar.

- Do not take aspirin if you have gout or if you take blood thinners (anticoagulants).

- Do not take aspirin for a hangover. Aspirin used with alcohol increases your risk for stomach irritation.

- High doses may result in aspirin poisoning (salicylism). Stop taking aspirin and call a health professional if any one of these symptoms occurs:

  - Ringing in the ears

  - Visual disturbances

  - Nausea

  - Dizziness

  - Rapid, deep breathing

Other Aspirin Uses

In addition to relieving pain and inflammation, aspirin is effective against many other ailments. Because of the danger of side effects and the interactions aspirin may have with other medications, do not try these uses of aspirin without a doctor's supervision.

- **Heart attacks and strokes**: Aspirin in low but regular doses helps prevent heart attacks and strokes in certain people. Doses as low as 30 mg per day have helped. Aspirin may also help as a first aid measure for heart attacks. Chewing ½ tablet may be enough to help. See page 55.

- **Stomach and colon cancer**: Some studies have shown that taking 1 aspirin tablet per day can reduce the risk of cancers in the digestive system.

- **Migraines**: Regular, low-dose aspirin use may reduce the frequency of migraines.

Other Pain Relievers

Ibuprofen (the active ingredient in products such as Advil and Nuprin), **ketoprofen** (in products such as Orudis KT and Actron), and **naproxen sodium** (in products such as Aleve) are other nonsteroidal anti-inflammatory drugs (NSAIDs). Like aspirin, these drugs relieve pain and reduce fever and inflammation. Also like aspirin, they can cause nausea, stomach irritation, and heartburn. People who take blood thinners (anticoagulants) should use these drugs with caution.

Acetaminophen (the active ingredient in products such as Tylenol) reduces fever and relieves pain. It does not have the anti-inflammatory effect of NSAIDs, such as aspirin and ibuprofen, but it also does not cause stomach upset and other side effects.

The product's package label will tell you how many milligrams (mg) of medicine are in each pill; how much you should take; and how often you should take it. Do not exceed the dosage limits, and follow the instructions on the package if you have health problems that may make it unsafe for you to take the usual dosage of a product.

Syrup of Ipecac

For any poisoning, call your doctor, emergency department, or poison control center immediately!

Syrup of ipecac is a drug used to induce vomiting when a poison has been swallowed.

In most cases of poisoning, the best treatment is to get the substance out of the victim's stomach as quickly as possible. Syrup of ipecac is excellent for this. Also see page 65.

However, making someone vomit can sometimes be harmful. Do not use ipecac when a person has swallowed any of the items listed under "Poisons" on page 349. Give water to dilute the poison without inducing vomiting.

Dosage for Ipecac

Do not give ipecac to children younger than 1 year of age. For anyone older than 1, give 1 tablespoon. After giving the ipecac, have the person drink at least 12 ounces of water, which is essential to ensure vomiting. Try to keep the person walking around.

Repeat the dose of ipecac in 20 minutes if the person has not yet vomited. Repeat only once. When the person vomits, have the person lie on his or her side with the mouth lower than the chest, so that vomited material will not enter the airway. If the person leans over a toilet, be sure the chest is lower than the stomach.

The vomiting caused by ipecac is very violent. Ipecac should not be used in the following situations:

- If a woman is more than 5 months pregnant.
- If the victim has a history of heart disease.
- If the child is younger than 1 year of age.

• If the victim might choke on the vomited material or inhale it into the lungs. This can happen if the person:

- Is over 65.

- Has taken Valium or another drug that may cause unconsciousness.

- Is drunk.

- Is drowsy or lethargic.

Keep ipecac on hand and replace it every 5 years if you haven't used it. It will remain effective for 1 year after it has been opened.

Poisons

Do not induce vomiting:

• Dishwasher detergent

• Gasoline, kerosene

• Drano

• Oven cleaner

• Oil-based paints

• Furniture polish

• Cleaning solutions

• Antifreeze

Induce vomiting:

• Dishwashing liquid

• Plant food

• Aspirin and other medications

• Ink

• Fingernail polish remover

• Rat poison

Prescription Medications

There are thousands of different prescription medications used to treat hundreds of different medical-conditions. Your doctor and your pharmacist are your best sources of information about your prescription medications.

Guidelines for taking every kind of prescription medication could fill several books. Common types covered here include antibiotics, minor tranquilizers, and sleeping pills.

Antibiotics

Antibiotics are drugs that kill bacteria. They are effective against bacteria only and have no effect on viruses. Therefore, antibiotics will not cure the common cold, flu, or any other viral illness. Unless you have a bacterial infection, it's best to avoid the possible adverse effects of antibiotics, which may include:

• **Side effects**, including **allergic reactions**. Common side effects of antibiotics include nausea, diarrhea, and increased sensitivity to sunlight. Most side effects are mild, but some, especially allergic reactions, can be severe. An allergic reaction can be life-threatening. If you have any unexpected reaction to an antibiotic, tell your health professional before another antibiotic is prescribed.

- **Secondary infections**. Antibiotics kill most of the bacteria in your body that are sensitive to them, including the bacteria that help your body. Antibiotics can destroy the bacterial balance in your body, leading to stomach upset, diarrhea, vaginal infections, or other problems.

- **Bacterial resistance**. When antibiotics are used too often, bacteria change so that the antibiotics are no longer effective against them. This makes bacterial infections more difficult to treat.

When you and your health professional have decided that an antibiotic is necessary, carefully follow the instructions for taking the prescription.

- Take the whole dose for as many days as prescribed, unless you have unexpected side effects (in which case, call your health professional). Antibiotics kill off many bacteria quite quickly, so you may feel better in a few days. However, if you stop taking the antibiotic too soon, the weaker bacteria will have been eliminated, but the stronger ones may survive and flourish.

- Be sure you understand any special instructions about taking the medication. The instructions should be printed on the label, but double-check with your doctor and pharmacist.

- Store antibiotics in a cool, dry place. Check carefully to see if they need refrigeration.

- Never give an antibiotic prescribed for one person to someone else.

- Do not save leftover antibiotics, and do not take an antibiotic prescribed for another illness without a health professional's approval.

Medication Guidelines

The following are basic guidelines for taking prescription and non-prescription medications:

- Use medications only if non-drug approaches are not working.

- Know the benefits and side effects of a medication before taking it.

- Take the minimum effective dose.

- Never take a drug prescribed for someone else.

- Follow the prescription instructions exactly or let your doctor know why you didn't.

- Keep medications tightly capped in their original containers, and store them as directed.

- Do not take medications in front of small children. Children are great mimics. Don't oversell the "candy" taste of children's medicines or leave children's vitamins accessible to children.

- Add a consumer's guide to medications to your home health library.

Minor Tranquilizers and Sleeping Pills

Minor tranquilizers (such as Valium, Librium, Xanax, and Tranxene) and sleeping pills (such as Dalmane, Restoril, and Ambien) are widely prescribed. However, these drugs can cause problems, including memory loss, addiction, and injuries from falls caused by drug-induced unsteadiness.

Minor tranquilizers can be effective for short periods of time. However, long-term use is often of limited value and introduces the risk of addiction and mental impairment.

Sleeping pills may help for a few days or a few weeks, but using them for more than a month generally causes more sleep problems than it solves. For other approaches, see page 314.

If you have been taking minor tranquilizers or sleeping pills for a while, talk with your doctor about reevaluating your need for the medication or reducing your dosage. If you have experienced any unsteadiness, dizziness, or memory loss, tell your doctor.

Medication Problems

Several kinds of adverse medication reactions can occur:

Side effects. Side effects are predictable but unpleasant reactions to a drug. They are usually mild, but they can be inconvenient. In some cases, they are more serious.

Adverse Drug Reactions

Side effects, drug-drug and food-drug interactions, overmedication, and addiction may cause:

- Nausea, indigestion, and vomiting.
- Constipation, diarrhea, or problems with urination.
- Dry mouth.
- Headache, dizziness, ringing in the ears, or blurred vision.
- Confusion, forgetfulness, disorientation, drowsiness, or depression.
- Difficulty sleeping, irritability, or nervousness.
- Difficulty breathing.
- Rashes, bruising, and bleeding problems.

Don't assume any symptom is a normal side effect that you have to suffer with. Call your doctor or pharmacist any time you suspect that your medicines are making you sick.

Allergies. Some people have severe, sometimes life-threatening reactions (called anaphylaxis) to certain medications. See page 141 for signs of an allergic reaction.

Drug-drug interactions. These occur when two or more prescription or nonprescription drugs mix in a person's body and cause an adverse reaction. The symptoms can be severe and may be improperly diagnosed as a new illness.

Drug-food interactions. These occur when medications react with food. Some drugs work best when taken with food, but others should be taken on an empty stomach. Some drug-food reactions can cause serious symptoms.

Overmedication. Sometimes the full adult dose of a medication is too much for small people and those over age 60. Too much of a drug can be very dangerous.

Addiction. Long-term use of some medications can lead to dependency, and severe reactions may occur if the medications are withdrawn suddenly. Narcotics, tranquilizers, and barbiturates must be taken very carefully to prevent addiction. See page 304.

Save Money on Medications

Nonprescription and prescription medications can be very expensive. Here are some ways to cut your medication costs:

- Buy generic nonprescription products. They are chemically equivalent to brand-name drugs but are usually cheaper. Ask your doctor if generic forms of your prescription medications are available and appropriate for you.

- Shop around and compare prices at several pharmacies. Prices can vary widely. It may be worth paying a little more if you know and trust the pharmacist.

- Ask your doctor for samples of newly prescribed medications, or ask your pharmacist to fill only the first week's worth of pills. If the medication has to be changed later, you will have saved paying for the full prescription.

- Consider buying expensive drugs that you use regularly from mail-order or Internet pharmacies if they charge less. The only disadvantage is that you will not have a partnership with a local pharmacist.

Home Medical Tests

Many common medical tests are now available in home kits. Combined with regular visits to your health professional, home tests can help you monitor your health and, in some cases, detect problems early.

Home medical tests must be very accurate (over 95 percent) to be approved by the Food and Drug Administration (FDA). However, they must be used correctly to give such accurate results. Follow the package directions exactly. If you have questions, ask your pharmacist or call the toll-free phone number on the product label.

Home medical tests are especially helpful if you have a chronic condition that requires frequent monitoring, such as diabetes, asthma, or high blood pressure. Ask your doctor which home medical tests would be appropriate for you. Some common tests are described next.

Blood Glucose Monitoring

If you have diabetes, you may already monitor your blood sugar levels using a finger prick and a test strip or an electronic monitor.

This test should always be used under a doctor's supervision. Never adjust your insulin dose based on a single abnormal test, unless your doctor has specifically instructed you to do so.

Check with your doctor if you have symptoms of abnormal blood sugar levels, even if the test is normal. See page 237.

Blood Pressure Monitoring

If you have high blood pressure, it is important to monitor your blood pressure frequently. With a little instruction, you can easily monitor your blood pressure at home.

By checking your blood pressure at home, when you are relaxed, you will be able to track changes resulting from your home treatment and medications.

- Do not make any changes to your medications based on your home blood pressure readings without consulting your doctor.

- Check your blood pressure at different times of day to see how rest and activities affect it. For regular readings, check it at the same time every day. Blood pressure is usually lowest in the morning and rises during the day.

- For the most accurate reading, sit still for 5 minutes before taking your blood pressure.

- Have your blood pressure cuff device adjusted (calibrated) yearly.

Tests for Blood in Stool

The fecal occult blood test can detect hidden blood in your stools, which may indicate colon cancer or other problems. This test is inexpensive and easy to do, but it may not be able to detect colon cancer as well as other screening tests can. Your doctor may recommend a more accurate screening test for colon cancer called a flexible sigmoidoscopy. See page 98.

Home Pregnancy Tests

If you become pregnant, it is important that you know right away. The quickest way to find out is with a home pregnancy test. Home pregnancy tests are inexpensive and very reliable when done correctly. Some tests can show positive results within a few days of the first missed period. Use a test that has simple instructions and follow them exactly. Mistakes can lead to false results.

If the result is positive, schedule an appointment with your doctor to confirm the result.

Even if the pregnancy test result is negative, it is a good idea to see your doctor to confirm the results. Treat yourself as if you are pregnant until you know for sure.

Home Medical Records

Your home health center is a good place to keep your family's medical records. A 3-ring binder or wire-bound notebook with dividers for each member of the family is helpful. Each person should have a cover sheet listing:

- Diagnosed chronic conditions (arthritis, asthma, diabetes, high blood pressure, etc.).

- Any known allergies to drugs, foods, or insects.

- Information that would be vital in an emergency, such as whether the person has a pacemaker or a hearing aid, has diabetes or epilepsy, or is deaf or blind.

- Name and phone number of primary doctor.

Other important information that should be included:

- An up-to-date list of medications that includes name of drug, purpose, dose, instructions, name of doctor who prescribed the drug, and date prescribed.

- Immunization records: childhood immunizations, tetanus, influenza, and pneumonia.

- Health screening results: blood pressure, cholesterol, vision, and hearing.

- Records of major illnesses and injuries, such as pneumonia, bronchitis, and broken bones.

- Records of any major surgical procedures and hospitalizations.

- Records listing major diseases in members of your family: heart disease, stroke, cancer, or diabetes.

Health Information at Home

Getting good health information is the key to making good health decisions. If the information you need is not in this book, keep looking. Here's how:

On the Internet. Follow the instructions on the back cover of this book to get to the Healthwise® Knowledgebase. With over 100 times the information in the book, the Healthwise Knowledgebase has accurate, unbiased, and frequently updated information on almost all health problems. It is written in language most people can understand. And, it is free. If you have Internet access, go to this site first.

If you don't find everything you need in the Healthwise Knowledgebase, don't give up. There is plenty of reliable information out there if you know where and how to look for it. See Five Tips for Finding Good Web Sites on page 355.

On the phone. Many hospitals and health plans have nurse call centers that can respond to your health questions. Local offices of national organizations like the American Cancer Society, American Heart

Association, Arthritis Foundation, or American Diabetes Association can help connect you with information resources in your area. Check your phone book.

At your library or bookstore.
Research librarians at public libraries spend a good part of their time helping people find information. Ask for their help if you are trying to learn more about a health problem. Libraries can also be a good place to use the Internet if you don't have a computer at home. Be aware that the information found in books and magazines is not guaranteed to be any more accurate than that found on the Internet. Use some of the tips for finding good Web sites as a guide for finding helpful books.

Health information you find on the Internet or in books or magazines should never replace the medical expertise and experience of a health professional. Discuss what you find with your doctor to learn if and how it relates to your particular situation.

Five Tips for Finding Good Web Sites

As a source of health information, the Internet has two major drawbacks. First, there is little to no regulation of what gets published. Misleading, contradictory, inaccurate, and even fraudulent health information is all over the Internet. Second, the amount of information available on the Internet can make your search overwhelming and time-consuming.

With so much information out there, how do you separate the good from the bad? We hope these guidelines will help you find information you can trust.

1. Don't rely on search engines. Instead, go to trusted sources recommended by your health professional, hospital, or health plan. If you have to use a search engine, be sure to follow the other four tips closely.

2. Don't trust the information on a health Web site unless the site clearly indicates:

- Who wrote and reviewed the information.

- When the information was last updated.

- What sources and references the information is based on. (Look for a bibliography or reference list.)

If information is missing, be skeptical of the site's reliability.

3. Check the site's privacy policy. It should tell you that your personal information will not be given to any third party without your explicit permission. Web sites displaying the URAC Health Web Site Accreditation seal should be safe.

4. Check the site ownership or sponsorship. Web sites displaying the URAC Health Web Site Accreditation seal should indicate any influence that the owner or sponsor has on the site's content.

5. Watch out for these clues that a Web site is of questionable quality:

- Heavy use of personal testimonies without references to good research.

- Unsupported claims of a "secret" or "revolutionary" cure.

- Promotion of a specific drug, dietary supplement, medical device, or other product.

- Requirement of a financial investment.

Your final test should be the common sense test. If information doesn't make sense to you, don't trust it without first talking with your health professional. Never make a health care decision based solely on what you read on the Internet.

Index

A

Abdominal pain 79
  after eating 91
  between meals or at night 87, 92, 100
  burning beneath the breastbone 87
  cramping 81
  generalized 81
  in children 228
  in lower right abdomen 81
  in upper right abdomen 92, 94
  localized 81
  lower abdominal/pelvic pain
    (females) 255, 260, 264
  lower abdominal/pelvic pain
    (males) 269, 270, 271, 273
  menstrual cramps (dysmenorrhea) 259
  rigid or tender abdomen 37
  with bloating and gas 91
  with fever 81, 92
  with unexpected vaginal bleeding 255
Abdominal problems, see Digestive and
  urinary problems 79
Abrasion
  corneal 63
  skin (scrapes) 69
Abstinence, sexual 276, 282
Abuse, drug or alcohol 29, 304
Abusive behavior 317
Accidental needle stick 284
Accidental tooth loss 34
Acetaminophen 348
Achilles tendon injury 127, 130
Acid reducers 341
  heartburn and 88
  ulcers and 101
ACL (anterior cruciate ligament) 131
Acne 195
Acquired immunodeficiency syndrome
  (AIDS) 281
Acupuncture 330
  treatment for back pain 116
Addiction 352
  alcohol or drug 304
Adenoids 166, 167
  adenoidectomy 167
  adenoiditis 166
  ear infections and 166, 167
Adrenaline kit, for stings 61
Advice nurses 8
Aerobic exercise 286
Affirmations 319
AIDS (acquired immunodeficiency
  syndrome) 281
Al-Anon 306
Alcohol use
  alcoholism 304
  moderate 305
  problems 304
Alcoholics Anonymous 306
Allergic reaction 60, 143

Allergies 141
  anaphylactic shock 143
  antihistamines and 345
  asthma and 146
  atopic dermatitis and 198
  food 144
  insect bites and stings and 60
  medications for 343
  milk (lactose intolerance) 300
  rashes and 209
  shots 143
Alopecia areata 214
Alternative medicine, see Complementary
  medicine
Anal, also see Rectal
  fissure 97
  itching 96, 234
Anaphylactic shock 60, 143
Anger and hostility 307, 317
Angina 152
Animal bites 35
Anorexia nervosa 312
Antacids 341
  heartburn and 88
  ulcers and 101
Anterior cruciate ligament (ACL) 131
Antibiotics 349
  diarrhea and 86
  nausea and vomiting and 95
Antidiarrheals 343
Antihistamines 345
Anti-inflammatories 346, 347
  heartburn and 88
  ulcers and 100
Antioxidant vitamins 294
Anxiety 308
Apnea 170, 314
Appendicitis 81
Arthritis 121, 127, 133
  back pain and 109
  common types of (chart) 122
  jaw pain and 137
  neck pain and 117
Ask-the-Doctor Checklist 2
Aspirin 346
  asthma and 146
  bruises and 44
  hearing loss and 183
  heart attack and 347
  heartburn and 88
  nosebleeds and 62
  Reye syndrome and 221
  ringing in the ears and 186, 347
  ulcers and 100
Asthma 146
  action plan for 147, 148
Atherosclerosis 240
Athlete's foot 205
Atopic dermatitis 198
Aura, before headache 190

Nosebleeds 62
Numbness and tingling
    after an injury 75
    in arm or hand 117, 120
    in fingers or hands 128, 129
    in genital or rectal area 115
    in hands or feet 238
    in heel or foot 131
    in leg 132
    in leg or foot 109
Numbness, on one side of body 76
Nurse practitioners 8
Nursing, see Breast-feeding
Nutrition 23, 293
    Food Guide Pyramid 295
    for children 302
    guidelines 293, 294, 295

O

Obesity 24
Objects
    in the ear 63
    in the eye 63
    in the nose 64
Office visits, preparing for 6
Optimism, health and 318
Oral contraceptives 275, 276
Orchitis 273
Orthostatic hypotension 177
Osteoarthritis 121, 122
Osteoporosis 135
    back pain and 109
    calcium and 136
    hormone therapy and 256
    menopause and 257
    vitamin D and 136
Otitis externa, see Swimmer's ear 184
Otitis media, see Ear infections 179
Ovarian cancer 264
Ovarian cyst 80, 81
Overeating, compulsive 313
Overmedication 352

P

Pain
    abdominal 79
    between navel and breastbone 100
    breast 246, 249, 261
    burning beneath the breastbone 87
    calf 133
    chest 152, 153
    chronic 320
    during ejaculation 269
    during sexual intercourse 255, 262, 265, 278
    during urination (females) 106, 262, 265
    during urination (males) 106, 269, 270
    ear 179, 181
    elbow 125
    eye 171, 175

    foot 122, 123, 127, 130
    groin 89
    hand 128
    heel 127, 130
    hip 124, 127
    in back, side, groin, or genital area 106
    in cheek, upper teeth, forehead, or behind eyes 164
    in scrotum or testes 273
    jaw 137
    knee 124, 127, 131
    leg 133
    muscle 133
    neck 117
    pelvic/lower abdominal (females) 255, 260, 264
    pelvic/lower abdominal (males) 269, 270, 271, 273
    prostate 269
    rectal 82, 83, 96, 97
    scrotum or groin 89
    scrotum or testes 272, 273, 274
    shooting down one arm 120
    shoulder 124, 126
    side (flank) 106
    stomach, see Abdominal pain
    teeth 164
    testicular 272
    wrist 125, 128
Pain relievers 346
Painful periods 254, 259
Panic disorder 308
Pap test 250
Paralysis, on one side of body 76
Patellar tendinitis 131
Patellofemoral (kneecap) pain 131
Pelvic exam 250
Pelvic infection 255, 259
Pelvic inflammatory disease (PID) 279, 280
Penis
    circumcision 217
    cleansing of 267
    discharge from 278
Peptic ulcer 100
Periods, see Menstrual problems
Pertussis vaccine 17
Phlebitis 133
Phlegm 157
Phobias 308
Phototherapy, for seasonal affective disorder 311
Physical exams, frequency of 20
Physical therapy, for back pain 116
Physician assistants 8
Physician, see Doctor
Phytochemicals, in foods 302
Piles, see Hemorrhoids 96
Pimples 195
    on eyelid 175
Pinched nerve 117
Pinkeye (conjunctivitis) 173
Pinworms 233
Pipe smoking, quitting 26
Plantar fasciitis 127, 130

V

Vaginal
bleeding, severe 255
discharge 250, 255, 262, 265, 278
dryness 256, 257, 258
infection (vaginitis) 262
itching 262, 265
Vaginitis 262
recurrent 238, 263
yeast 265
Vaporizer 338
Varicella (chickenpox) 220
vaccine 220
Vasectomy 276, 277
Vein, inflammation of 133
Venereal disease (VD), see Sexually transmitted diseases 278
Vertebrae 107, 331
Vertigo 176
Violence 317
Viral gastroenteritis 86
Viral infections 156
Vision problems, also see Eye problems
PRK and LASIK surgeries 176
surgery for 176
Vision, also see Eye problems
blurred 165, 174, 175
blurred, does not clear with blinking 76
blurred, with difficulty swallowing 99
blurred, with sudden eye pain 175
screening, frequency of 21
visual disturbances, headache and 190
Visualization 319
Vitamin D, osteoporosis and 136
Vitamins 299
supplements 299
Vomiting 95
bloody 88, 96, 227
dehydration and 84, 225, 227
eating disorders and 312
head injury and 53
in children 225
morning sickness 252
persistent, with drowsiness, hyperventilation, and behavior changes 221
poisoning and 66, 349
syrup of ipecac 348
with abdominal pain and fever 81, 91, 92
with sleepiness, lethargy, stiff neck 162
with stiff neck, headache, fever 162

W

Warts 213
genital 279
plantar 213
Wasp stings 60
Water in ear, how to remove 184

Weakness 139
bone (osteoporosis) 135
in arm or hand 117
in arms 120
in hand 128, 129
in leg or foot 109, 115, 120
on one side of the body 76
Weapons, safety 31, 317
Weight and height, screening, frequency of 21
Weight gain, unexplained 310
Weight loss
also see Eating disorders 312
unexplained 94, 150, 238, 310
Weight management 23
high blood pressure and 243
high cholesterol and 243
tips 24
Well-baby visits 22
Wheezing
after an insect sting 60, 145
with asthma 146
with bronchitis 149
Whiplash 117, 120
Winter blues (seasonal affective disorder) 310, 311
Withdrawal method (birth control) 276
Withdrawal symptoms
alcohol dependence 305, 306
drug dependence 305
Women's health 245
World Wide Web, using to find health information 6, 354
Worrying 308
Wounds, puncture 67
Wrist pain 125, 128

Y

Yeast infections 262, 265
Yellow jacket stings 60
Yoga 335